For Reference Only

This volume must not
be removed from the Library
without the express permission
of the Librarian

University of Central Lancashire Library
Preston PR1 2HE
Telephone: 01772 892279

Atlas of Tooth- and Implant-Supported Prosthodontics

Atlas of Tooth- and Implant-Supported Prosthodontics

Lawrence A. Weinberg, DDS, MS, FACD, FICD

Islandia, New York

Quintessence Publishing Co, Inc

Chicago, Berlin, Tokyo, Copenhagen, London, Paris, Milan, Barcelona, Istanbul, São Paulo, New Delhi, Moscow, Prague, and Warsaw

To my loving wife, Carolyn

Library of Congress Cataloging-in-Publication Data

Weinberg, Lawrence A., 1928-
  Atlas of tooth- and implant-supported prosthodontics / Lawrence A. Weinberg.
       p. ; cm.
  Includes bibliographical references.
  ISBN 0-86715-427-6 (hbk.)
 1. Dental implants—Atlases. 2. Prosthodontics—Atlases.
  [DNLM: 1. Dental Prosthesis—methods—Atlases. 2. Dental Implantation—methods—Atlases. WU 507 W423a 2003] I. Title.
  RK667.I45 W445 2003
  617.6'9—dc21
                                                          2002154522

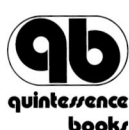

©2003 Quintessence Publishing Co, Inc

Quintessence Publishing Co, Inc
551 Kimberly Drive
Carol Stream, IL 60188
www.quintpub.com

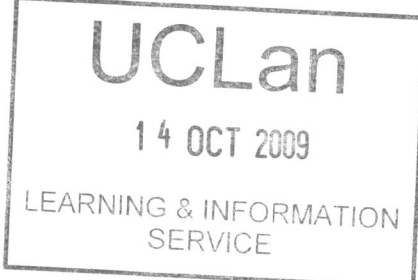

All rights reserved. This book or any part thereof may not be reproduced, stored in a retrieval system, or transmitted in any form or by any means, electronic, mechanical, photocopying, or otherwise, without prior written permission of the publisher.

Editors: Lisa C. Bywaters and Kathryn O'Malley
Cover and Internal Design: Dawn Hartman
Production: Dawn Hartman and Susan Robinson

Printed in China

Table of Contents

Preface **vii**

1. Esthetic Planning and Tooth Preparation for Porcelain Laminates and Full Crowns **1**

2. The Semi-adjustable Articulator: Concept, Modification, and Clinical Application **13**

3. Esthetic, Functional, and Vertical Dimension Planning for Complete-Arch Prostheses **27**

4. Biomechanics of Tooth- and Implant-Supported Prostheses **47**

5. Reduction of Implant Loading via Therapeutic Biomechanics **67**

6. Three-dimensional Guidance System for Implant Placement **85**

7. Clinical Procedures for Complete-Arch Osseointegrated Prostheses **107**

8. Clinical Procedures for Tooth- and Implant-Supported Overdentures and Fixed-Retrievable Prostheses **121**

9. Clinical Problems **141**

10. Occlusion and Centric Relation Evaluation **181**

11. Clinical Techniques for Occlusal Adjustment **201**

Index **219**

Preface

The objective of this atlas is to describe practical, step-by-step clinical procedures for tooth- and implant-supported prosthodontics that will improve long-term success. The concepts and clinical techniques presented are directed primarily at solving practical clinical problems associated with tooth- and implant-supported prosthodontics. Although it was necessary to use photographs of various specific implant systems throughout the text, the descriptions of the required armamentaria deliberately have been made as generic as possible, enabling the principles and techniques discussed to be applied to any implant system.

It is my opinion that once implants have been successfully osseointegrated—regardless of the surface or design—and the prosthesis completed, the determining factor for long-term success is the degree of occlusal loading to the supporting bone. The same can be said for natural tooth–supported prostheses; however, the biomechanical principles associated with each approach are completely different. This is a result of the difference between the respective supporting systems, ie, the stiffness of the osseointegrated interface versus the flexion of the periodontal ligament interface.

This text presents new biomechanical concepts associated with the differential mobility of natural teeth and implants. These new concepts are needed to understand and visualize the interactions of occluding surfaces of prostheses and how they generate and distribute forces to the supporting bone through the periodontal ligament or osseointegrated interfaces. This is especially important in cases where natural teeth and implants are used in the same or opposing arch, or within the same prosthesis.

A new paradigm also is suggested for diagnosis and treatment, calling for pre-planning of implant placement that considers the biomechanical factors and force distribution in order to decrease implant and/or tooth loading. This process of remediation of each biomechanical factor in the physiologic chain of events, called *therapeutic biomechanics*, is designed to diminish the cumulative result (ie, occlusal overload). To maximize the advantages of therapeutic biomechanics, a three-dimensional guidance system for implant placement is recommended. This system accurately integrates the planned occlusion with the residual bone topography.

The use of natural teeth and implants in the same or opposing arch requires the introduction of another new paradigm, called *differential occlusal loading*. This process requires *differential occlusal adjustment*, a new technique that distributes the forces of occlusion more equitably between implants and natural teeth.

I would like to acknowledge the scientific and personal contributions of my mentors, Dr Clyde Schuyler (occlusion) and Dr Jerome M. Schweitzer (complete-mouth restoration), which have structured in large measure the body of knowledge upon which this work is based. Very special appreciation is given to my son, Richard, for his instruction on the scanning and editing of 35-mm slides and for his development of a technical process for the conversion of my drawings into electronic files for commercial printing. Without his contributions, there would be no atlas.

The surgical skills and clinical insights contributed by Drs Burt Langer and Charles Berman clarified my understanding of the surgical process, much to the benefit of my patients. I am also extremely grateful to Dr Frank V. Celenza for his friendship and the knowledge he has shared since our collaboration as instructors at New York University College of Dentistry in the mid-1960s.

Special appreciation is also given to my classmate and friend, Dr Charles Weiss, who has made a recognized lifelong contribution to the field of implantology, and who never stopped encouraging my literary efforts since our graduation in 1952. Many of my colleagues have made direct contributions to this work that cannot be detailed here other than in the grateful mention of their names: Drs Jack Chastain, David Gelb, Bernard Kruger (chapter 6), Lynn Lager, Edmond Mukamal, Neil Starr, Robert Weller, and Joel Gluck. There can be no prostheses without the expertise of laboratory technicians; therefore, I am grateful for the many years of personal friendship and expertise of Ray Selle, CDT.

I would also like to express my appreciation to the editorial and production staff of Quintessence Publishing Co, Inc for their expertise and extra effort in the layout and editing of the manuscript.

There is no literary undertaking that occurs without paying the price of *time*. That essential ingredient is always at the expense of one's family. I am grateful beyond words to my wife, Carolyn, who never wavered from total commitment and support for this project. I also would like to acknowledge the lifetime moral support and inspiration provided by my brother, Richard.

1 Esthetic Planning and Tooth Preparation for Porcelain Laminates and Full Crowns

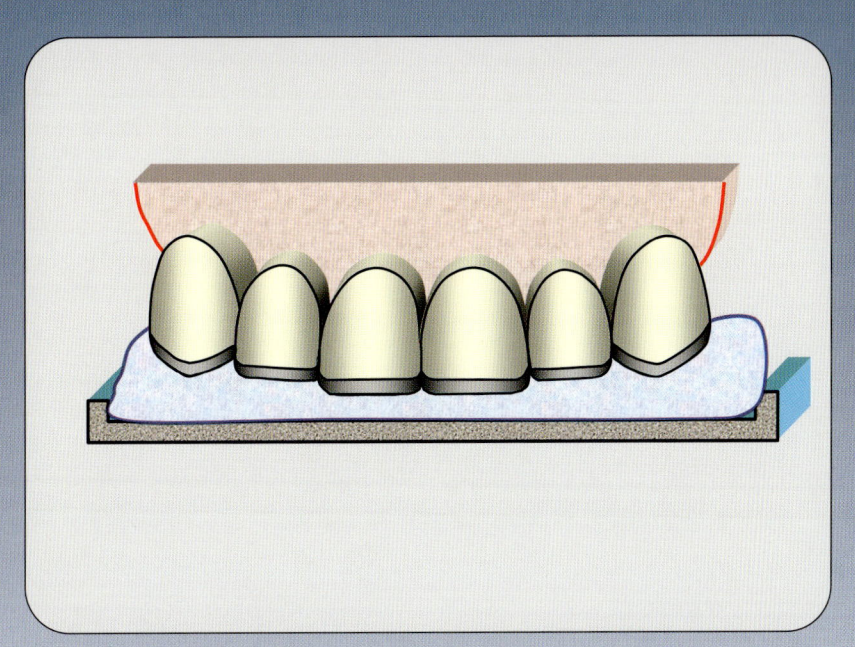

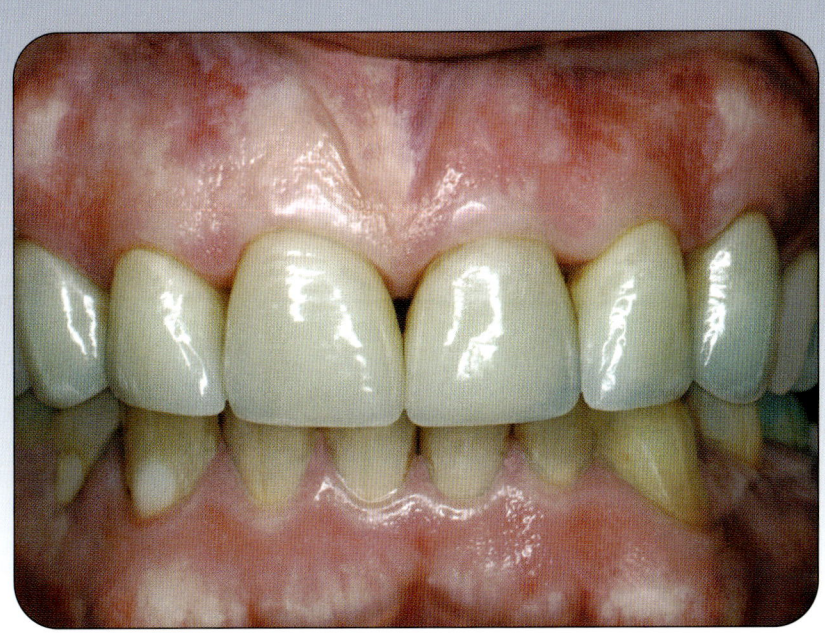

This chapter focuses on esthetic planning and tooth preparation for anterior porcelain laminates[1-5] and anterior full-crown restorations.[6-8] A technique to plan, control, and transfer the esthetics from the planning cast through the final restoration will be presented, followed by a step-by-step clinical procedure for tooth preparation.

Esthetic Laminate Planning

One of the most critical esthetic factors to be considered is the incisal edges of the planned restoration and their control during all clinical and laboratory procedures. Natural teeth have an esthetic gingival taper that provides space for the gingival papillae (Fig 1-1). Failure to remove sufficient tooth structure in the labial-proximal area will result in a restoration that appears square and unesthetic (see Fig 1-1). Sometimes the anatomic smile line should be reproduced without change (Fig 1-2). In this case, heavy-bodied elastomeric impression material (or plaster) may be used in an altered mandibular stock tray to obtain an occlusal index (Fig 1-3). The elastomeric material is trimmed to the occlusal edges of the teeth with care to preserve the labial incisal line angle (Fig 1-4).

Incisal reduction

Controlled reduction of the incisal edges of the teeth is obtained by frequent replacement of the occlusal index. In this manner, the exact incisal reduction of each tooth is revealed by the distance between the incisal edges of the prepared teeth and the elastomeric impression (Fig 1-5). Thus, controlled incisal reduction of all teeth is required to reproduce the existing esthetics and anatomic smile line (Fig 1-6).

Corrective esthetics

Usually the incisal edges of the teeth require lengthening, shortening, or recontouring (Fig 1-7). After these alterations are made on the cast (Fig 1-8), it is necessary to have a means of recording the planned esthetics, transferring that information to the mouth to guide incisal reduction, and then transferring it back again to the final casts to ensure three-dimensional replication of the planned restorations.

Esthetic Laminate Planning

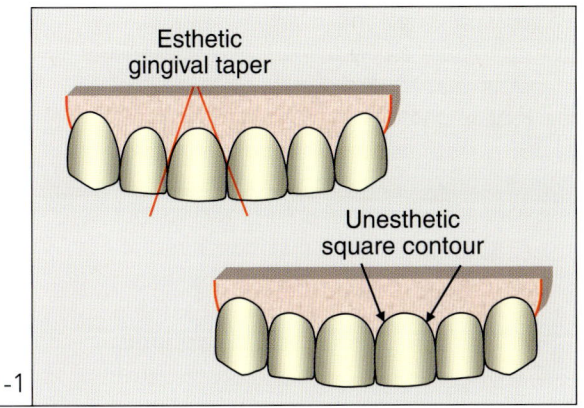

1-1

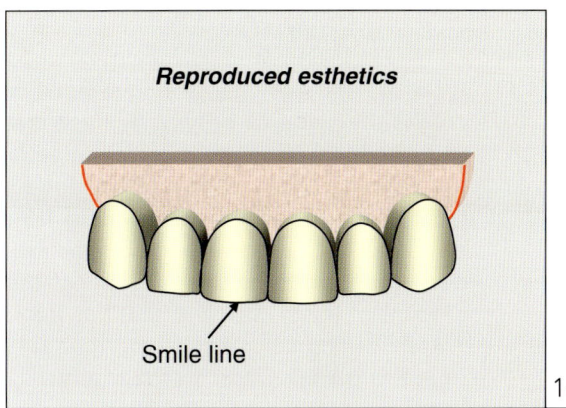

1-2

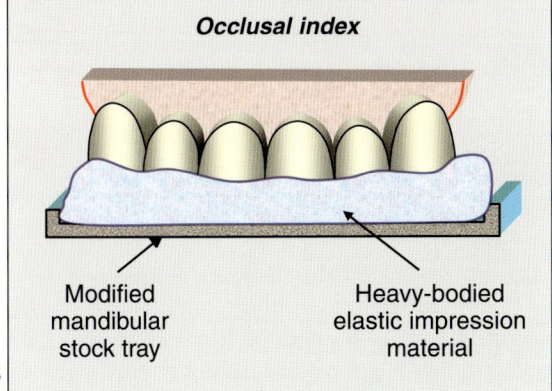

1-3

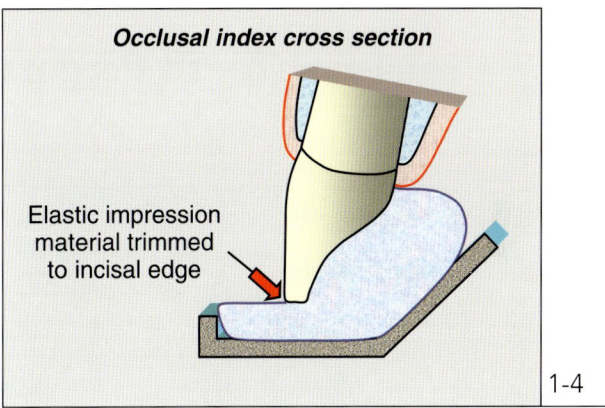

1-4

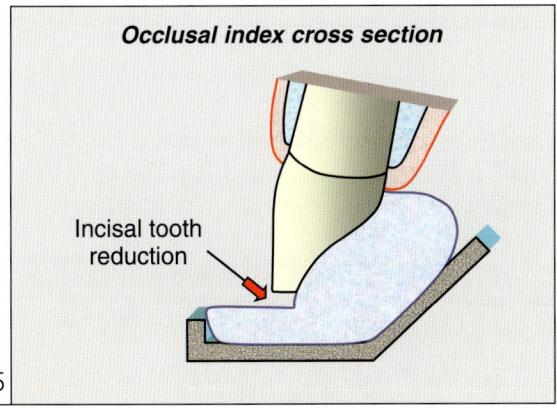

1-5

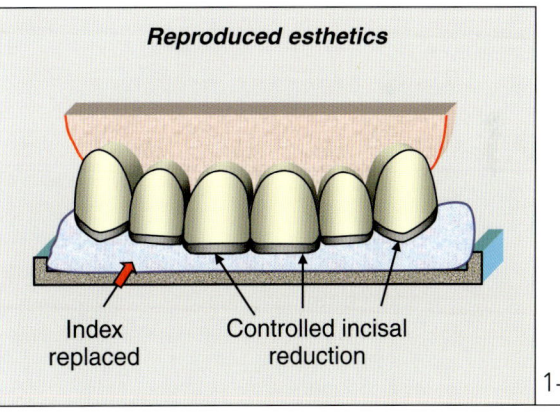

1-6

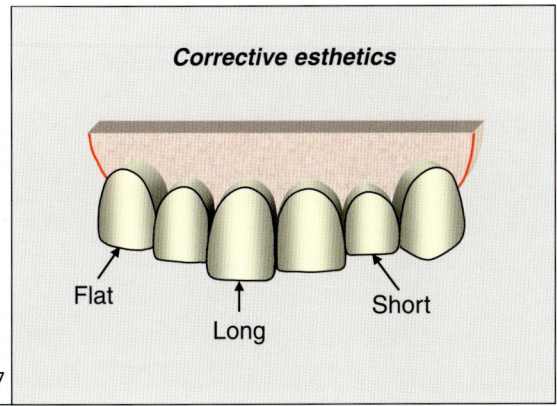

1-7

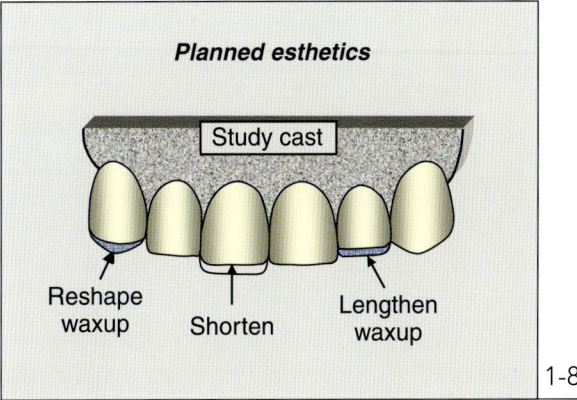

1-8

Esthetic transfer

After the esthetic changes have been made on the planning cast, the transfer process is the same as previously described (see Figs 1-3 and 1-4). An occlusal index of heavy-bodied impression material (or plaster) is obtained in a mandibular stock tray that has been modified by reducing the labial flange so as to allow the premolars to be included for stability (Fig 1-9). The impression material is trimmed to, but not beyond, the incisal edges of the teeth (Fig 1-10). Controlled incisal tooth reduction is accomplished by reseating the occlusal index, which reveals the exact amount of tooth structure that has been removed relative to the planning cast (Fig 1-11). This process provides a means of transferring the planned incisal esthetics from the planning cast to the mouth.

Laminate Tooth Preparation

Esthetic objectives

From the labial view, natural anterior teeth are tapered toward the coronal portion, as described above. However, from the proximal view, the labial enamel surfaces of the maxillary anterior teeth do not form a straight line. The body and incisal third are in the frontal plane of the patient, while the gingival third is inclined lingually and roughly parallels the root surface (Fig 1-12). If this two-plane relationship is not reproduced in the preparation, then the restoration cannot reproduce the esthetics without adding increased bulk proximally and labially. Furthermore, when there is gingival recession, the two-plane relationship becomes exaggerated.

Tooth preparation

The first step of tooth preparation is to reduce the incisal edge approximately 1.0 mm following the controlled procedure previously described (see Figs 1-3 to 1-11). The two-plane labial surface is reproduced by a uniform 0.5-mm reduction of enamel in two separate steps. First, the shoulder is prepared with a #701 (unused) carbide bur at or slightly below the free margin of the gingiva (Fig 1-13). It is positioned parallel to the gingival third, as shown in Fig 1-12.

It is important to extend this gingival preparation to the proximal midline and up to the contact area (Fig 1-14); otherwise, the laminate will be bulky and unesthetic in this critical area. The proximal reduction is extended incisally while maintaining the contact point. The gingival contour is completed with a tapered diamond stone held in the same gingival plane (Fig 1-15). The incisal third is reduced with a tapered diamond stone held parallel to the incisal plane (Fig 1-16). To ensure an even reduction of 0.5 mm, it is clinically helpful to use one of the depth-controlling diamond stones (held in the same plane) before using the tapered diamond stone.

Laminate Tooth Preparation

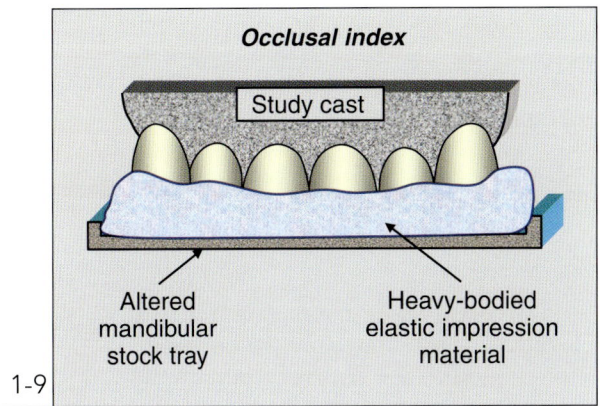

1-9 Occlusal index — Study cast; Altered mandibular stock tray; Heavy-bodied elastic impression material

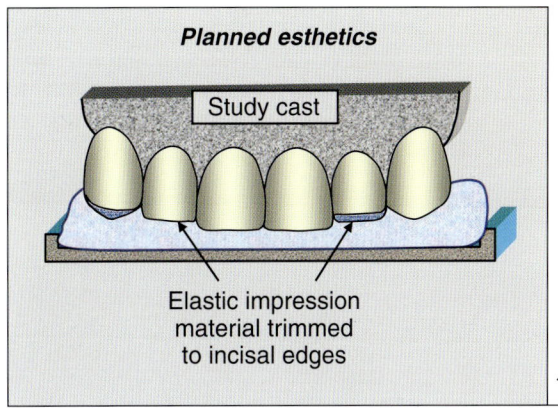

1-10 Planned esthetics — Study cast; Elastic impression material trimmed to incisal edges

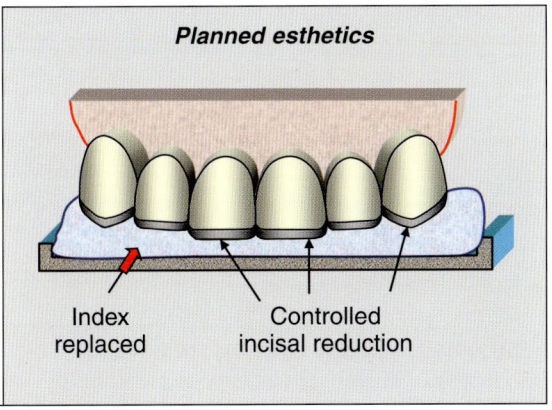

1-11 Planned esthetics — Index replaced; Controlled incisal reduction

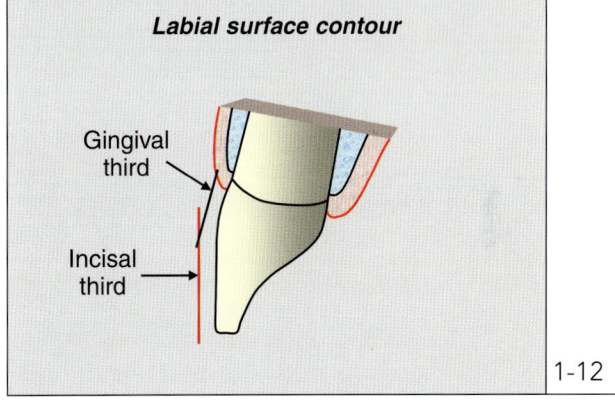

1-12 Labial surface contour — Gingival third; Incisal third

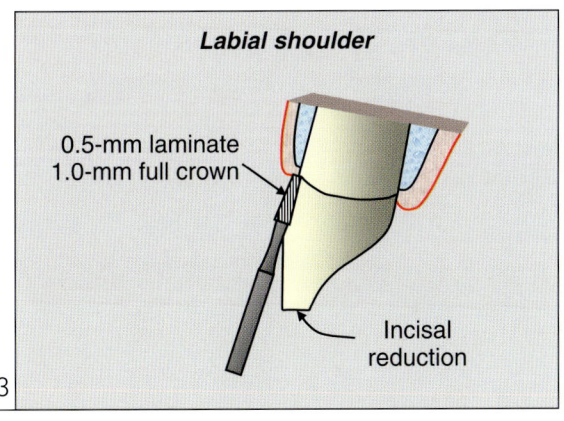

1-13 Labial shoulder — 0.5-mm laminate 1.0-mm full crown; Incisal reduction

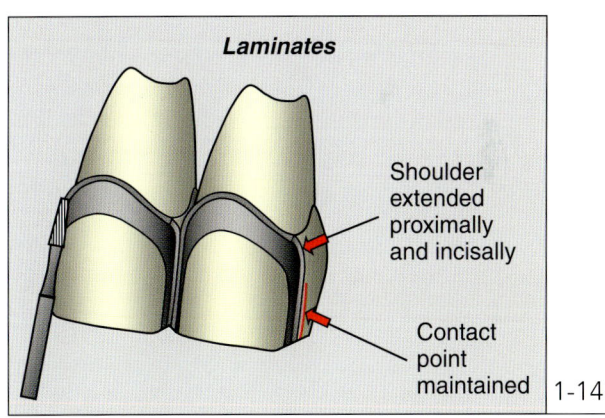

1-14 Laminates — Shoulder extended proximally and incisally; Contact point maintained

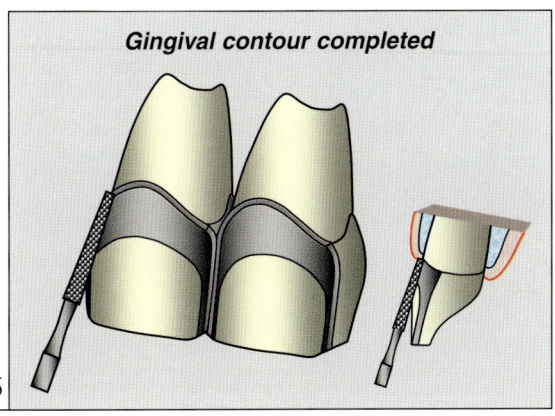

1-15 Gingival contour completed

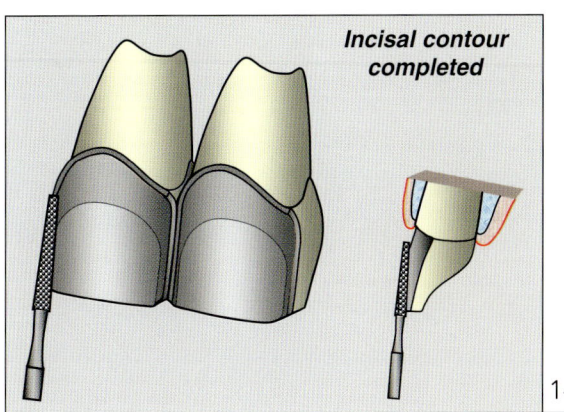

1-16 Incisal contour completed

5

The labial incisal line angle is rounded to the lingual line angle (Fig 1-17), and the labial surfaces are blended (Fig 1-18). Rounding of the incisal surface is critical to ensure that light refracts as it passes through the laminate in the incisal area (see Fig 1-17). The purpose of this procedure is to provide a blended transition in the color from the body to the incisal edge.

Maximum esthetic laminates

Because an even thickness of enamel was removed, when the porcelain laminate is bonded to the tooth (Fig 1-19), maximum esthetics results, facilitating the reproduction of normal anatomy and color in the restoration (Fig 1-20). For example, an unhappy patient presented with anterior maxillary laminates that were square and much longer than her original natural teeth (Fig 1-21). Six anterior maxillary laminates were fabricated following the procedure just described. Note that the gingival contours are tapered to provide a more natural appearance (Fig 1-22). The color was created to match her remaining natural teeth.

Anterior Full-Crown Preparation

Esthetic objectives

The esthetic anatomic objectives and transfer procedures for full coverage are similar to those for porcelain laminates. However, since the restoration is prepared totally around the tooth, the clinical problems are different. The most difficult esthetic challenge is to find enough space for metal, opaque, and porcelain within the original anatomic configuration of the natural tooth. This problem is magnified in the critical proximal area because underpreparation results in a bulky, unesthetic restoration, while overpreparation can lead to future pulpal exposure in the preparation when the proximal surfaces are being tapered.

Anterior Full-Crown Preparation

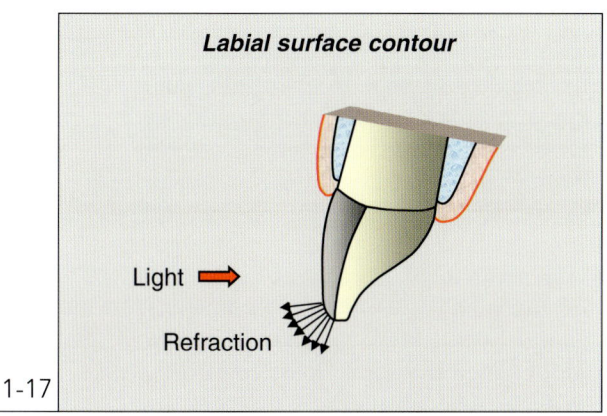

Labial surface contour

Light → Refraction

1-17

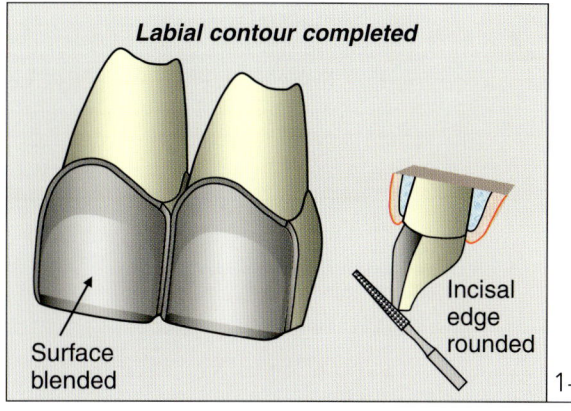

Labial contour completed

Surface blended

Incisal edge rounded

1-18

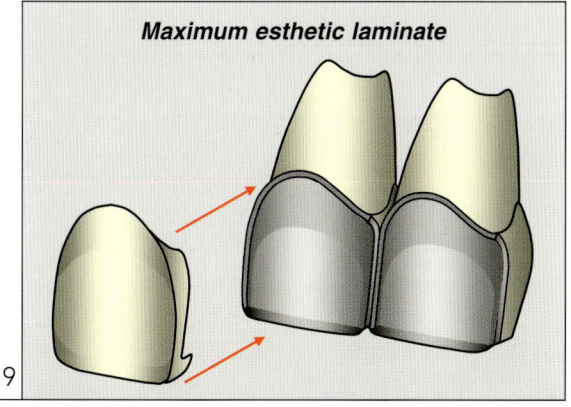

Maximum esthetic laminate

1-19

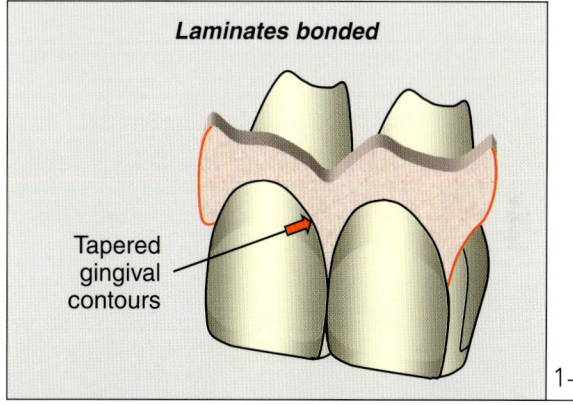

Laminates bonded

Tapered gingival contours

1-20

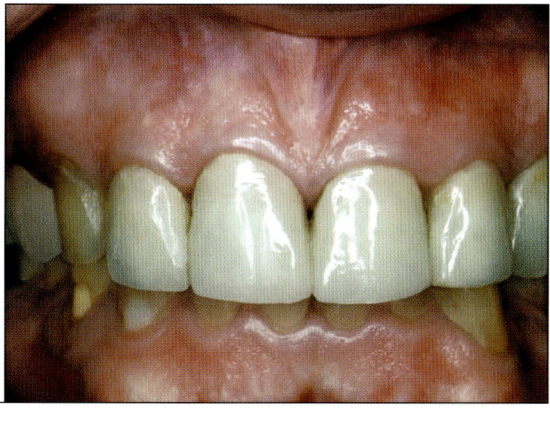

1-21

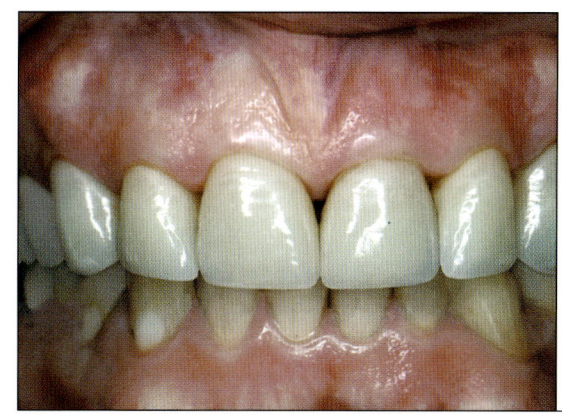

1-22

Tooth preparation

The clinical procedure is similar to that for porcelain laminates in terms of the orientation of the instruments and their chronologic application. The first step is incisal reduction, which is pre-planned and controlled with the occlusal index as before, but this time reduction will be a minimum of 2.0 mm (Fig 1-23). No lingual reduction is done at this time. A new #701 bur is used to prepare a 1.0-mm shoulder approximately 1.0 mm below the free margin of the gingivae and is held parallel to the gingival third of the labial surface (see Fig 1-23). The shoulder is extended proximally to the midline, carefully following the contour of the gingiva, which usually traverses toward the incisal, as shown in Fig 1-23. The danger here is in moving directly toward the lingual without following the gingival contour. Since the root tapers toward the apex, the thickness of the shoulder also diminishes. This can produce many clinical and esthetic problems. For example, if the preparation is immediately too far subgingival, an esthetic proximal contour is prevented, and if a 1.0-mm shoulder is created, overpreparation can lead to pulpal exposure when attempting to create tapering proximal surfaces.

The #701 bur is extended to the lingual in the dentinoenamel junction without producing a proximal taper (Fig 1-24). Due to the shortness of the #701 bur, the shoulder preparation proceeds incisally as well as lingually 1.0 mm (Fig 1-25). As the tapered diamond stone progresses proximally, it should produce a very slight taper on the proximal surfaces (see Fig 1-25).

Parallelism

The lingual surface is prepared with a slight taper relative to the labial-gingival third (see Fig 1-25). The recommended inclination of the gingival third seemingly produces an undercut. However, it should be noted that an undercut can only be created relative to a path of insertion established by the opposing lingual surface. Therefore, if the lingual surface has a slight taper relative to the labial third, then the path of insertion becomes slightly inclined lingually without producing an undercut. Most clinicians prepare the lingual surfaces of the anterior teeth with more than sufficient taper relative to the labial gingival third to avoid any undercut problem. The inclusion of posterior abutments with anterior teeth is discussed later.

The incisal third is reduced with the tapered diamond stone positioned parallel to that surface as shown in Fig 1-26. Many clinicians prefer to start with a long, depth-controlling diamond for enamel removal to prevent overpreparation. The body-incisal portion is then finalized before the corners are slightly rounded (see Fig 1-26). Over-rounding can cause pulpal exposure as well as a tendency for the casting to rotate on the abutment, leading to eventual loosening. Since the proximal taper has been completed previously, very little reduction is required. Occlusal clearance is best provided lingually with a round stone, which will facilitate an even thickness of restorative material (Fig 1-27). Because of the tapered topography of anterior teeth when viewed proximally, care should be taken to preserve the lingual wall near the gingival margin and to avoid excessive taper of the proximal walls to ensure a resistance form and thereby prevent subsequent loosening of the casting.

Anterior Full-Crown Preparation

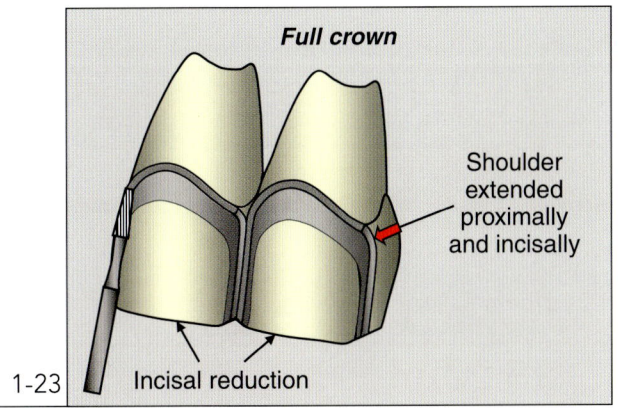

1-23

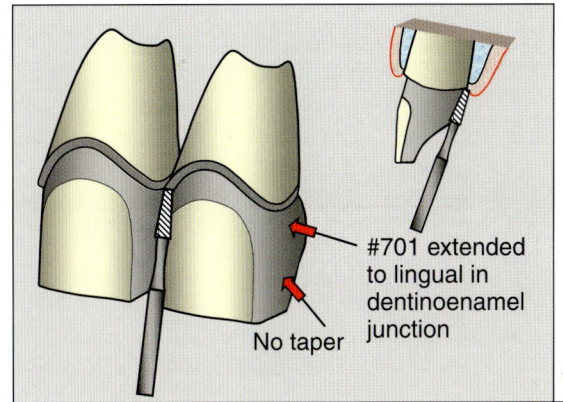

1-24

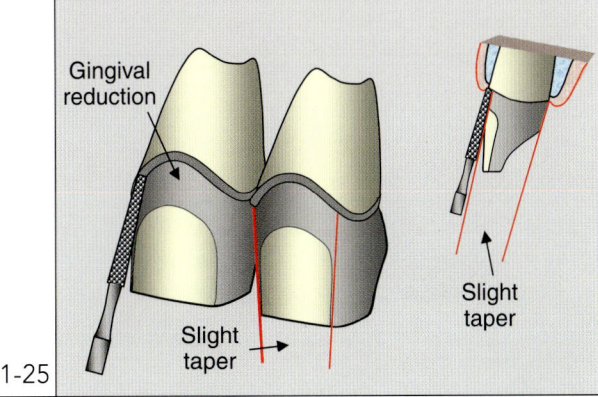

1-25

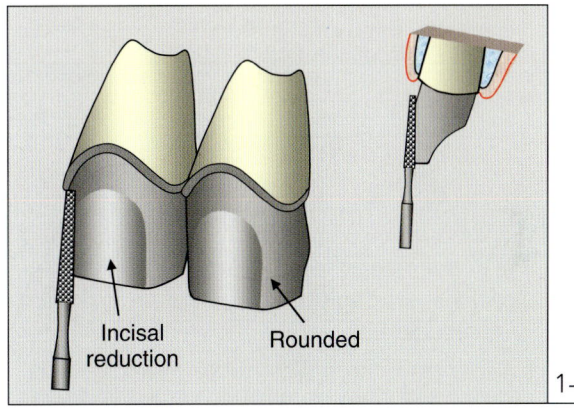

1-26

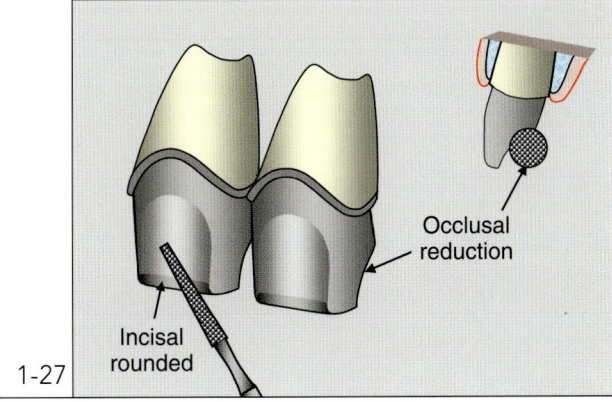

1-27

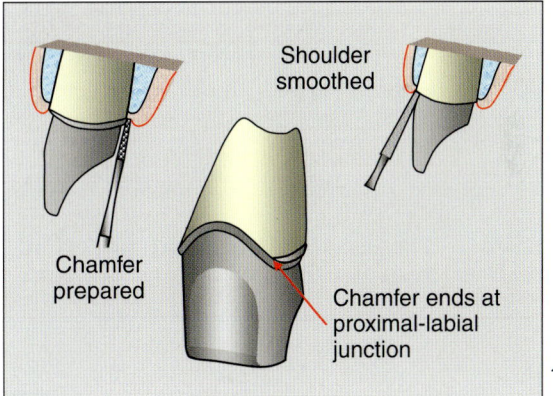

1-28

Modified chamfer

A full 1.0-mm chamfer produces approximately 1.0 mm of metal exposure at the gingival margin. Although this can produce an esthetic problem anteriorly, it is often unavoidable when the structural integrity of the tooth is compromised. Otherwise, a modified chamfer preparation that does not include the labial portion of the shoulder can be used. The first step in a modified preparation is to smooth the labial shoulder with the square-end portion of a fine finishing stone (Fig 1-28). The chamfer is prepared on the lingual and proximal surfaces, ending at the proximal-labial junction. The impression can be obtained in any material because the slightly lingually inclined path of insertion is harmonious with the labial root surface (see Fig 1-25).

1 Esthetic Planning and Tooth Preparation for Porcelain Laminates and Full Crowns

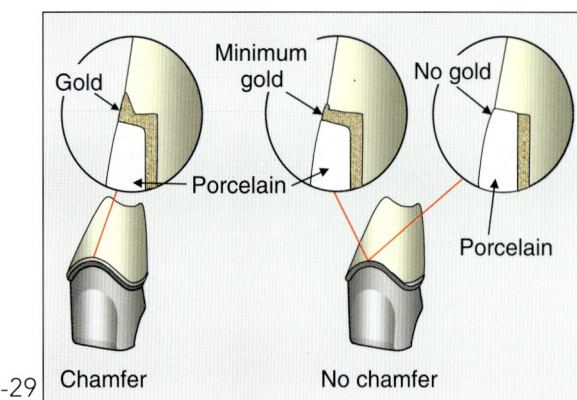

1-29

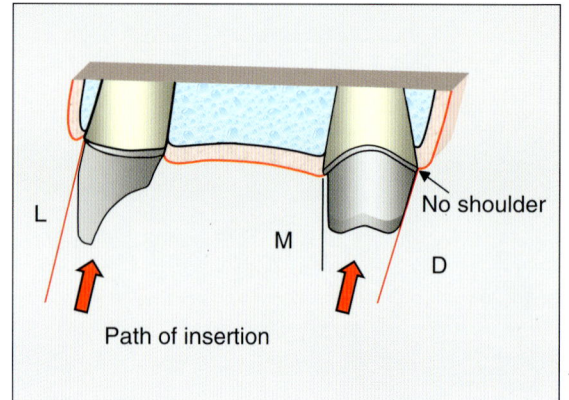

1-30

Metal finish lines

With a standard full-chamfered preparation, the exposed labial metal is at least 1.0 mm thick (Fig 1-29). A full chamfer may be required because of a tooth's poor structural integrity or because a tooth that has undergone root canal therapy with a post is susceptible to lateral force. In many cases, gingival recession gradually leads to undesirable esthetics. Two alternative procedures can be used, both of which involve a modified chamfer preparation that has a smooth labial shoulder without a chamfer. The chamfer is prepared on the lingual and proximal surfaces and ends at the proximal-labial junction. However, to use these alternatives successfully, it is necessary to make the impression at least 1.0 mm beyond the shoulder.

The first of these alternatives is to place a reduced collar on unprepared tooth structure over the labial shoulder, resulting in minimal gold (see Fig 1-29). The wax-up is created with a 1.0-mm collar to ensure proper casting. The labial metal collar is then reduced to 0.5 mm after the final glaze. The 0.5-mm labial collar is placed on unprepared tooth structure; however, a meticulous impression of this root area first must be made and duplicated on the die.

The second alternative is to provide no metal on the shoulder and to abut the porcelain directly to the shoulder.[6] This procedure is obviously more esthetic but highly technique sensitive.

Framework finishing for maximum esthetics

The sole purpose of a square shoulder in the preparation is to provide sufficient gingival space for metal, opaque, and porcelain without excessive bulk. Usually the technician waxes up with excess bulk in the gingival area and obliterates the shoulder contours. After casting and assemblage, the shoulder then has to be cut out of the metal in the gingival area to provide the required space, as described above. This is often left incomplete for fear of penetration of the metal and/or because of time constraints. Ideally, the metal framework should be a uniform thickness of 0.5 mm, which is difficult to accomplish and usually uneven.

Another critical area is the incisal tip of the casting. The labial incisal edge is rounded (see Fig 1-27) to provide the space necessary for metal, opaque, and porcelain. If insufficient space is provided, a whitish dot of the incisal opaque shows through the porcelain. To prevent this, the technician usually makes the porcelain thicker over the entire labial surface, resulting in an oversized and therefore unesthetic restoration.

Anterior Full-Crown Preparation

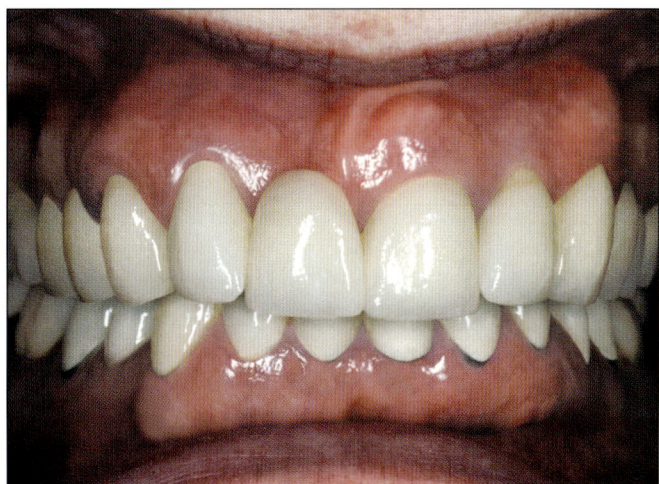

1-31

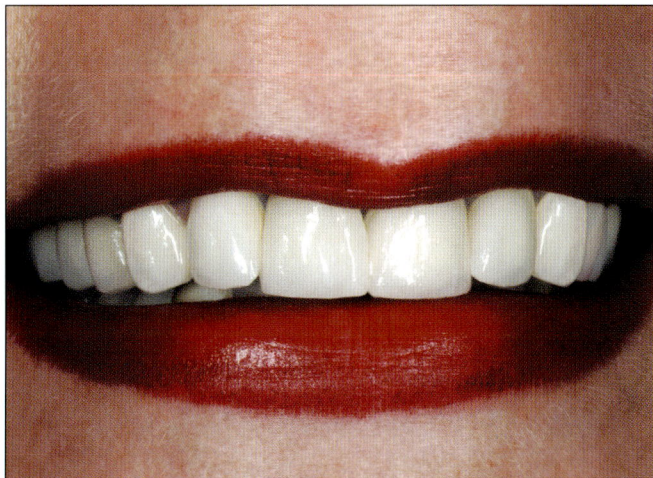

1-32

Parallelism

When posterior teeth are included in the restoration, parallelism need not be a problem. Because the path of insertion of the anterior restorations is inclined slightly lingually (see Fig 1-25), all that is required is to provide slightly more inclination to the distal proximal surfaces of all the posterior abutments to be in harmony with the path of insertion established anteriorly (Fig 1-30). No distal shoulder is advised to prevent pulpal involvement. The mesial proximal surfaces should be made nearly vertical (Fig 1-30) to provide basic retention when combined with the slightly exaggerated distal proximal surfaces.

Esthetic refinements

Tapered gingival contours in combination with the gingival papillae provide the maximum esthetics (Fig 1-31). The lateral incisors are overlapped with longer central incisors, which have minimal rounding of the incisal corners (Fig 1-32). This provides a natural appearance, resembling the esthetics of the patient's own natural teeth. The mandibular prosthesis in Fig 1-32 is 10 years old and reveals a slight exposure of gingival gold on a few margins due to the requirement of a full chamfer on all the preparations to maintain the integrity of the abutments. Note the proximal labial line angles, rather than grooves, between the anterior teeth. The proximal line angle configuration requires another biscuit bake after the initial contouring and establishment of occlusion. The porcelain is added to the proximal "grooves" and contoured with a sharp scalpel-like instrument while in the powder stage, thus creating a sharp line angle after the biscuit bake. These proximal line angles are not contoured with a disc after firing, since this would create unsightly grooves. (See chapter 3 for the step-by-step clinical procedure.)

Summary

Regardless of the restoration, maximum esthetics requires pre-planning, controlled incisal reduction, adequate tooth preparation to permit the restorative material to duplicate normal anatomy, and a three-dimensional occlusal index for the technician.

References

1. Buonocore MG, Matsui A, Gwinnert AM. Penetration of resin dental materials into enamel surfaces with reference to bonding. Arch Oral Biol 1968;13:61–70.
2. Jurim A. McAndrews-Northern Dental Laboratory. Personal communication, 1981. Patent applied for, April 1983, granted 1986, #4,632,660.
3. Horn H. A new lamination: Porcelain bonded to enamel. NY State Dent J 1983;49:401–403.
4. Starr M, Weller R. Nutra-bond II etched porcelain facings (veneers) and Kerr porcelite etched porcelain veneer cement. Technique and materials manual, 1983.
5. Weller R. New insights into porcelain laminates. Dent Today 1997;16:50–53.
6. Shillingburg HT Jr, Kessler JC. Recent developments in dental ceramics. Quintessence Dent Technol 1985;9:89–92.
7. Chiche GL. A common denominator to veneers and all-ceramic crown restorations. Pract Periodontics Aesthet Dent 1998;10:964.
8. Lang SA, Starr CB. Castable glass ceramics for veneer restorations. J Prosthet Dent 1992;67:590–594.

2 The Semi-adjustable Articulator: Concept, Modification, and Clinical Application

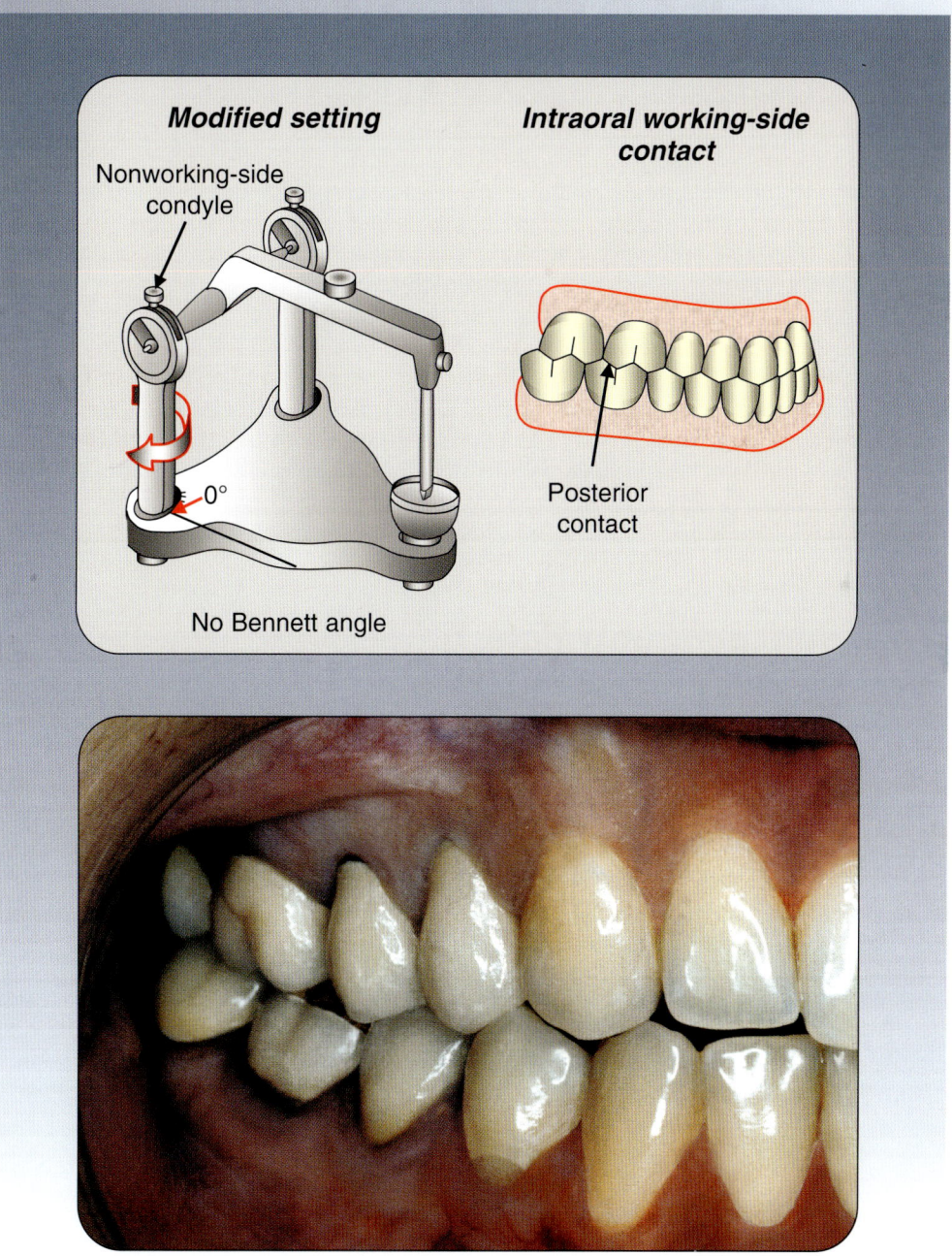

Over time, use of the dental articulator for fixed prostheses has ranged from three-dimensional recordings[1] to a straight-line hinge. Semi-adjustable articulators were originally designed primarily for complete denture fabrication.[2,3] Centric relation records were obtained with a facebow transfer for mounting,[4] and protrusive check bites were used to set the instrument for protrusive condylar inclination.[3] Hanau suggested the formula

$$\frac{H}{8} + 12$$

to calculate the medial inclination of the nonworking condylar movement (Bennett angle)[3] (Fig 2-1), where H is the protrusive condylar inclination. The derivation of this formula is unknown.

During the so-called golden age of gnathology,[5,6] three-dimensional records known as pantographs were obtained and transferred to three-dimensional articulators that had adjustable intercondylar distances, curved condylar paths, individual Bennett side shift, and an arcon condylar articulation (condylar ball on the lower member and the condylar path on the upper member).[5,6] Unfortunately, there were practical clinical drawbacks to the procedure as well as added expense. The technique could only be applied to complete-mouth restorative dentistry, and it took so long to complete that in most cases full-mouth cast gold acrylic veneer provisional restorations were required.

Gnathologic occlusions could only be created in gold. With the advent of esthetic porcelain-fused-to-gold (alloy) restorations, the conceptual arguments over gnathologic principles became academic. Thus, while gnathologic concepts significantly enhanced understanding of occlusion and the concepts of articulators,[7,8] there was no practical occlusal application to unilateral or single-arch prostheses. This left a tremendous void between three-dimensional gnathologic articulators and the straight-line hinge articulator upon which most fixed prostheses are constructed.

Reproducing Equivalent Physiologic Movement on a Semi-adjustable Articulator

The semi-adjustable articulator is a practical tool for constructing a prosthesis in the laboratory that will require a minimum of occlusal adjustment when seated intraorally. In short, it is a labor-saving device that *decreases* chair time to obtain the desired occlusion. This chapter describes the concept of the semi-adjustable articulator, its modification, and its clinical application.

Physiologic mandibular movement

During lateral mandibular movement, the nonworking-side condylar movement is downward, forward, and medial (see Fig 2-1). The downward inclination is obtained from the protrusive condylar inclination, with the forward component as a straight linear movement. For the sake of accuracy, it should be noted that during gnathologic tracings each of these components, as well as the arcon articulation, has a separate inclination and curvature.[7] However, each of these potential discrepancies has been calculated mathematically and found to be clinically insignificant.[7–9]

Working-side condylar movement has been described as rotation and simultaneous lateral shift (see Fig 2-1).[3] Some clinicians dispute the existence of a lateral mandibular side shift, and maintain it is an artifact in gnathologic tracings due to operator manipulation.[10] A study of the lateral Bennett shift has revealed variations.[11]

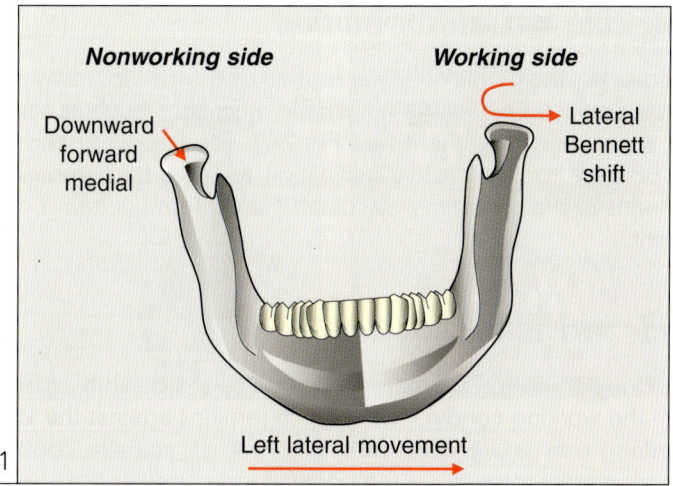

2-1

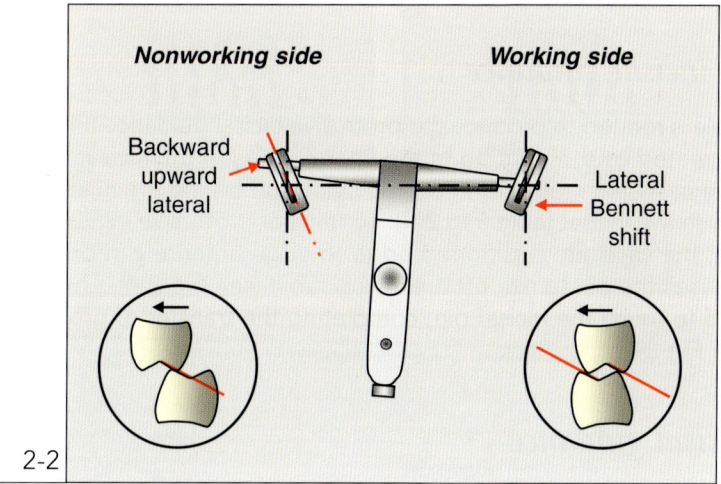

2-2

Articulator imitation of physiologic movement

With most standard articulators in use today, the condylar ball is attached to the upper member and the slot portion is part of the lower member. However, with an Arcon articulator, this relationship is reversed.[7] Since both designs produce exactly the same motion, the standard configuration is preferred only for its convenience of handling.[7] However, the direction of the motion on the standard articulator is the reverse of physiologic motion: The upper member moves while the lower member is stationary. For example, to imitate the left lateral physiologic motion shown in Fig 2-2, the upper member of the articulator moves in the opposite direction, that is, toward the patient's *right* side. Note also the working- and nonworking-side tooth relationships for orientation.

Working-side occlusion

If there is no Bennett shift to the working condylar movement[10,11] and the incisal guidance is 30 degrees, then all the working cusp inclines will be 30 degrees (see Fig 2-7).[8,14] In this case, the only difference between all the working cusp inclines will be their length. The more posteriorly the working cusp inclines are located along the arch, the shorter they will be as influenced by the working condylar rotation. Conversely, the working cusp inclines located closer to the anterior incisal guidance will be longer than the posterior cusp inclines.

When the working condyle rotates with a lateral shift of 0 degrees, the working cusp incline at the midpoint is the average of the two extreme guidances, or 15 degrees (Fig 2-7).[12,13] As the *location* of the working cusp incline moves toward the (anterior) incisal guidance, it is influenced more by that inclination and therefore will increase. Conversely, as the location of the working cusp incline shifts posteriorly toward the condyle with a lateral Bennett shift, the cusp inclination will decrease.[12,13]

Clinical significance

The 15-degree increase that is generated by a rotating working condyle (with no lateral Bennett shift) at the midpoint cusp incline is extremely important clinically. For a 3-mm cusp, the 15-degree increase produces a 0.8-mm increase in cusp height (Fig 2-8).[8,14] The significance of this finding is described below.

Modification of Articulator Settings

Clinical results with normal settings

For a 24-degree (average) condylar inclination, the Hanau formula[3] would call for a 15-degree medial rotation of the nonworking-side condylar post (Fig 2-9). Long-term clinical experience indicates that these settings produce a posterior opening on the working side (negative error), which cannot be corrected by occlusal adjustment.

Clinical results with modified settings

To eliminate all lateral Bennett shift, the nonworking-side condylar post is turned laterally to 0 degrees (Fig 2-10). When these restorations are seated intraorally, working-side contact is provided posteriorly (see Fig 2-10), and only minor occlusal corrections are required. The clinical example in Fig 2-11 shows four individual posterior porcelain-fused-to-gold restorations fabricated on the Hanau articulator with the modified settings just described. Simultaneous posterior contact (group function) is shown on the articulator in right lateral position.

When the restorations are seated intraorally, as shown in Fig 2-12, notice that the occlusal relationships are the same as they were in the laboratory. The point here is that regardless of the clinician's personal concept of occlusion, the semi-adjustable articulator can be modified to provide an accurate spatial relationship in the laboratory as in the mouth. Thus, the modified semi-adjustable articulator can be used as a practical, labor-saving device for unilateral, bilateral, or full-arch prosthodontics (see chapter 3).

Modification of Articulator Settings

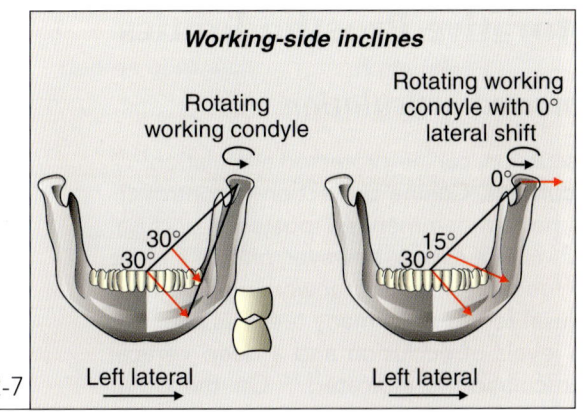

2-7

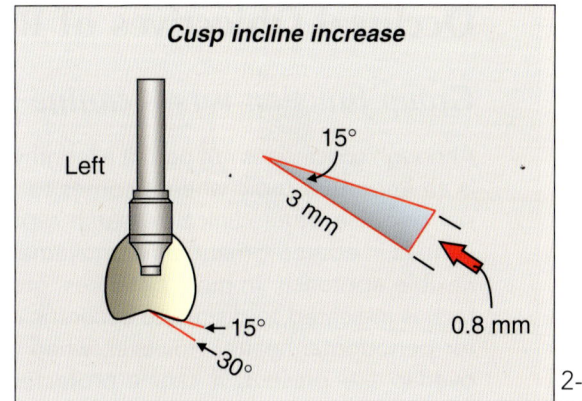

2-8

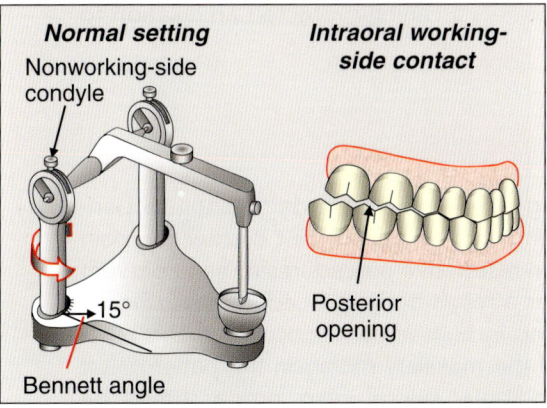

2-9

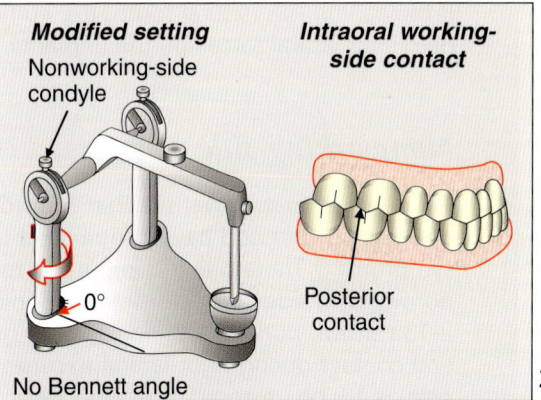

2-10

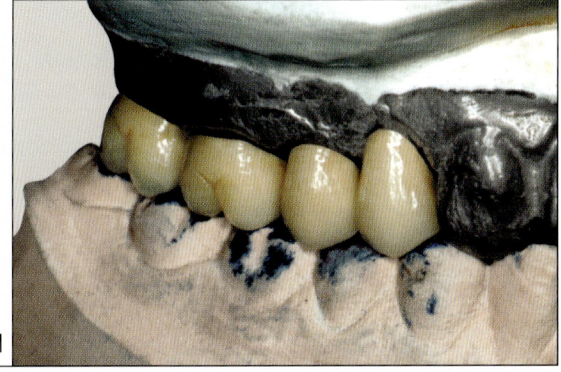

2-11

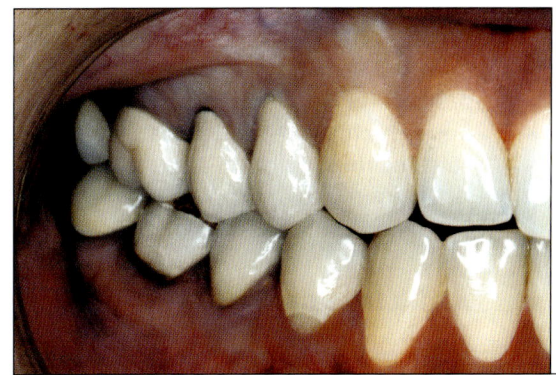

2-12

19

Incisal guidance modification for a modified occlusal anatomy

Standard incisal guidance
With standard incisal guidance, the motion of the incisal pin meets in a sharp angle as it moves from right to left laterally (Fig 2-15). As a result, the incisal guidance carves the standard anatomy, in which the cusp inclines meet in a sharp line angle.

Modified incisal guidance
In order to produce a posterior horizontal fossa of 1.5 mm, the incisal edges of the incisal pin are beveled approximately 1.5 mm (Fig 2-16). Bilateral movement of the incisal pin on the plane produces a motion that flattens in the middle before advancing up the inclines (see Fig 2-16). This produces a reverse form in the maxillary fossae, that is, a horizontal fossa of 1.5 mm.

Protrusive guidance

Physiologic variation in centric relation[27–30] also requires freedom of movement anteriorly. Anterior freedom of movement is provided by judicious occlusal adjustment, using the two-colored marking system (Fig 2-17). To provide this freedom, the incisal table is rotated to 0 degrees. Once this freedom of movement is ground into the restorations, the incisal table is returned to its original inclination (Fig 2-18). Using the two-color marking system once again, the protrusive excursion is adjusted while maintaining centric contact.

Occlusal harmony with a modified occlusal anatomy

A modified occlusal anatomy containing a horizontal fossa of 1.5 mm requires bilateral occlusal adjustment.[26] The opposing occlusion must be pre-adjusted to contain corresponding fossae using a procedure similar to that described for Fig 2-13b. Otherwise, centric occlusion will be lost on the affected cusps.

For example, standard working-side inclines are shown in Fig 2-19. Right working-side movement of the modified incisal guidance carves half of the horizontal fossa and the maxillary buccal cusp incline of the restoration (Fig 2-20). The maxillary lingual (slope) surface is reduced by the mandibular lingual cusp incline (see Fig 2-20).

When the modified incisal guidance moves in the opposite nonworking-side direction, the mandibular buccal cusp incline reduces the maxillary lingual cusp incline (Fig 2-21). When the casts are returned to the centric occlusion position, there is a loss of the maxillary centric-maintaining lingual cusp (Fig 2-22). This was one of the clinical problems associated with the functionally generated path technique previously discussed.

Occlusal Objectives of Restorative Prosthodontics

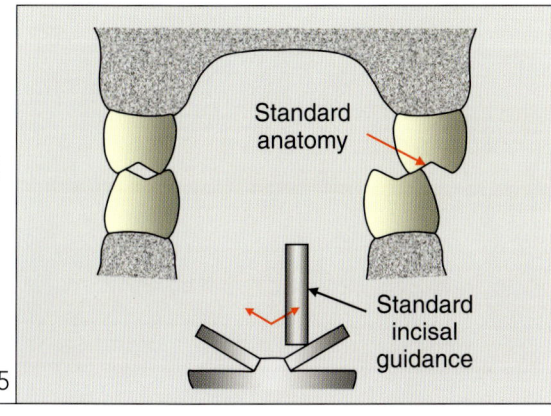
2-15

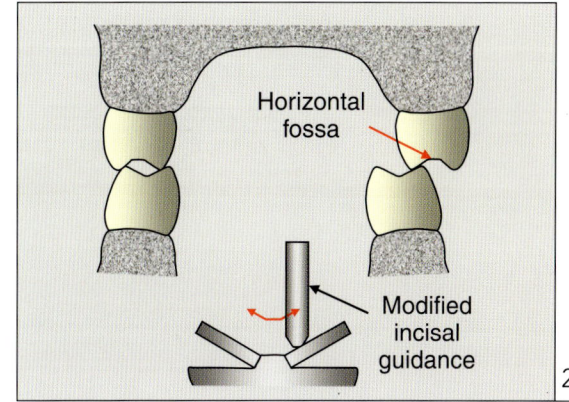
2-16

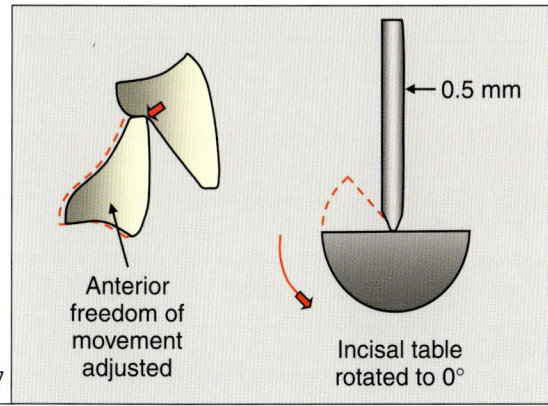
2-17

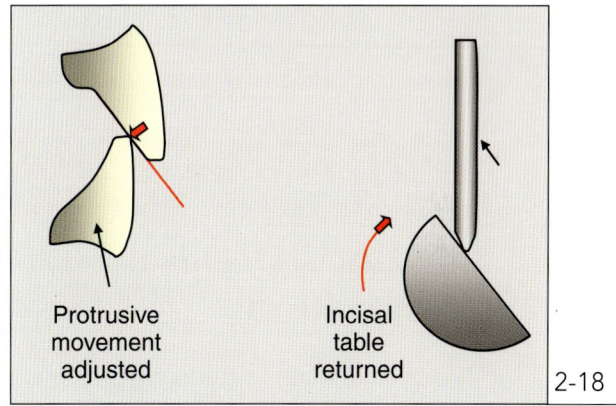
2-18

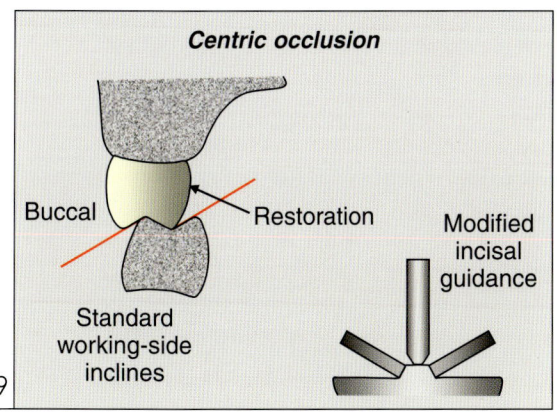
2-19

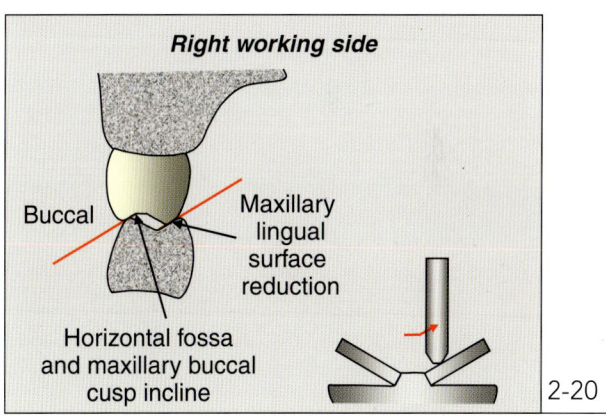
2-20

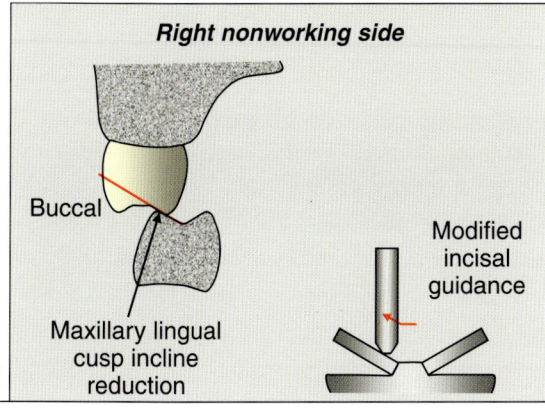
2-21

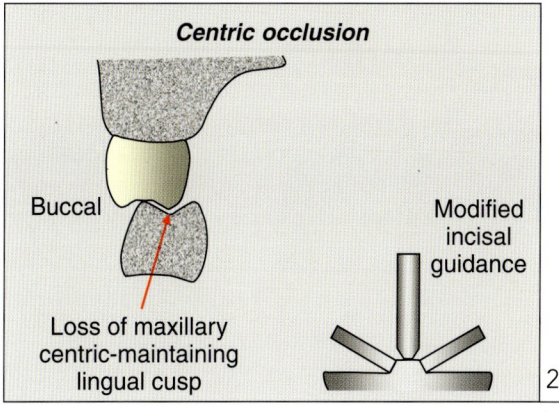
2-22

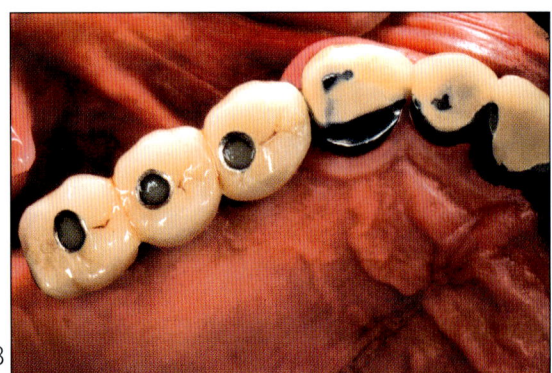
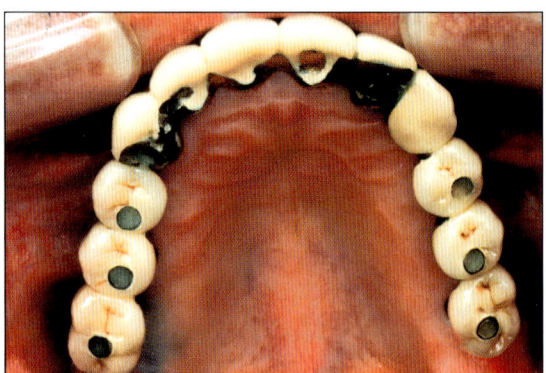

2-23   2-24

Modified Occlusal Anatomy with Existing Restorations

Modified occlusal anatomy will not be in harmony with adjacent natural teeth or other traditionally restored dentition. By definition, the 1.5-mm horizontal fossa requires corrective grinding of adjacent occlusal surfaces in the entire arch (and opposing occlusion) to be in harmony. This process, which is described in chapter 5, may be easily accomplished with a two-color marking system.

Figure 2-23 shows a three-unit, implant-supported prosthesis seated adjacent to a pre-existing toothborne prosthesis. The lingual contacting areas in the pre-existing fixed prosthesis have been occlusally adjusted with the two-color marking system to preserve centric contact. Any perforations in the metal can be repaired with an appropriate filling material. In Fig 2-24, bilateral posterior implant-supported prostheses are adjacent to a pre-existing anterior toothborne fixed prosthesis. The lingual surfaces of the anterior restoration have been corrected to be in harmony with the posterior modified centric occlusal anatomy. (Nine-year postoperative radiographs of both cases are shown in chapter 5, Figs 5-31, 5-32, and 5-37 to 5-40.)

Summary

The relationship of the incisal guidance, condylar paths, and cusp inclines provide the basis for the modification of standard semi-articulator settings that facilitate its practical clinical application. A modified centric occlusal anatomy, containing 1.5-mm horizontal fossae, can be accomplished with a simple incisal guide pin modification.

References

1. McCullum BB. Fundamentals involved in prescribing restorative remedies. D Items Interest 1939;61:522–535,641–648,724–736,852–856,942–950.
2. Gysi A, Clapp GW. Practical application of research results in denture construction (mandibular movements). J Am Dent Assoc 1929;16:199–223.
3. Hanau RL. Full Denture Prosthesis, ed 4. Buffalo: Hanau Engineering, 1930:39.
4. Snow G. The philosophy of mastication. Dent Cosmos 1900;42:531–535.
5. Stuart CE, Stallard H. Principles involved in restoring occlusion to natural teeth. J Prosthet Dent 1960;10:304.
6. Granger ER, Lucia V, Hudson W, Celenza F, Pruden W Jr. Hinge axis committee. Presented at the 5th Scientific Meeting of the Greater New York Academy of Prosthodontics, New York, Dec 1959.
7. Weinberg LA. Arcon principle in the condylar mechanism of adjustable articulators. J Prosthet Dent 1963;13:263–268.
8. Weinberg LA. An evaluation of basis articulators and their concepts. J Prosthet Dent 1963;13:622–644,645–663,873–888,1038–1054.
9. Weinberg LA. An evaluation of the face bow mounting. J Prosthet Dent 1961;11:32–42.
10. Landa J. Critical analysis of the Bennett movement. J Prosthet Dent 1958;8:709–726.
11. Issacson D. A clinical study of the Bennett movement. J Prosthet Dent 1958;8:641–649.
12. Cohen R. The relationship of anterior guidance to condylar guidance in mandibular movements. J Prosthet Dent 1956;6:758–767.
13. Schuyler CH. Factors of occlusion applicable to restorative dentistry. J Prosthet Dent 1953;3:772–782.
14. Weinberg LA. Incisal and condylar guidance in relation to cuspal inclination in lateral excursions. J Prosthet Dent 1959;9:851–862.
15. D'Amico A. The canine teeth—Normal functional relation of the natural teeth of man. J South Calif Dent Assoc 1958;26:6–23,49–60,127–142,175–182,194–208,239–241.
16. D'Amico A. Functional occlusion of the natural teeth of man. J Prosthet Dent 1961;11:899–915.
17. Weinberg, LA. Occlusal equilibratrion in eccentric positions. NY State Dent J 1957:23:310–312.
18. Weinberg LA. The prevalence of tooth contact in eccentric movements of the jaw: Its clinical implications. J Am Dent Assoc 1961;62:403–406.
19. Yurkastas AA, Emerson WH. A study of tooth contact during mastication with artificial dentures. J Prosthet Dent 1954;4:168–174.
20. Brewer AA, Hudson DC. Application of miniaturized electronic devices to the study of tooth contact in complete dentures. J Prosthet Dent 1961;11:62–72.
21. Schweitzer JM. Masticatory function in man. J Prosthet Dent 1961;11:625–647.
22. Weinberg LA. A cinematic study of centric and eccentric occlusions. J Prosthet Dent 1964;14:290–293.
23. Weinberg LA. Functional and esthetic planning for full coverage. J Am Dent Assoc 1963;66:42–53.
24. Posselt U. Temporomandibular joint syndrome and occlusion; Research committee report. Am Equilibration Soc Compend 1963-64;7:51.
25. Mann A, Pankey L. Oral rehabilitation II. Reconstruction of the upper teeth using a functionally generated path technique. J Prosthet Dent 1960;10:151–162.
26. Weinberg LA. Reduction of occlusal loading using a modified centric occlusal anatomy. Int J Prosthodont 1998;11:55–69.
27. Grasso J, Sharry J. The duplicability of arrow-point tracing in dentulous subjects. J Prosthet Dent 1968;20:106–115.
28. Kantor M, Silverman S, Garfinkel L. Centric relation recording techniques: A comparative investigation. J Prosthet Dent 1972;28:593–600.
29. Calagna L, Silverman S, Garfinkel L. Influence of neuromuscular conditioning on centric relation registrations. J Prosthet Dent 1973;30:598–604.
30. Celenza FV. The centric position: Replacement and character. J Prosthet Dent 1973;30:591–598.

3 Esthetic, Functional, and Vertical Dimension Planning for Complete-Arch Prostheses

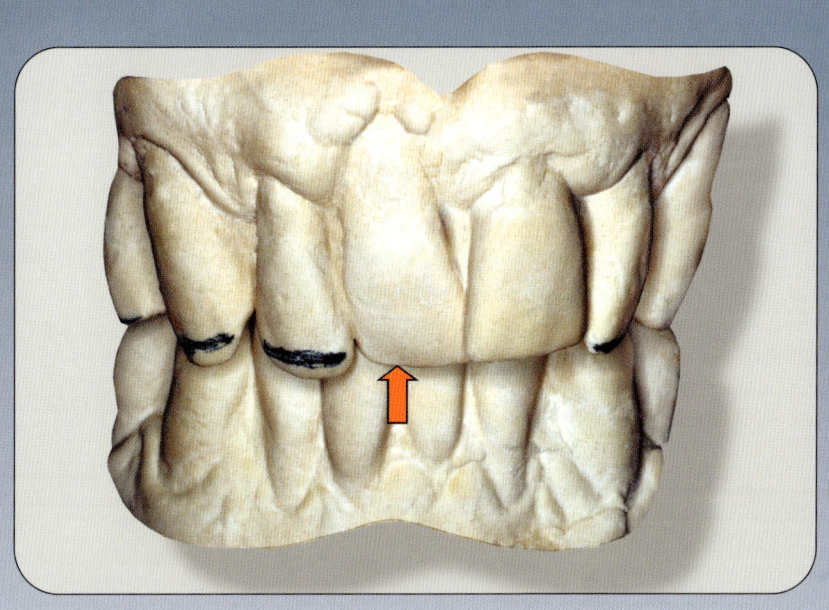

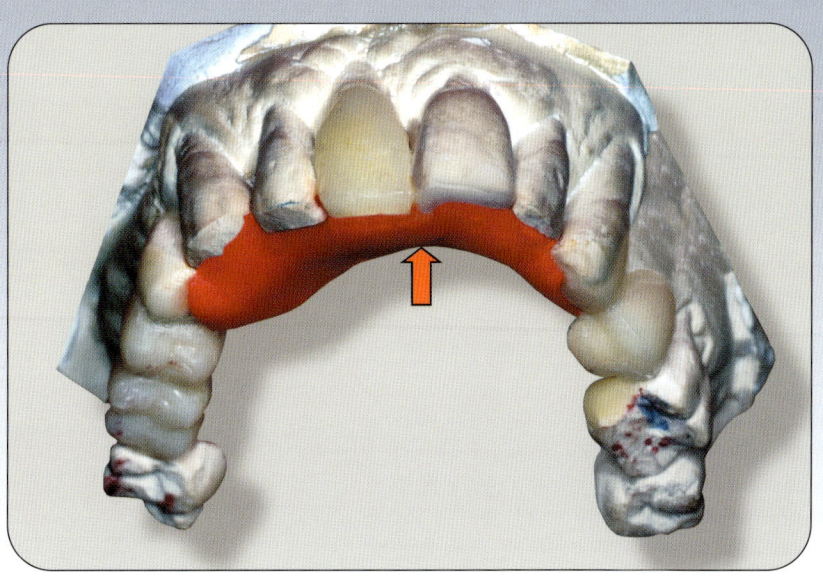

Esthetic, functional, and vertical dimension planning should precede any restorative procedures for complete-arch or complete-mouth prostheses. When tooth preparations are not made relative to an overall esthetic and functional plan, the result may be too much or not enough tooth structure removal. Since the preparations dictate the final results, optimum esthetics and functional relationships cannot be obtained. Moreover, the patient has no time to adjust to the planned esthetics and functional relationships, sometimes requiring remakes. Once tooth structure is removed, the original centric relation and vertical dimension landmarks are obliterated. A therapeutic trial of functional relationships is indicated to reduce the risk of temporomandibular joint dysfunction problems. This chapter presents a practical esthetic and functional planning technique that can be used effectively for a prosthesis of any size.

Esthetic and Functional Planning Outline

The starting point for esthetic planning is ensuring that the smile line (ie, the incisal edges of the maxillary anterior teeth) parallels the interpupillary line. When necessary, this is corrected on mounted study casts and followed by correction of the posterior occlusal plane and setup of any missing teeth. These changes are then transferred to the natural teeth *before* tooth preparation. The teeth are then prepared using the corrected casts to fabricate the provisional restorations. This procedure provides for a clinical trial of the esthetics and functional planning before the final restorations are completed.

Esthetic and functional corrections

A patient presented with rampant caries and poor oral hygiene following years of neglect (Fig 3-1). Before any long-term treatment was discussed, soft tissue treatment, caries removal, and oral hygiene instruction were provided (Fig 3-2). Study casts were then mounted on a semi-adjustable articulator with a facebow to orient the casts to the true horizontal plane (interpupillary line), which required correction. Hand articulation completed the mounting (Fig 3-3). (Centric relation and vertical dimension will be discussed later in this chapter.) The elongated anterior teeth were marked for shortening, and linguoversion of the maxillary right central incisor (*arrow*) was noted (see Fig 3-3). The anterior maxillary teeth were shortened as indicated, the maxillary right central incisor was reshaped, and the posterior occlusal plane was corrected to complete the waxup (Fig 3-4).

Transfer of esthetic changes

Before any abutment preparations were undertaken, all anterior maxillary and mandibular esthetic changes on the cast were transferred to the mouth using Duralay (Reliance, Worth, IL) lingual indexes. Figure 3-5 shows the corrected maxillary cast with a Duralay lingual index trimmed to the corrected anterior teeth. The elongated maxillary anterior teeth were then shortened intraorally to the level of the Duralay lingual index (Fig 3-6). Figure 3-7 shows the smile line before treatment; note the marked tilt of the incisal edges of the teeth. The after-treatment view reveals a marked improvement in the anterior esthetics of the natural teeth *before* restorative procedures have been initiated (Fig 3-8). The mandibular anterior teeth have been treated with the same indexing procedure.

Esthetic and Functional Planning Outline

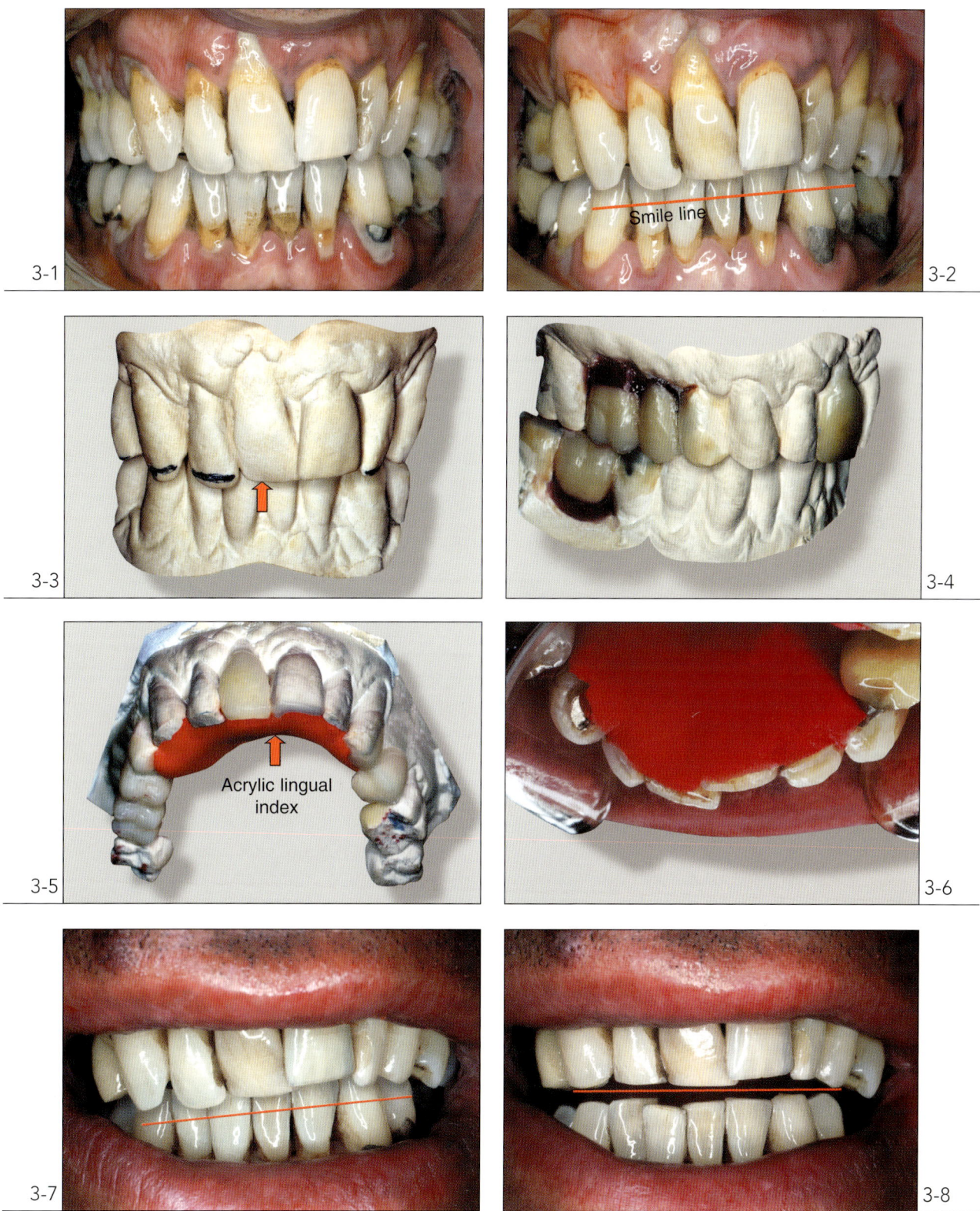

3 Esthetic, Functional, and Vertical Dimension Planning for Complete-Arch Prostheses

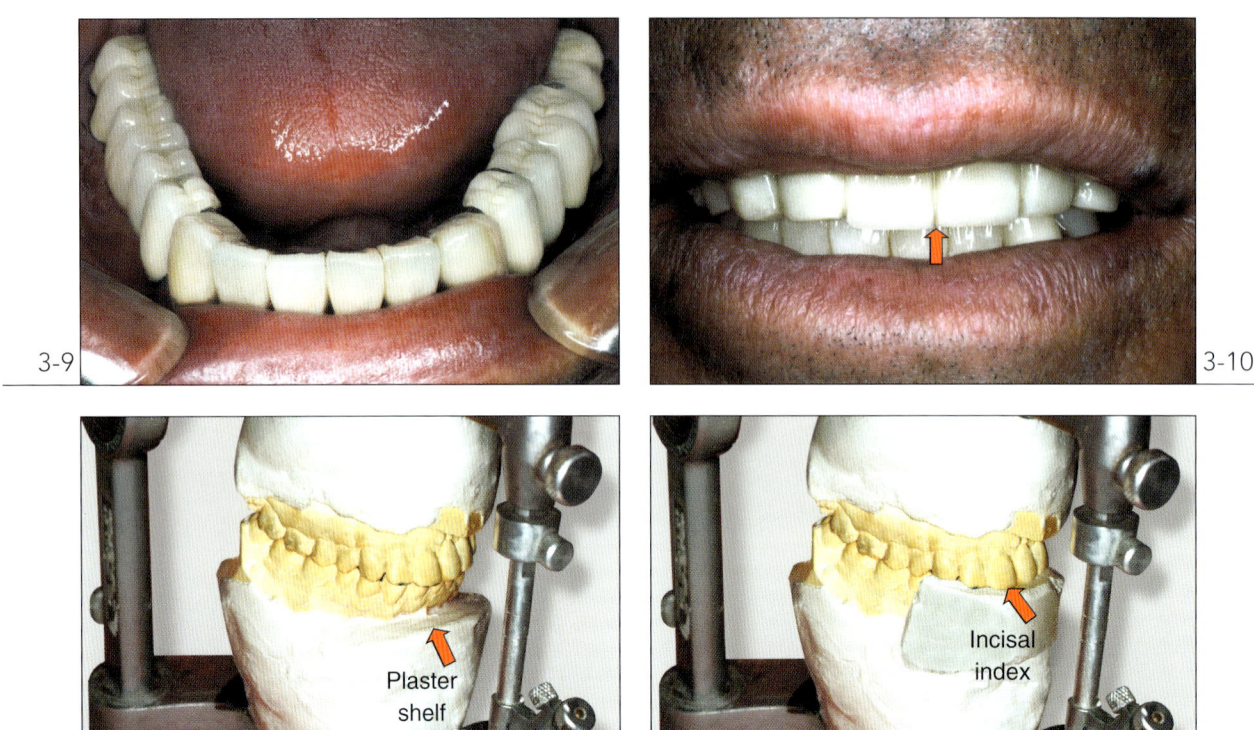

3-9

3-10

3-11 Plaster shelf

3-12 Incisal index

It is the author's view that unless this or a similar procedure is followed, the technician will find it virtually impossible to create acceptable restorations, resulting in inefficiency, frustration, and the need for remakes. The concept of performing an incisal index that will be transferred to the final working casts (also discussed in chapter 1) will ensure complete control of the esthetics from the planning cast through the provisional restorations and into the final restorations.

Although the esthetics of a restoration are judged on the appearance of the maxillary arch (both anteriorly and posteriorly), the mandibular arch is constructed first. This is because the occlusion functions as an inverted mortar and pestle, where the sides of the mortar function as the guiding inclines while the pestle itself is in motion. For example, the anterior overlap is exactly like the inverted mortar and pestle, where the incisal guidance for protrusive, right, and left lateral excursions serve as the mortar's surface and the mandibular anterior teeth act as the pestle. The normal buccal overlap of the maxillary posterior teeth functions in a similar way. (The mandibular lingual molar cusp inclines are the exception; however, these inclines often are not restored in lateral function.) All occlusal corrective procedures are presented in chapter 11.

Provisional restorations

Once the anterior esthetics and posterior occlusal planes are corrected, the provisional mandibular restorations can be constructed one quadrant at a time. As outlined previously (see Figs 3-3 to 3-8), a full-arch impression of the mandibular study cast will facilitate the *exact replication* of centric relation, centric occlusion, and the original vertical dimension, even though esthetics and the occlusal plane have been corrected. As each quadrant is prepared and provisional restorations are provided, the remaining two quadrants serve as constant occlusal references. This approach facili-

Esthetic and Functional Planning Outline

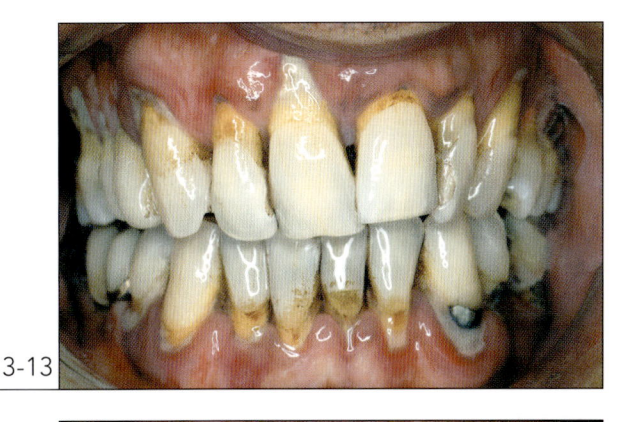

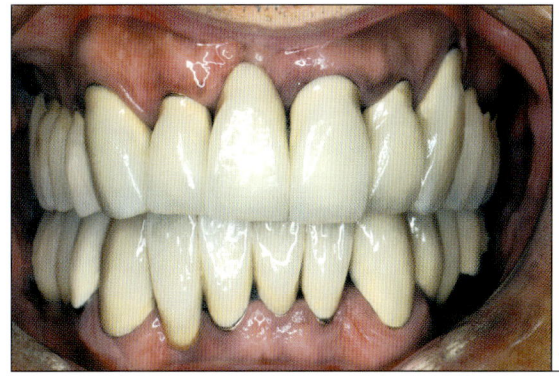

3-13

3-14

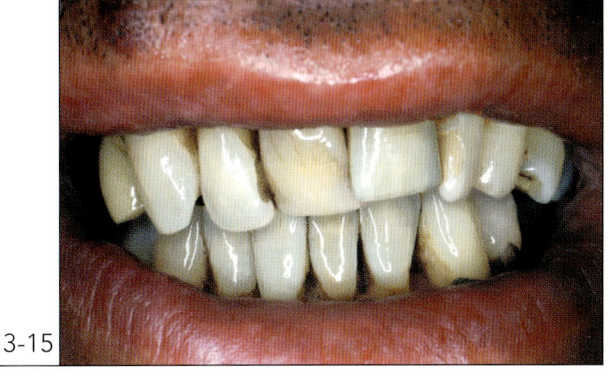

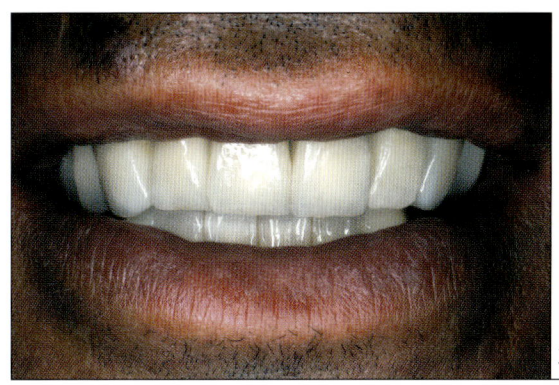

3-15

3-16

tates the completion of the final mandibular restoration (Fig 3-9) in conformity with the original esthetic and functional planning.

Since centric relation and the vertical dimension have been maintained, and since the desired esthetics have been "planned into" the construction of the mandibular arch, the maxillary prosthesis should provide no unexpected surprises. The posterior maxillary teeth are prepared in quadrants, and provisional restorations are constructed using a full-arch impression of the maxillary planning cast. Next, the maxillary anterior teeth are prepared and provisional restorations are created, again using a full-arch impression of the maxillary planning cast (Fig 3-10). The maxillary anterior provisional restorations should be constructed with great care because they will serve as the model for the final restorations. In the author's experience, autocuring acrylic shells created in the laboratory (*arrow*) provide an excellent means of duplicating the planned esthetics (see Fig 3-10). (The complete clinical procedure is presented later in this chapter.) Any final changes in the smile line or individual tooth position should be performed intraorally in the provisional restoration.

A maxillary study cast of the completed provisional maxillary restorations is obtained. It is mounted on the articulator by manual articulation with the completed mandibular cast (Fig 3-11). A plaster shelf, or indexing of the buccal muscle border in the anterior area, provides a seat for an incisal index (see Fig 3-11). Plaster or polysiloxane modeling putty provides an incisal index that should be trimmed to (but should not obliterate) the incisal edges of the teeth (Fig 3-12). The incisal index provides a three-dimensional guide for the definitive maxillary restorations.

The study casts of the maxillary provisional restorations and the definitive mandibular prosthesis provide a means of transferring the planned esthetics and incisal guidance back to the articulator for use with the final maxillary working cast.

The before-treatment retracted appearance shown in Fig 3-13 can be compared to the final retracted appearance in Fig 3-14. The before-treatment and after-treatment smiles are shown in Figs 3-15 and 3-16 respectively.

Determining the Vertical Dimension

The vertical dimension (VD) of occlusion[1] is the distance between the chin and nose points when the teeth are in maximum occlusion (Fig 3-17, *red arrows*). The vertical dimension of rest is the distance between the same two points when the mandible is in the physiologic rest position (see Fig 3-17). The physiologic rest position varies as to postural tonicity,[2–4] mitotic reflex,[5–10] and gravity-elasticity.[11]

Physiologic rest position

The variability of the physiologic rest position is due to the maze of proprioceptors contributing to mandibular posture. The joint capsule receptors, which help establish joint-position sense,[5–10] the muscle spindles (stretch reflex),[16–20] and the proprioceptors in the periodontal membrane and oral mucosa[16–18] all interact to establish the physiologic rest position.

Originally, the rest position was thought to be stable throughout life.[19] Subsequent research has shown it to vary[20-22] according to head position,[23,24] loss of teeth,[25–28] environmental changes,[29,30] and insertion of dentures.[31,32] Thus, the position sense of the physiologic rest position is monitored by proprioceptor reflex stimuli from the joints, muscles, periodontal membranes, and oral mucosa.

Speaking space

The speaking space is the minimum vertical distance between the teeth during speech—that is, the distance between the vertical dimension of physiologic rest and the vertical dimension of occlusion (maximum intercuspation) (see Fig 3-17). Electromyography studies on the speaking space are beyond the scope of this presentation; however, long-term studies show that muscle length will tend to re-establish itself. For instance, Ramfjord and Blankenship[33] placed pins in the alveolar bone of the anterior maxilla and mandible of adult monkeys and opened the vertical dimension 7 mm anteriorly with the placement of posterior onlays (Fig 3-18). Within 36 months, the anterior pins had almost returned to their original vertical dimension (VD) and the posterior teeth had intruded into the bone to permit closure (see Fig 3-18).

The following clinical observations can be made based on the results of vertical dimension research. *(1)* Opening the vertical dimension beyond the speaking space (Fig 3-19) will usually cause reflex clenching by the patient, resulting in the long-term intrusion of teeth (*arrows*) and a return to the original muscle length (Fig 3-20). *(2)* The vertical dimension of rest varies within the same patient. *(3)* There is no known physiologic norm for the speaking space. *(4)* Exaggerated physiologic wear of the teeth (Fig 3-21) does not necessarily indicate a "lost vertical dimension" that should be restored. *(5)* When the speaking space is minimal (2 mm), the restorations should not increase the vertical dimension of occlusion regardless of occlusal wear; in the present case (Fig 3-22), the physiologic eruption kept pace with the occlusal wear. Therefore, the premolar-to-premolar restorations conformed to the existing vertical dimension.

Since the physiologic rest position varies within each patient and the speaking space varies from patient to patient, occlusal wear alone cannot be used as a criterion for raising the vertical dimension. First, a minimum of 2 mm of speaking space must be maintained. Second, clinical judgment combined with a thorough clinical trial with an acrylic occlusal onlay or provisional restoration (at the planned new vertical dimension) is recommended before the final prosthesis is fabricated.

Determining the Vertical Dimension

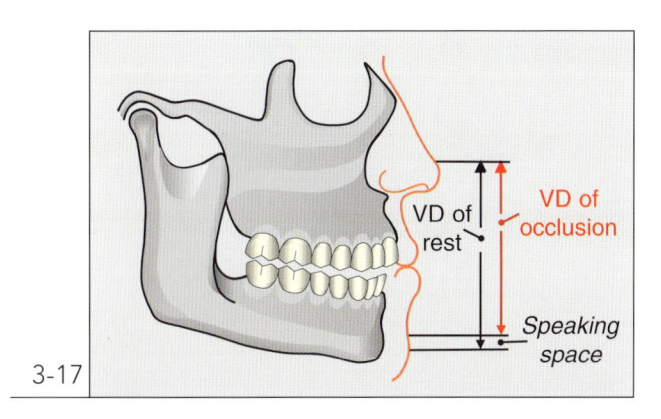

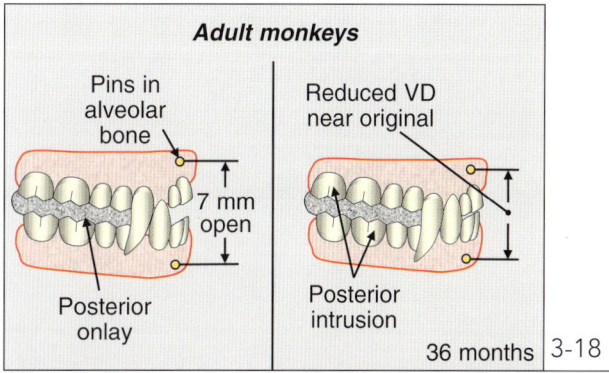

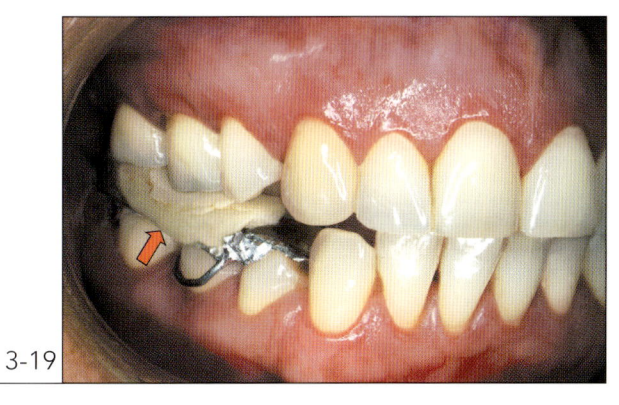

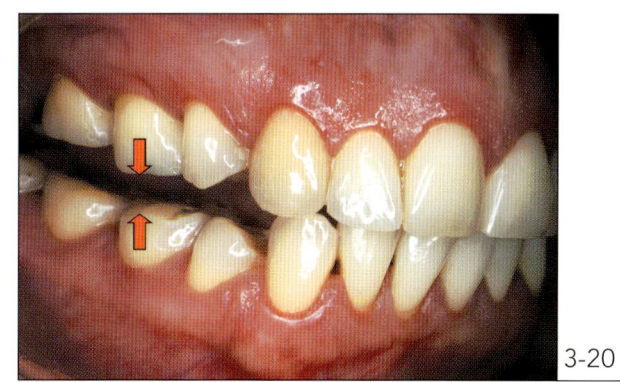

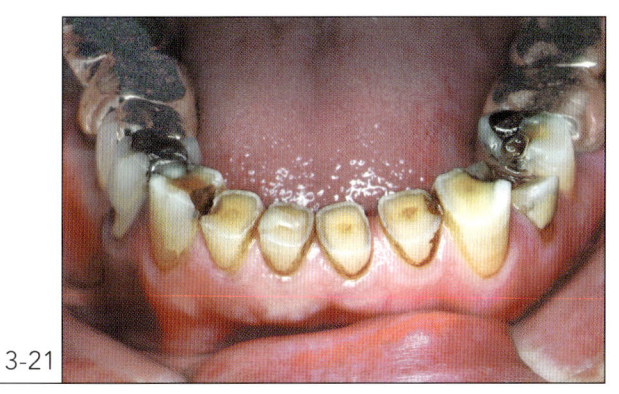

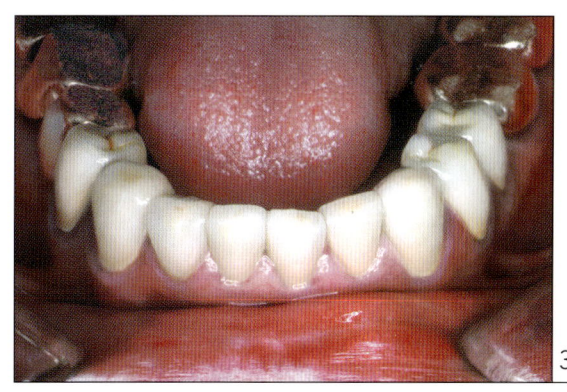

3-17

3-18

3-19

3-20

3-21

3-22

Clinical Procedure for Increasing the Vertical Dimension

Evaluation

The patient shown in Fig 3-23 presented with a severe vertical overlap, extensive wear of the posterior teeth into dentin (*arrow*), and perforation of the gold on the lingual surface of the canine (Fig 3-24). The speaking space was exaggerated and clinical judgment indicated that a 1.5-mm opening at the first molar could easily be tolerated.

Planning casts

The casts were mounted with a facebow and hand articulated because centric relation and centric occlusion coincided (Fig 3-25). The incisal guidance was transferred as described in chapter 2. The incisal pin was then opened to provide 1.5 mm of opening at the first molar. (Duralay was added to the top of the incisal pin to prevent inadvertent change; see Fig 3-43). Autocuring acrylic stops were painted on the posterior occlusal surfaces (*arrows*), and the anterior teeth were waxed up (Figs 3-26 and 3-27). Anterior contact was provided on the lingual surfaces of the waxup, as indicated by the blue marks in Fig 3-27.

Transfer of the esthetics

An alginate impression of the planning casts was obtained, and autocuring acrylic was painted into the anterior portion to produce thin shells (Fig 3-28, *arrow*). Care must be exercised during this process to achieve a minimum degree of thickness (Fig 3-29). The posterior acrylic occlusal onlays were then positioned bilaterally to the patient's teeth to transfer the planned vertical dimension. Next, the six anterior teeth were prepared and lubricated, and soft acrylic was placed into the shells and seated over the preparations. The jaws were occluded until the posterior stops made contact (Fig 3-30, *arrows*). The anterior prosthesis was then finished, and the occlusion was checked. This process transferred the esthetics, the planned vertical dimension, and the centric occlusion.

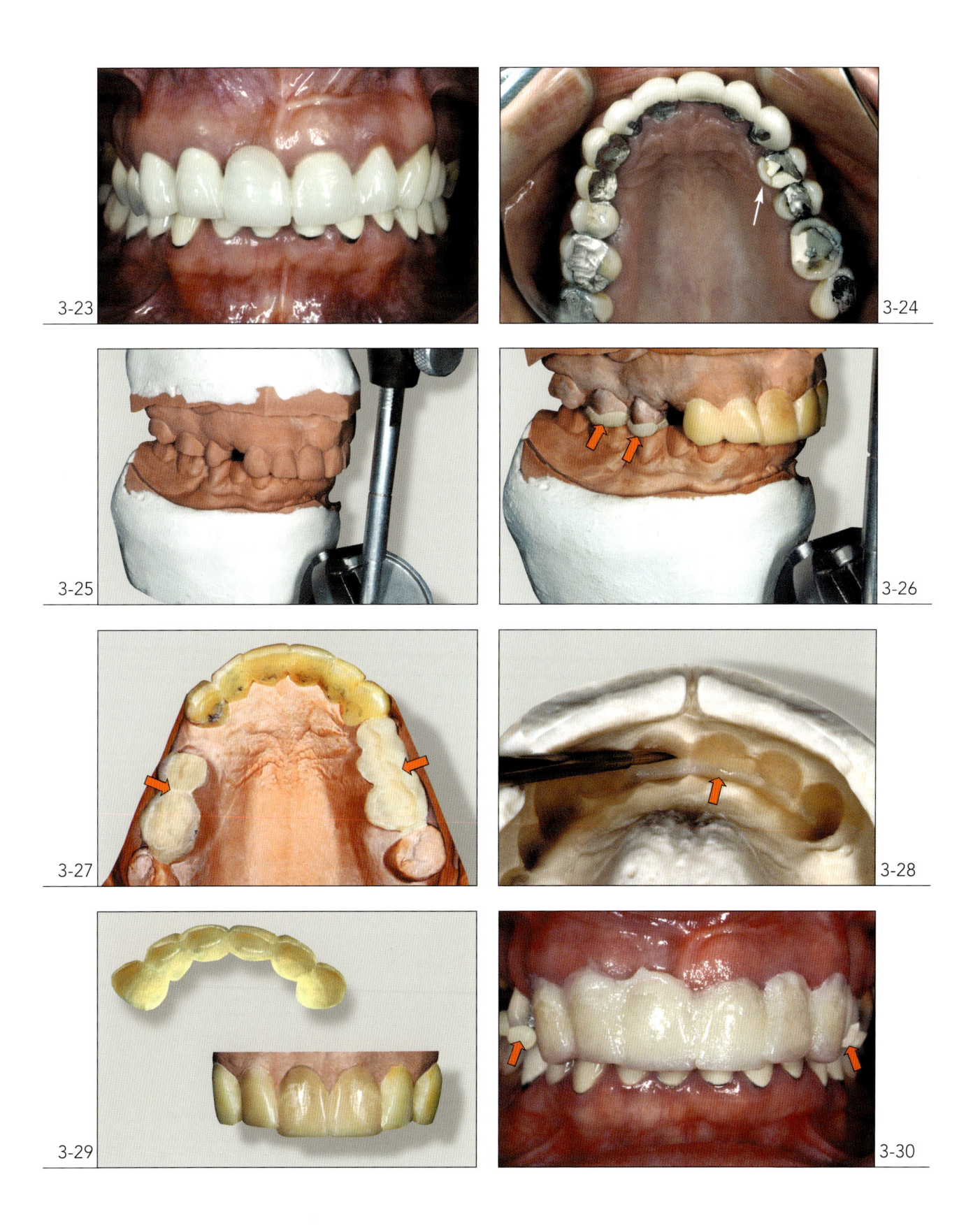

Clinical Procedure for Increasing the Vertical Dimension

3-23

3-24

3-25

3-26

3-27

3-28

3-29

3-30

Posterior preparations

The posterior teeth were prepared on one side (Fig 3-31). Using an impression of the planning maxillary cast, only one posterior provisional prosthesis was fabricated at a time. (Some clinicians prefer the shell technique posteriorly as well.) The impression was then filled with soft acrylic and seated intraorally. The occlusion was adjusted using the anterior acrylic prosthesis and acrylic stops on the opposite posterior side as guides. This process was then repeated for the opposite posterior quadrant. The appropriate occlusal clearance was confirmed in each quadrant before impressions were obtained (Fig 3-32).

Master Impression and Centric Occlusion Transfer Record

Impressions

Some clinicians prefer elastic impression materials for the crown preparations and stone dies while others prefer compound tube impressions and plated or resin dies. In either case, the centric record should be obtained at the vertical dimension of occlusion using Duralay copings in quadrants to capture the exact planned vertical dimension and centric occlusion.

Compound tube impression technique

The posterior provisional restoration is removed on one side, and Duralay copings are seated on the preparations. The copings should not be in occlusal contact. Duralay is painted over the copings, the opposing teeth are lubricated, and the patient is asked to close (Fig 3-33). The anterior and opposite posterior provisional prostheses provide occlusal guidance at the planned vertical dimension. After the acrylic polymerizes, the sharp edges are removed, the occlusion is checked for accuracy (*arrow*), and the transfer of the planned vertical dimension is confirmed by placing an Artus occlusion strip (Artus, Englewood, NJ) between the anterior provisional prostheses (Fig 3-34). With the strip in place, the patient is instructed to apply continued occlusal pressure so that it cannot be pulled through anteriorly. If the strip freely slides through, the record has increased the vertical dimension and the process should be repeated after occlusal reduction of the acrylic record. The procedure is then repeated on the opposite posterior side (Fig 3-35). Finally, the anterior provisional prosthesis is removed and the process repeated once again (Fig 3-36).

Master impression for compound tube technique

An overall elastomeric impression or impression plaster can be used for the master impression. The author prefers to use a practical full-arch plaster impression technique, including an assemblage model for metal coping soldering, to provide accurate assemblage. Despite its accuracy, most clinicians avoid plaster because it is difficult to handle. With the special two-piece impression technique described below, fracture of the impression is routinely avoided.

Master Impression and Centric Occlusion Transfer Record

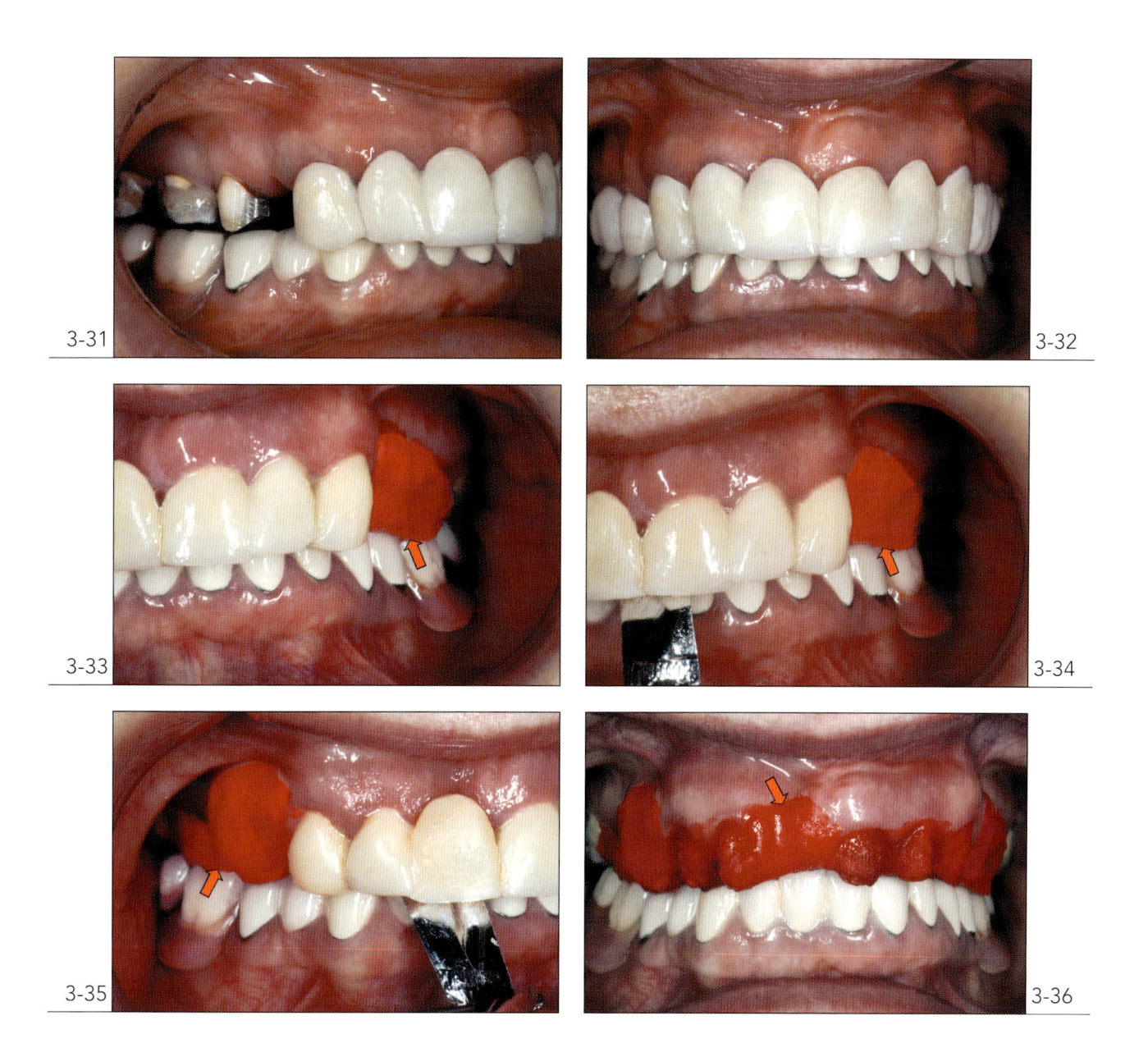

3-31

3-32

3-33

3-34

3-35

3-36

37

Plaster labial flange

A piece of baseplate wax is trimmed to create an arch form and heated. The patient is instructed to occlude into the wax, leaving a 5- to 6-mm border (Fig 3-37, *arrows*). The incisal edges of the copings should penetrate the wax 2 to 3 mm, and the patient should be instructed to remain occluded. Impression plaster is then mixed and placed on the labial portion of the arch from the distal of each canine. The lip is pulled over the soft plaster and baseplate wax, and the plaster trimmed (Fig 3-38, *arrows*). After the plaster sets, the wax is removed, exposing the Duralay centric record and the 5- to 6-mm occlusal edge (*arrows*) of the plaster labial index (Fig 3-39). This edge is lubricated to facilitate later separation.

Occlusal index

To avoid excess plaster posteriorly, an oversized *lower* plaster tray is used to obtain the occlusal index (Fig 3-40). It can be trimmed and bent lingually to suit the patient's anatomy. The objective is to obtain *only* an occlusal index without engaging excessive undercuts and to avoid the posterior palatal area to prevent gagging. However, the impression must be in one piece without fracturing, which is easy with the following technique.

The impression plaster is mixed to a soft, whipped cream consistency and loaded into the tray. Before seating the tray, the clinician should wait until the plaster reaches a cream cheese consistency. The thick consistency of the plaster prevents excessive seating of the tray (see Fig 3-40, *arrows*). While the occlusal index is obtained, digital pressure is applied toward the lingual to the labial plaster flange to prevent its movement. The occlusal index should be removed during the initial set *before* the plaster sets completely to ensure removal in one piece. If the plaster is in the "crumbly" stage, the unwanted undercuts will drag and the occlusal index can be removed in one piece. The consistency of the plaster is the key to performing this procedure.

Copings and centric occlusion records seated

The posterior buccal and lingual plaster is trimmed to within 2 mm of the occlusal index, and the Duralay acrylic records are seated. The anterior Duralay record is seated and the labial plaster index is snapped into position (Fig 3-41, *arrows*). All of the records are secured with sticky wax to ensure no movement. Modeling clay is used to block out any unwanted undercuts. The impression is boxed and poured in stone.

The technique described above, although primarily designed for plated dies, can be used for any assemblage for full-mouth impressions to provide extremely accurate master casts and centric relation records at the vertical dimension of occlusion.

Centric records for elastic impression technique

If an elastic impression is used for the final cast, individual Duralay copings are made on the stone (or epoxy) dies without full extension to the finish lines. Extra care should be taken to prevent breakage. The process of securing the centric record in quadrants is the same as previously described. The Duralay centric occlusion records over the stone (or epoxy) dies are used for mounting on the articulator.

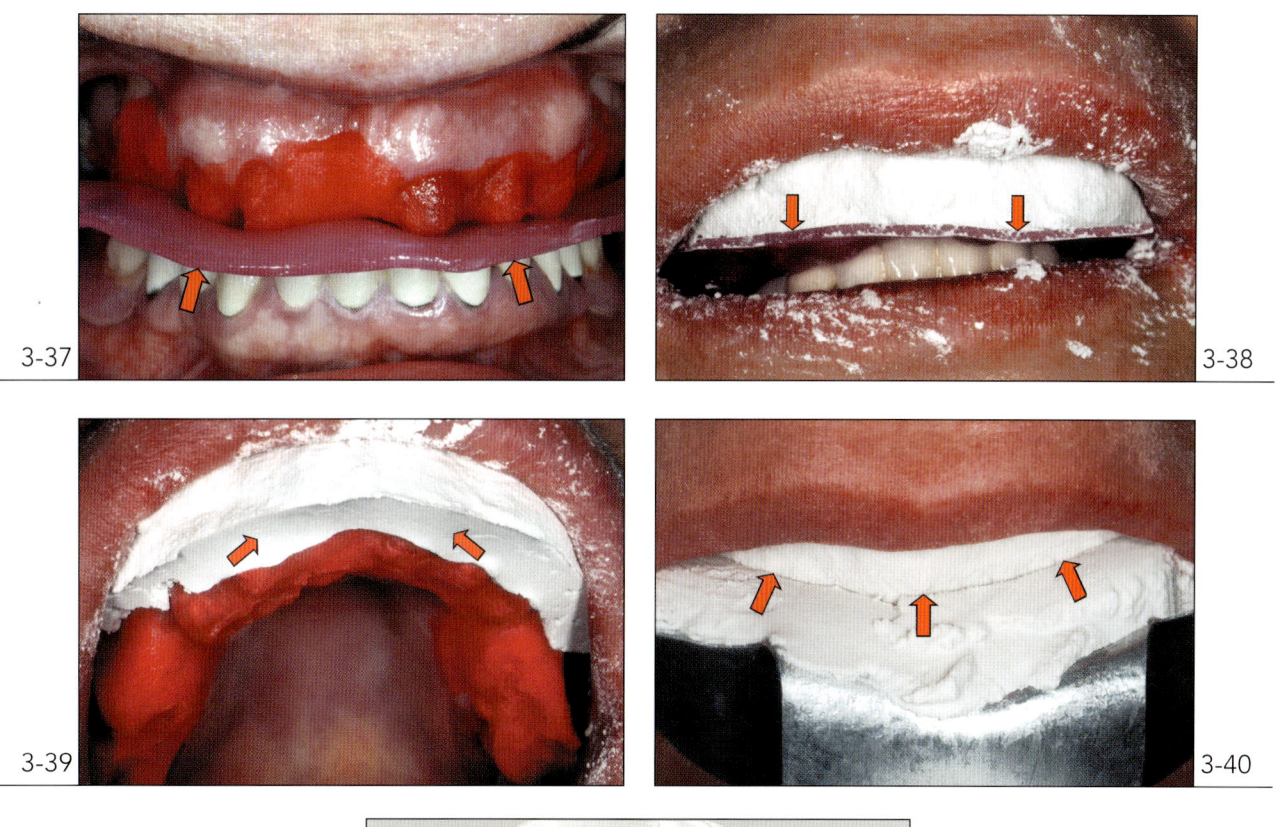

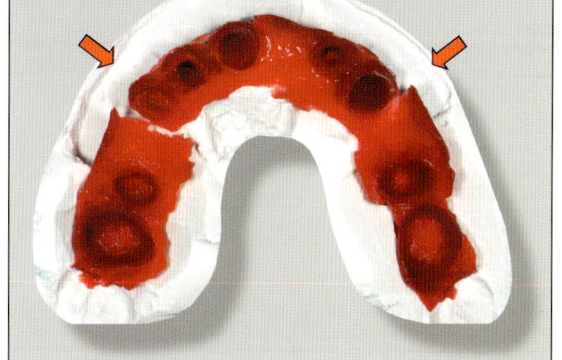

Master Impression and Centric Occlusion Transfer Record

3-37

3-38

3-39

3-40

3-41

39

Mounting the casts

A facebow should be used to mount the maxillary cast on the articulator (Fig 3-42).[34] The incisal edges of the teeth should be approximately level with the notch on the incisal pin (see Fig 3-42, *arrow*). The mandibular cast is hand articulated with the maxillary cast and attached to the lower member of the articulator (Fig 3-43). It is extremely important to place Duralay on top of the incisal pin (*arrow*) to prevent any inadvertent change in the vertical dimension (see Fig 3-43). The occlusal records of the centric occlusion and vertical dimension should be permanently stored with the master cast for troubleshooting in the future.

Transfer of the Planned Esthetics

The master cast is removed from the articulator and replaced with a cast of the provisional restorations containing the planned esthetics (Fig 3-44). The anterior muscle border is notched, or a plaster table is created to provide an indexed base (see Fig 3-44, *arrows*). A separating medium is painted on the anterior portion of the mandibular cast, and a plaster (or polysiloxane) incisal index of the anterior teeth is obtained. It is carefully trimmed to preserve the incisal edges of the teeth (Fig 3-45, *arrow*).

Transfer of the Incisal Guidance

The casts are moved into protrusive position and the incisal table is rotated to touch the pin (*arrow*), which transfers the protrusive incisal guidance (Fig 3-46). Lateral incisal guidance (*arrow*) is transferred (Fig 3-47) as previously described in chapter 2.

Transfer of the Incisal Guidance

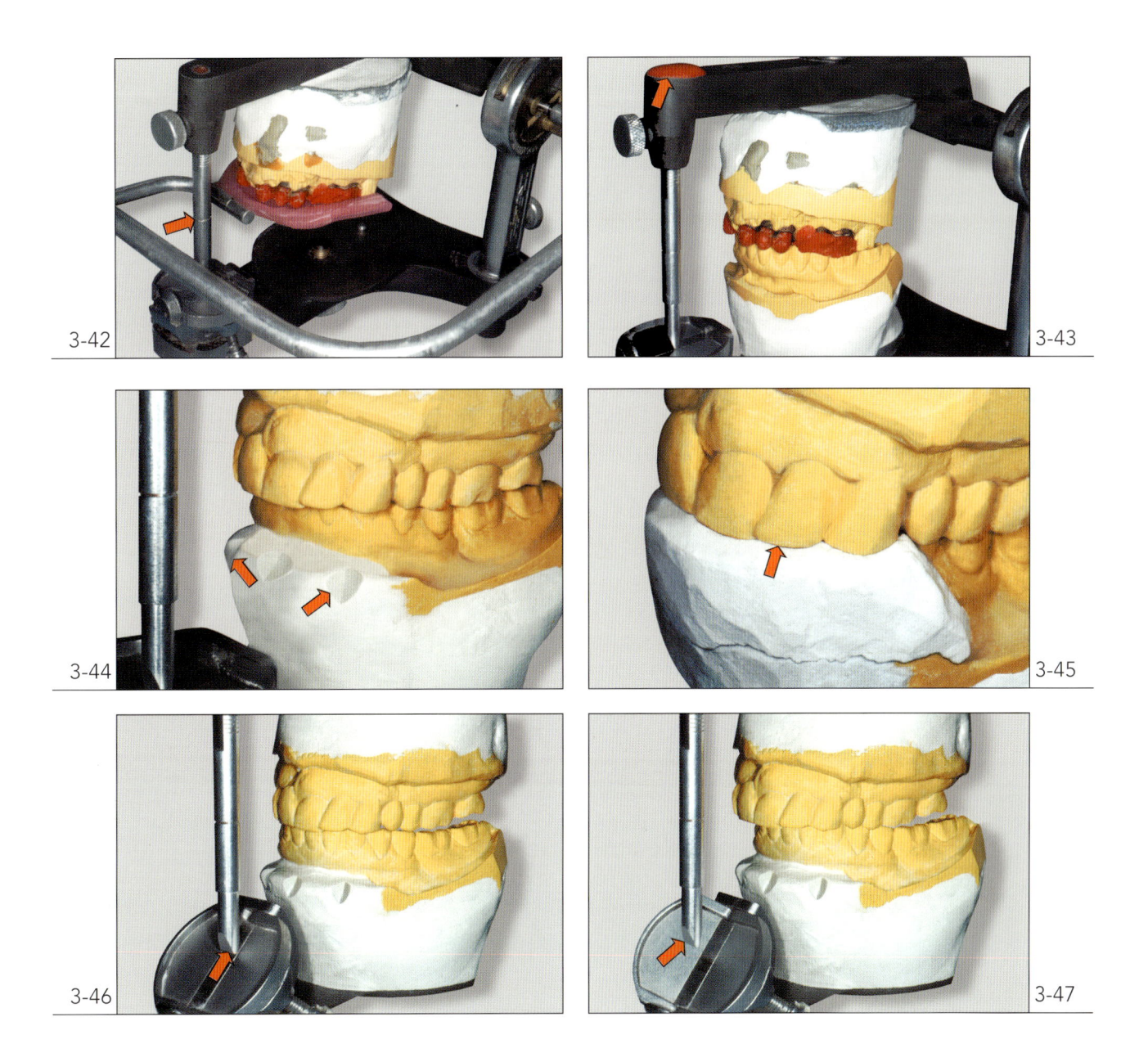

3-42

3-43

3-44

3-45

3-46

3-47

Waxup and castings

The position of the dies in relation to the incisal index serves as an exact physical blueprint for determining where the final restoration should end buccolingually and apico-occlusally (Fig 3-48, *arrows*). The waxups are completed to ensure maximum space for porcelain (*arrow*) to obtain ideal esthetics (Fig 3-49). The castings are then ready for intraoral assemblage impressions (Fig 3-50). Depending on the materials and technique used (stone/epoxy resin or plated dies), the assemblage procedure will vary slightly. The author prefers to try in the castings individually and assemble them in quadrants.

Centric remounting records

The objective of remounting records is to preserve the original centric occlusion and vertical dimension by using the provisional restorations as a guide to grind in a posterior assembled quadrant. Duralay is then painted over the assembled metal copings to record the centric occlusion at the planned vertical dimension. All pontic areas are recorded in Duralay. The Artus occlusion strips are again used to confirm the correct occlusal contact using the technique previously described (see Figs 3-33 to 3-36). The second posterior quadrant is seated and the process is repeated. Finally, the anterior quadrant is completed and the occlusion confirmed. The more care used here, the less the occlusal adjustment required later. The sharp edges are removed, and a full-arch, one-piece occlusal plaster index is obtained with a removable plaster labial flange as previously described (see Figs 3-37 to 3-41).

Remounting and fusing of the porcelain

An epoxy resin model is then made from the one-piece plaster occlusal index and remounted. (If elastic impressions and poured stone dies were used, a new master cast is usually required. Many clinicians prefer an elastomeric complete-arch impression over the assembled castings.) The plaster incisal index is still accurate because extra care was used to maintain the planned centric occlusion and vertical dimension. The porcelain is fused and tried in intraorally, and the occlusion is adjusted. Figure 3-51 shows the glazed porcelain on the epoxy resin master cast (*bottom*) along with the esthetics as originally planned in the waxup (*top*), which were transferred to the provisional restorations, then to the plaster incisal index, and finally into the porcelain restorations. Figure 3-52 shows the final occlusal view. (See Fig 3-56 for final intraoral esthetics.)

Transfer of the Incisal Guidance

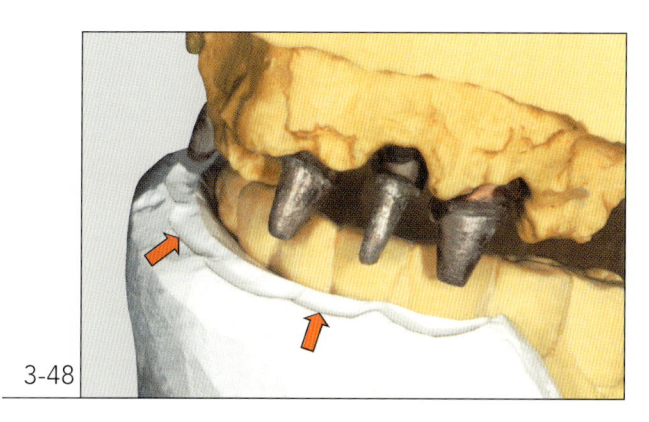

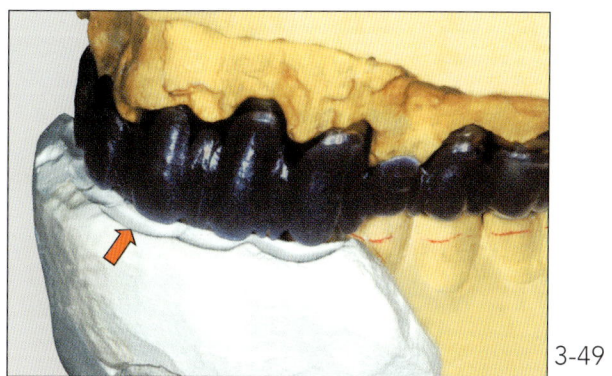

3-48

3-49

3-50

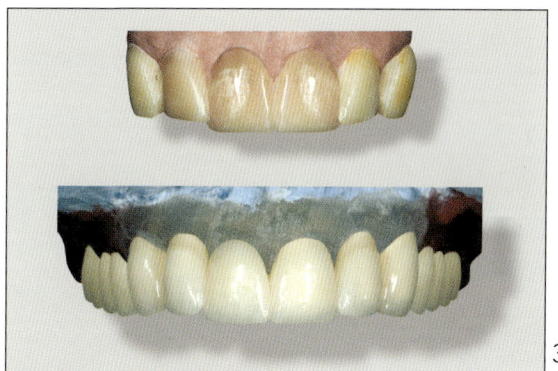

3-51

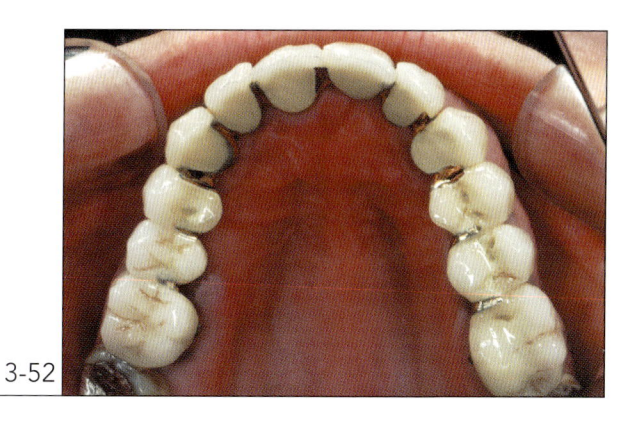

3-52

43

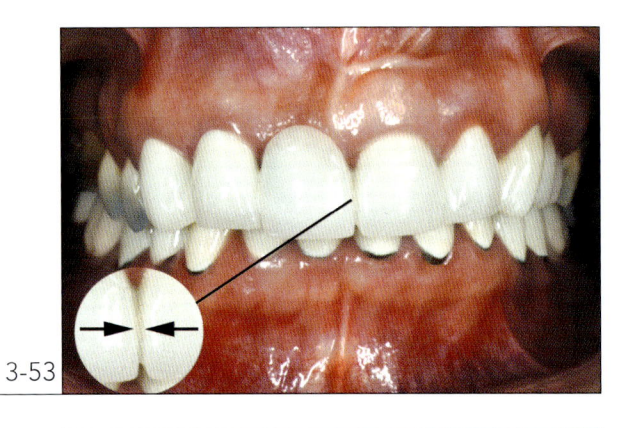

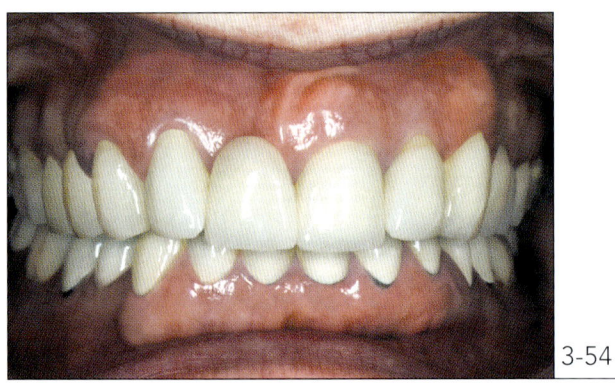

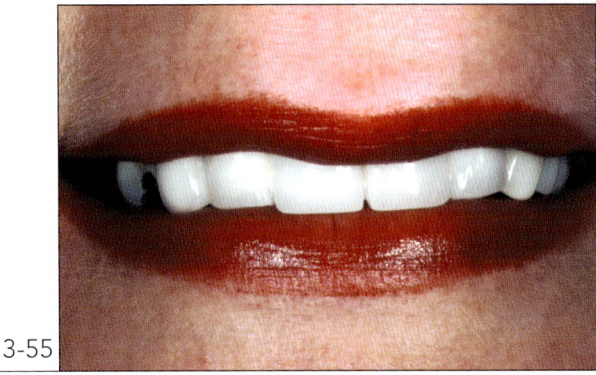

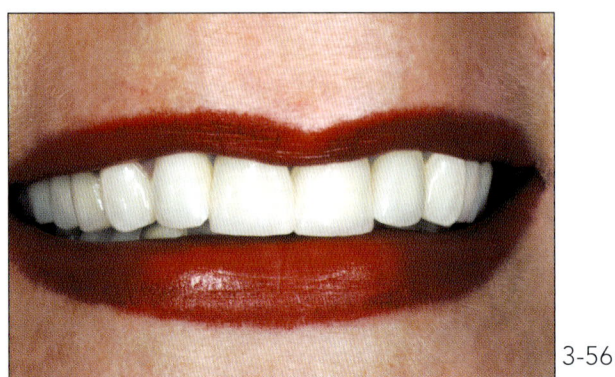

3 Esthetic, Functional, and Vertical Dimension Planning for Complete-Arch Prostheses

3-53

3-54

3-55

3-56

Preoperative and postoperative results

The preoperative esthetics and vertical dimension are shown in Fig 3-53. The final esthetics and restored vertical dimension are shown in Fig 3-54. Compare the unesthetic proximal grooves (*arrows*) in the enlargement in Fig 3-53 with the sharp proximal line angles in Fig 3-54, which, with the overlapped laterals, provide a realistic appearance. The before-treatment (Fig 3-55) and after-treatment (Fig 3-56) esthetics demonstrate a corrected smile line; a restored lip contour; and a natural,[1] life-like appearance.

Summary

Complete-mouth treatment focuses on esthetic and functional planning on the study casts. These corrections are transferred to the mouth by means of lingual Duralay indexes before any tooth preparations are initiated. Once confirmed, the corrections are transferred first to the provisional restoration and then to the final prosthesis. Similarly, when planning a change in vertical dimension, the clinician should confirm the corrections in the mouth using an acrylic occlusal onlay or provisional restoration before fabricating the final prosthesis. In addition, research has shown that the clinician must provide at least 2 mm of speaking space when altering the vertical dimension. Following these procedures, as demonstrated step by step in the clinical case presented at the end of the chapter, will provide a successful functional and esthetic result.

References

1. Weinberg LA. Vertical dimension: A research and clinical analysis. J Prosthet Dent 1982;47:290–302.
2. Schweitzer JM. Oral Rehabilitation. St. Louis: Mosby, 1964:514.
3. Moyers RE. Temporomandibular muscle contraction patterns in angle Class II Division I malocclusions: An electromyographic analysis. Am J Orthodont 1949;35:837–857.
4. Woelfel JB, Hickey JC, Rinnear L. Electromyographic evidence supporting the mandibular hinge axis theory. J Prosthet Dent 1957;7:361–367.
5. Sherrington CS. The integrative action of the nervous system. New Haven: Yale UP, 1952.
6. Szentagothai J. Anatomical considerations of monosynaptic reflex arcs. J Neurophysiol 1948;11:445.
7. Ramfjord SP, Ash MM. Occlusion. Philadelphia: Saunders, 1966.
8. Jerge CR. The function of the nucleus supratrigeminalis. J Neurophysiol 1963;26:379.
9. Kawamura Y, Majima T. Temporomandibular joint's sensory mechanisms controlling activities of the jaw muscles. J Dent Res 1964;43:150.
10. Kawamura Y, Nishiyama T. Projection of dental afferent impulses to the trigeminal nuclei of the cat. Jpn J Physiol 1965;16:584.
11. Yemm R, Berry D. Passive control in mandibular rest position. J Prosthet Dent 1969;22:30–36.
12. Ransjö J, Thilander B. Perception of mandibular position in cases of temporomandibular joint disorders. Odont Tidskr 1963;71:134.
13. Thilander B. Innervation of the temporomandibular joint capsule in man. Trans R Sch Dent Stockh Umea 1961;7:1–67.
14. Kawamura Y, Majima T, Kato I. Physiologic role of deep mechanoreceptor in temporomandibular joint capsule [in Japanese]. J Osaka Univ Dent Sch 1967;7:63–76.
15. Greenfield BE, Wyke BD. Reflex innervation of the temporomandibular joint. Nature (Lond) 1966;211:940.
16. Brill N. Relexes, registrations, and prosthetic dentistry. J Prosthet Dent 1957;7:341–360.
17. Corbin KB, Harrison F. Functions of the mesencephalic root of the fifth cranial nerve. J Neurophysiol 1940;3:423.
18. Atwood DA. A cephalometric study of the clinical rest position of the mandible. Part III: Clinical factors related to variability of the clinical rest position following removal of occlusal contacts. J Prosthet Dent 1958;8:698–708.
19. Thompson JR. The rest position of the mandible and its significance to dental science. J Am Dent Assoc 1946;33:151–180.
20. Coulombe JAR. A serial cephalometric study of the rest position of the mandible on edentulous individuals. J Can Dent Assoc 1954;20:536–543.
21. Thompson JR, Brodie AG. Factors in the position of the mandible. J Am Dent Assoc 1942;29:925–941.
22. Ricketts RM. A study of changes in temporomandibular relations associated with the treatment of Class II malocclusion (Angle). Am J Orthod 1952;38:918–933.
23. Mohl N. Head posture and its role in occlusion. N Y State Dent J 1976;42:17–23.
24. Walsh J. Neurophysiological aspects of mastication. Dent J Aust 1951;23:49–62.
25. Tallgren A. Changes in adult face height due to aging, wear, and loss of teeth, and prosthetic treatment. Acta Odontol Scand 1957;15(suppl 24):1–122.
26. Atwood DA. A cephalometric study of the clinical rest position of the mandible. Part I. The variability of the clinical rest position following the removal of occlusal contacts. J Prosthet Dent 1956;6:504–519.
27. Kallenbach TE. Factors in correcting jaw position relative to the abnormal temporomandibular joint. Dent Digest 1941;47:66,108,166,220.
28. Lammie GA, Storer R. Osborne J. The use of onlays in partial denture construction. Br Dent J 1956;100:33–42.
29. Perry HT, Lammie GA, Main J, Teuscherer GW. Occlusion in a stress situation. J Am Dent Assoc 1960;60:626–633.
30. Yemm R. Irrelevant muscle activity. Dent Pract Dent Rec 1968;19:51–54.
31. Berry DC, Wilkie JK. Lips and tongue behavior in relation to prosthetics. Dent Pract Dent Rec 1961;11:334–340.
32. Carlsson GE, Ericsson S. Postural face height in full denture wearers. A longitudinal x-ray cephalometric study. Acta Odontol Scand 1967;25:145–162.
33. Ramfjord S, Blankenship J. Increased occlusal vertical dimension in adult monkeys. J Prosthet Dent 1981;45:74–83.
34. Weinberg LA. An evaluation of the face-bow mounting. J Prosthet Dent 1961;11:32–42.

4 Biomechanics of Tooth- and Implant-Supported Prostheses

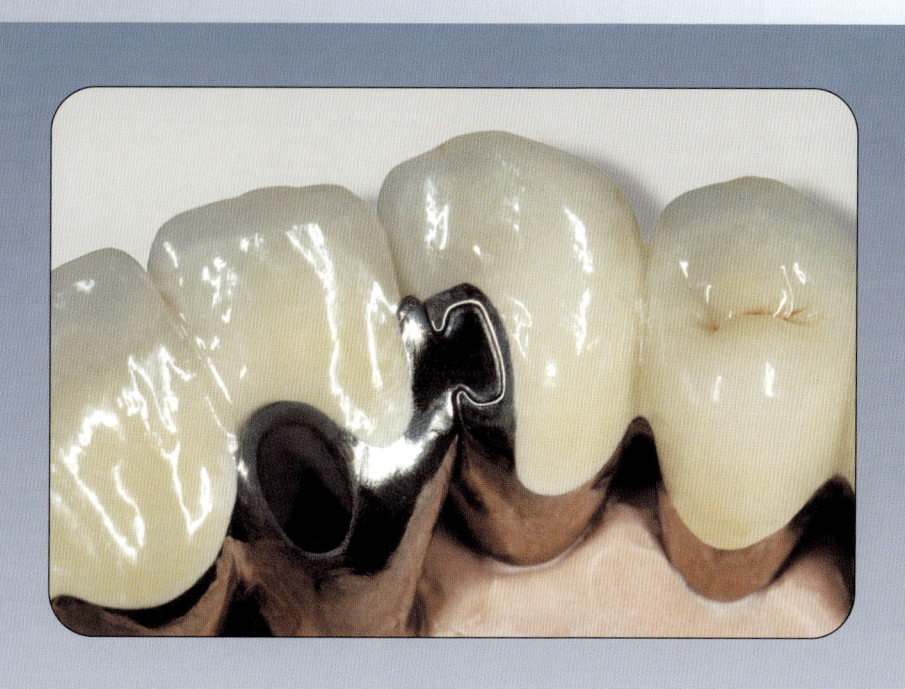

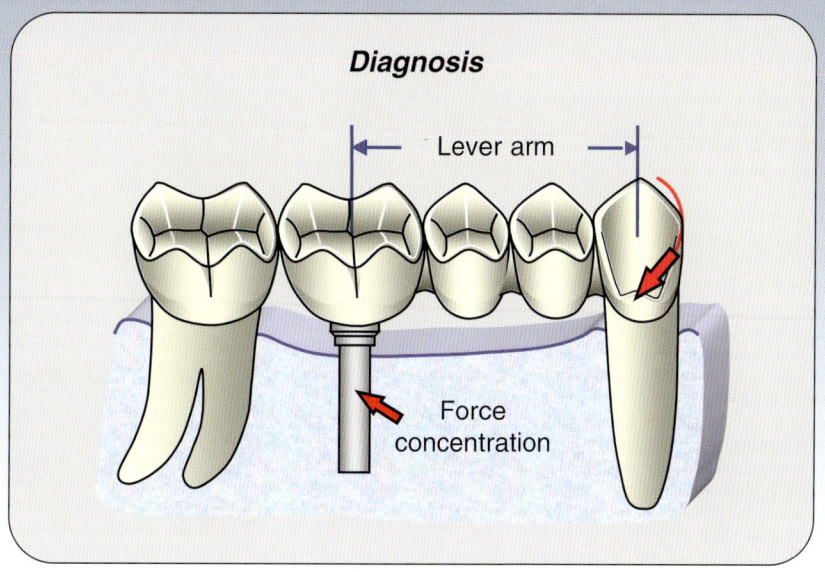

Diagnosis

Lever arm

Force concentration

4 Biomechanics of Tooth- and Implant-Supported Prostheses

The biomechanics of tooth-supported prostheses are completely different from those of implant-supported prostheses because the periodontal ligament permits flexion while the implant-osseous interface is stiff. Furthermore, when natural teeth and implants are used in the same prosthesis, the biomechanics are unlike those of either one alone. This chapter focuses on the fundamentals of biomechanics and the distribution of force to the supporting bone in common clinical situations.

Chewing Motion

Posselt[1] suggested that the chewing motion follows a teardrop configuration (Fig 4-1). As the stroke returns toward the starting position, the movement has both a vertical and a horizontal component. This means that the movement of the joints and mandible, as powered by the muscles, produce vertical and horizontal forces. However, biomechanics is not quite that simple because once the teeth contact, the shape of the contacting surfaces determines the direction of the resultant line of force. The force distribution to the supporting bone, its quantity, and its direction determine the longevity of the teeth (and/or implants) and of the restorations built upon them. Early on, some clinicians felt that the teeth did not penetrate the bolus except on deglutition.[2] However, even when a sinewy bolus reaches its maximum flow, it acts as a hydraulic system and distributes force as if the teeth contacted each other (Fig 4-2).[3]

Resultant force during occlusal contact

The fundamental basis for biomechanics is illustrated in Fig 4-2: When the teeth contact, a resultant line of force is produced perpendicular to the cusp inclination (*right*). Note that the force is inclined and away from the supporting bone. This produces a lever, which has a mechanical advantage and is potentially very damaging to the supporting bone. As the mathematician Archimedes once said, "Give me a lever and a place to put a fulcrum and I will move the world" (Fig 4-3). The mechanical advantage of a lever is proportionate to the distance from the applied force to the fulcrum (force arm) compared to the distance from the resultant force to the fulcrum (resultant arm).

Torque

When force is applied on a cusp incline, the resultant force (F) passes at a distance (D) from the center of rotation located in the apical third (Fig 4-4). Torque (moment) can be expressed as the force times the perpendicular distance to the resultant line of force. It can be visualized as the magnitude of the distance arm (see Fig 4-4, D) and resembles the force arm in a lever, the fulcrum being the center of rotation. The axiomatic expression for this is the longer the distance arm, the greater the torque. As noted above (see Fig 4-1), the original vertical and horizontal forces that are generated change direction dramatically as soon as tooth inclines occlude.

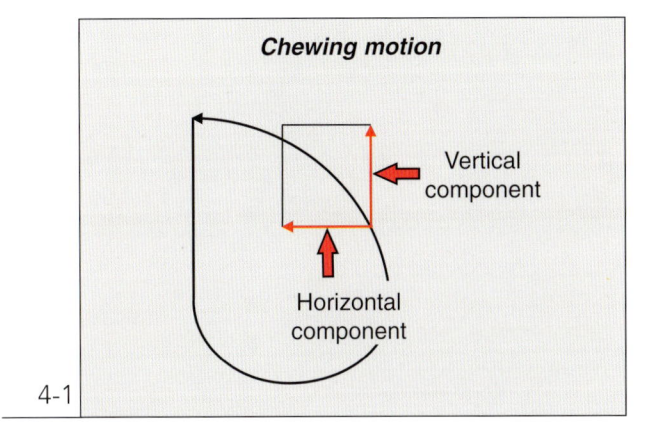

Chewing Motion

4-1 Chewing motion — Vertical component, Horizontal component

4-2 Forces during mastication (Limit of elasticity of bolus) — Forces during occlusal contact

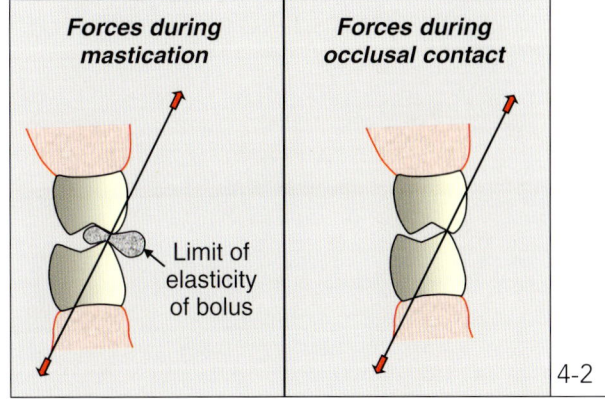

4-3 "Give me a lever and a place to put a fulcrum and I will move the world!"

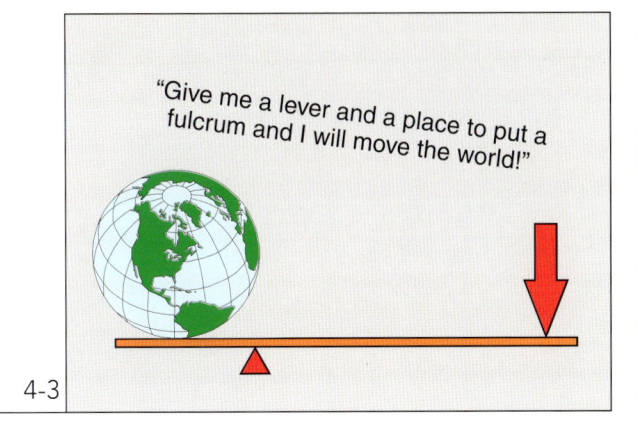

4-4 Summary — Cusp incline contact, Resultant line of force, Center of rotation, Torque

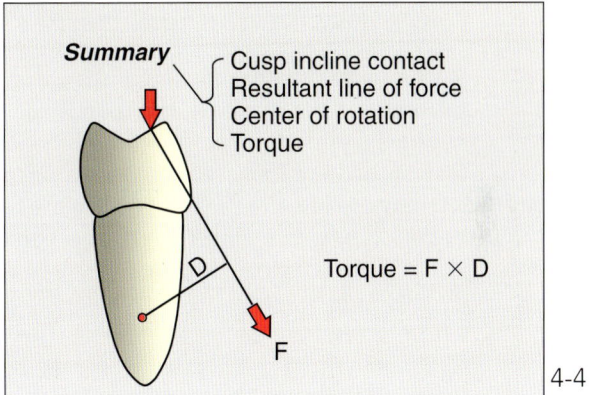

$$Torque = F \times D$$

Biomechanics

The study of biomechanics is therefore an analysis of the force distribution to the bone when teeth occlude. It is often observed clinically that lateral forces to the supporting bone are not tolerated as well as vertical forces.[4] Why is this? Because the lateral force acts as a lever arm, and the further away it is from the supporting bone the more torque that is developed. The objective of treatment should be to reduce torque and to direct resultant forces toward, rather than away from, the supporting bone as much as possible. This new approach, called *therapeutic biomechanics*, reduces loading on tooth- and/or implant-supported prostheses (see chapter 5).

Factors Influencing Force Distribution

Axial inclination, incline contact

If the teeth were oriented vertically and had a flat occlusion, maxillary and mandibular tooth contact would produce benign vertical force. However, natural teeth have axial inclination and cusp inclines and are rarely if ever oriented vertically over supporting bone. Anteriorly, the maxillary and mandibular teeth are inclined labially, with a vertical and horizontal overlap that is specific to each patient. For instance, when there is minimal vertical overlap, as illustrated in Fig 4-5 (*left*), vertical occlusal force (O) initiates labial rotation of the maxillary tooth around its center of rotation (CR) in the apical third.

Force distribution anteriorly

With minimal vertical overlap, the impact area (topography of the contacting surfaces) produces in the maxillary and mandibular teeth a resultant line of force (F) that is perpendicular to the impact area (see Fig 4-5, *center*). Because of topography, the upper resultant line of force falls at a great distance (D) from the center of rotation, producing high torque. On the other hand, the resultant line of force on the mandibular tooth passes very much closer (d) to the center of rotation, producing minimum torque. When there is a steep vertical overlap, the resultant line of force on the maxillary tooth (F) falls at an exaggerated distance (D) from the center of rotation, which produces extreme torque (see Fig 4-5, *right*). The torque on the mandibular tooth changes in direction toward the lingual. However, because the distance arm (d) is much shorter than on the upper, the torque is also much lower (see Fig 4-5, *right*).

Force distribution posteriorly

Figure 4-6 (*left*) illustrates vertical force on a buccal cusp incline, which produces an inclined resultant line of force (F) that is at a great distance (D) from the center of rotation of the tooth. As stated above, the torque is equal to force (F) times the perpendicular distance. Because of the resiliency of the periodontal ligament, the flexion distributes the force to all areas of the bone surrounding the tooth. The intensity and direction of the force distribution depend on the location relative to the center of rotation. When the cusp inclination is reduced, the resultant line of force (F) falls closer (d) to the center of rotation, reducing the distance arm and producing less torque (see Fig 4-6, *right*).

Force distribution with osseointegration

Clelland et al[5] and others,[6] using space-age computer models (three-dimensional finite element stress analysis), have shown that lateral and oblique loading on an implant concentrates the force distribution to the crestal bone and places maximum intensity at the level of the third screw thread (Fig 4-7). The finding of greatest significance is that there was *no force distribution along the remainder of the implant apically* (see Fig 4-7).

Factors Influencing Force Distribution

4-5

4-6 Force distribution — Torque = F × D — Reduced torque

4-7 Combined load bone only — Compression

4-8 Force distribution

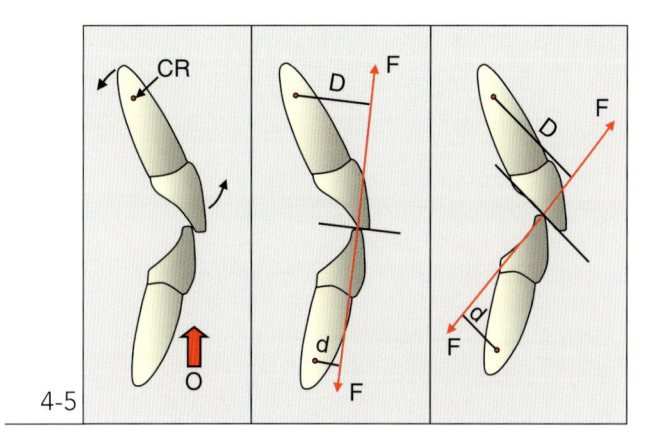

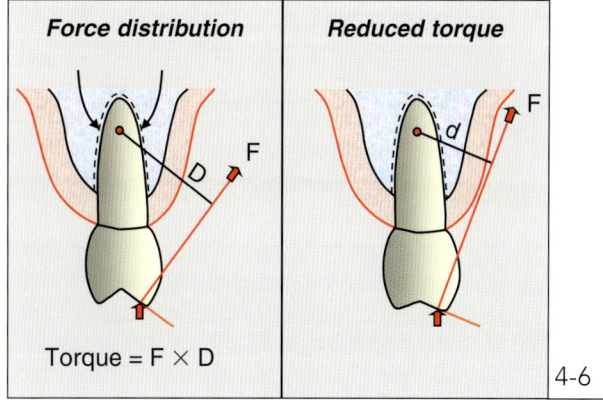

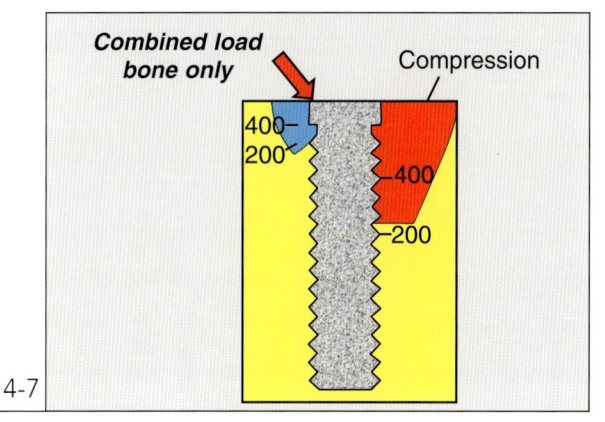

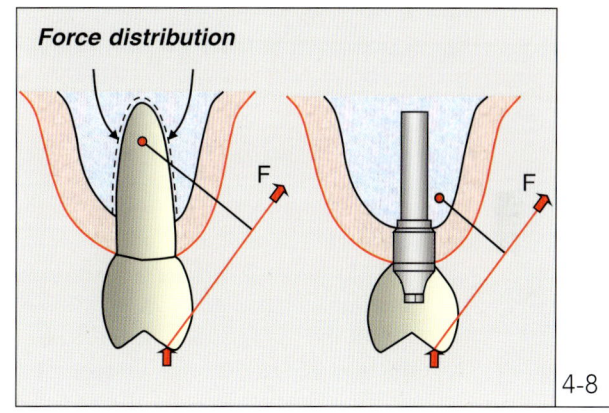

Comparing teeth and implants

The character of force distribution to bone is determined by the flexion (periodontal ligament) or stiffness (osseointegration) of the interface. When there are identical resultant lines of force produced by the occlusion, the periodontal ligament of a tooth *distributes* force to all of the surrounding bone (Fig 4-8), whereas the osseointegrated interface *concentrates* the force at the crestal bone.[5,6] The conclusion can be drawn that force distribution to bone by multiple tooth-supported prostheses is dramatically different from that of multiple implant-supported prostheses. It follows that when teeth and implants are used in the same prosthesis, the force distribution to bone is different from that of either one alone.

Principles of Force Distribution in Prostheses

System components

A multiple-supported prosthesis has three basic components: a vertical element (tooth or implant and restoration), a connecting element, and the supporting medium (Fig 4-9).[7] The distribution of force from one side to the other depends on the physical attributes of each element. For the sake of simplicity, we will assume that in all cases the connecting element is stiff.

If the supporting medium on both sides of the geometric structure shown in Fig 4-10 was flexible, such as dirt, lateral force applied to one side *(arrow)* would be distributed to the opposite side. The force distribution to the opposite side takes place because of the flexion of the dirt *on both sides* of the geometric structure.[7] Similarly, if the lateral force were applied at the right side *(arrow)*, it would be distributed to the opposite left side as well (Fig 4-11).[7]

Stiff and flexible supporting mediums

If the supporting medium at the site of the application of lateral force (Fig 4-12, *arrow*) was stiff, such as concrete, and the opposite supporting medium was flexible, there would be no force distribution to the opposite (right) side.[7] On the other hand, if lateral force *(arrow)* was applied to the side with the flexible supporting medium (Fig 4-13) rather than being distributed to both sides, force would be concentrated at the stiff concrete (left) side.[7] It is important to note that the lateral force will be exerted with a long, destructive lever arm (see Fig 4-13).[7] This hypothetical geometric system facilitates the establishment of a fundamental principle: Shared force distribution to another supporting member of a system depends on the flexion of both supporting mediums. If one supporting medium is stiff, the lateral force is concentrated only on that side.

Implants and teeth combined in a prosthesis

The osseointegrated interface is stiff (lateral force is concentrated at the crestal bone),[5,6] while the periodontal ligament imparts flexion that distributes force to all areas of the supporting bone.[8,9] Thus, when a lateral force is applied to the implant side of a combined prosthesis, no force is distributed to the opposite tooth side (Fig 4-14). This is similar to the hypothetical system illustrated in Fig 4-12. When lateral force is applied to the tooth side of the combined prosthesis, the force is not distributed to both sides but rather is concentrated at the implant side as a destructive, long lever arm (Fig 4-15). This corresponds to the hypothetical system illustrated in Fig 4-13.

Summary of implant force distribution

The osseointegrated implant–bone interface is stiff; therefore, lateral force is concentrated at the crestal bone at the level of the third screw thread (Fig 4-16),[5,6] and no force is distributed apical to the crestal bone level (see Figs 4-7 and 4-16).[5,6] The clinical implication is enormous: The length of the implant does not decrease the force distribution pattern exerted on it, unlike natural teeth, in which a longer root increases the force distribution to the supporting bone as a result of periodontal ligament flexion.[8,9]

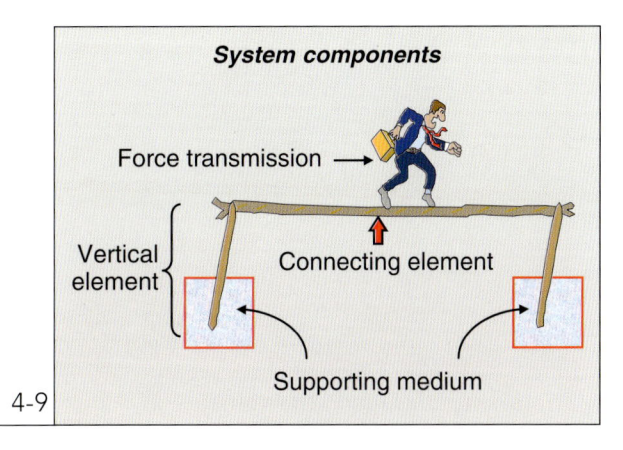

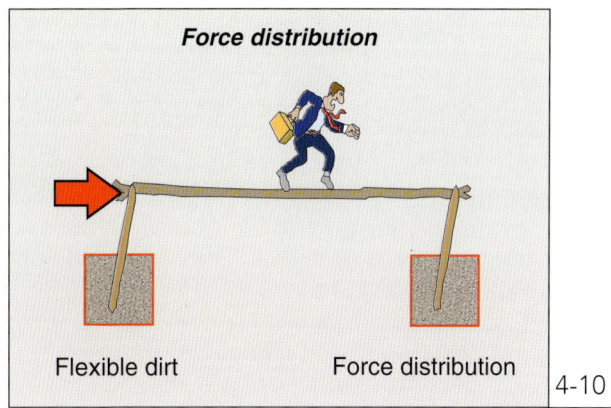

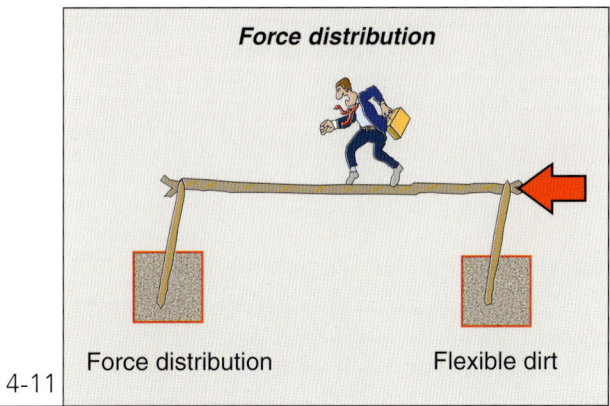

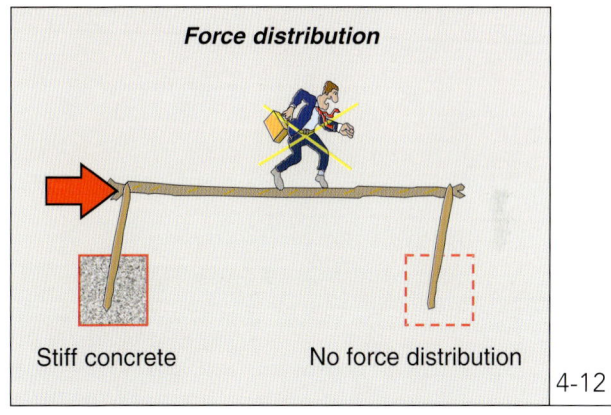

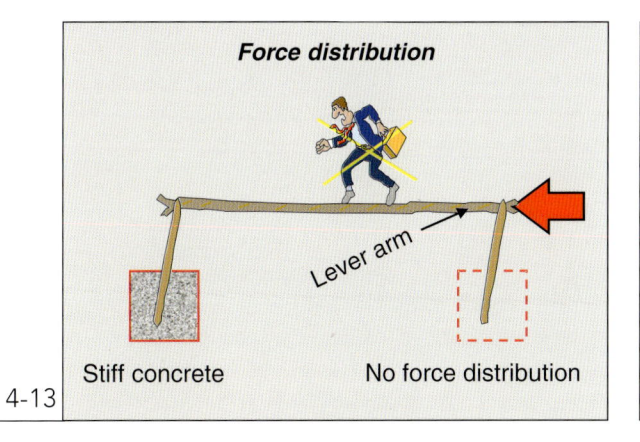

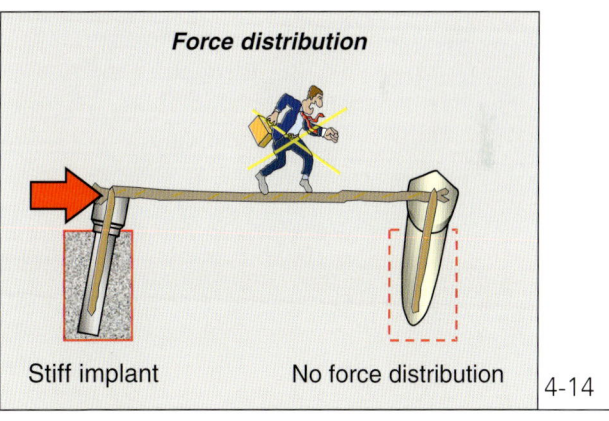

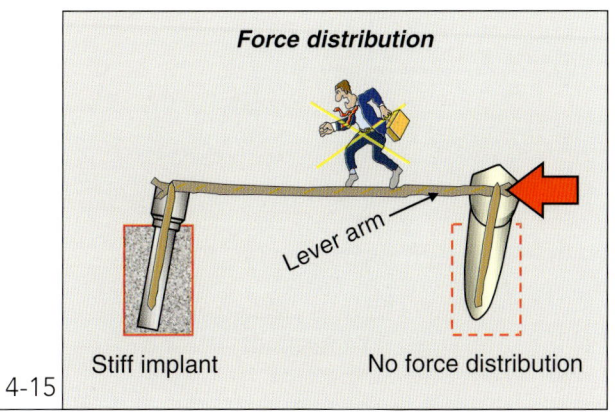

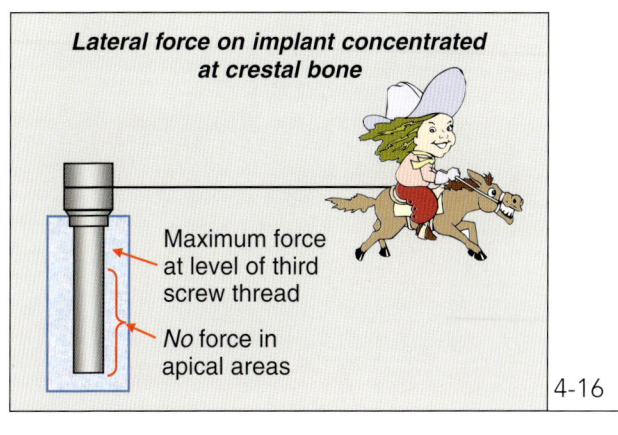

Principles of Force Distribution in Prostheses

4-9 **System components**: Force transmission, Vertical element, Connecting element, Supporting medium

4-10 **Force distribution**: Flexible dirt — Force distribution

4-11 **Force distribution**: Force distribution — Flexible dirt

4-12 **Force distribution**: Stiff concrete — No force distribution

4-13 **Force distribution**: Stiff concrete — No force distribution (Lever arm)

4-14 **Force distribution**: Stiff implant — No force distribution

4-15 **Force distribution**: Stiff implant — No force distribution (Lever arm)

4-16 **Lateral force on implant concentrated at crestal bone**: Maximum force at level of third screw thread; *No* force in apical areas

53

Force Distribution in Splinted Natural Teeth

Center of rotation effect

When posterior teeth are splinted by a fixed prosthesis, the force distribution is different from that of a single tooth.[10] Because of the stiff prosthesis, there is a vertical and horizontal center of rotation for the whole restoration since by definition a solid object can have only one vertical and one horizontal center of rotation. The force distribution pattern to the supporting bone depends on the location of the applied loading. For instance, if vertical force is applied on the lingual cusp incline of the anterior abutment (of splinted teeth), a lingually inclined resultant line of force will be initiated (Fig 4-17, *left*).[10] This will tend to initiate a horizontal rotation around the vertical center of rotation passing through the center abutment (see Fig 4-17, *right*).[10] The force will be distributed to all areas of the supporting bone.

Occlusal force on the cusp incline of the middle abutment will tend to initiate vertical rotation around the horizontal center of rotation passing through the apical third of all the teeth.[10] The force will be distributed to all areas of the supporting bone in the pattern shown in Fig 4-18. It should be noted that when teeth are in line as opposed to a cross-arch splint, there is relatively limited mutual support.

Mandibular cross-arch splint

With a mandibular cross-arch splint, the center of rotation passes through the apical third of the terminal abutments (Fig 4-19).[10,11] Occlusal force on the first premolar lingual cusp incline (or buccal slope) produces a lingually inclined resultant line of force, as illustrated in Fig 4-17 (*left*). However, the resultant line of force passes close to the center of rotation of the cross-arch splint, producing extremely little torque (see Fig 4-19).[10,11] This can happen only when the splint is in one piece. When an interlock rather than all solder joints is used, there is sufficient movement to allow each section to act as a straight-line splint, as in Figs 4-17 and 4-18. In this case there is no single center of rotation passing through the apical third of the terminal abutments, and the advantage of a cross-arch splint is thus lost.

Maxillary cross-arch splint

When a maxillary cross-arch splint is constructed, the center of rotation passes through the apical third of the terminal abutments (Fig 4-20).[10,11] Thus, when an occlusal force is applied to the buccal cusp incline, the resultant line of force passes buccally *away* from the center of rotation (see Fig 4-20).[10,11] This increases the torque as compared to that of the mandibular splint with the same configuration (see Fig 4-19). The protection of a cross-arch splint is therefore less effective on the maxillary arch compared to the mandibular arch, although the force is distributed to more teeth because of the flexion of the periodontal ligaments.

Force Distribution in Multiple-Implant Prostheses

Multiple-implant straight-line osseointegrated prosthesis

In a multiple-implant straight-line posterior prosthesis, when a force is applied to the lingual cusp incline (or buccal slope) of the anterior restoration, a lingually inclined resultant line of force is produced (Fig 4-21). Because of the stiffness of the osseointegrated interface, the force is concentrated at the site of loading at the crestal bone and is not effectively distributed to the other implants. It should be emphasized that

Force Distribution in Multiple-Implant Prostheses

Fig 4-17 Effect of center of rotation on force distribution

Fig 4-18 Horizontal center of rotation

Fig 4-19 Cross-arch splint — Minimum torque

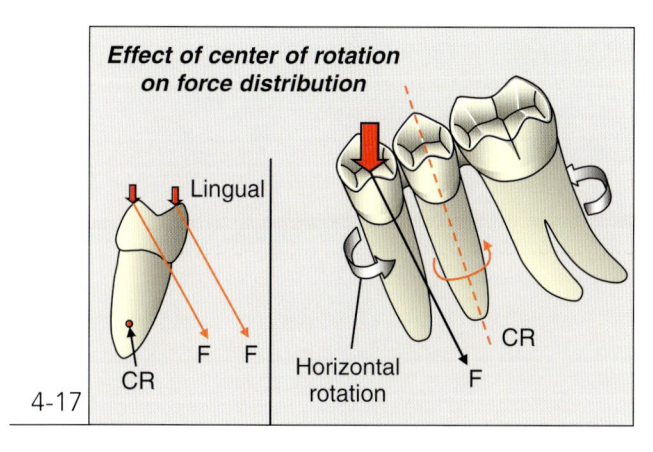

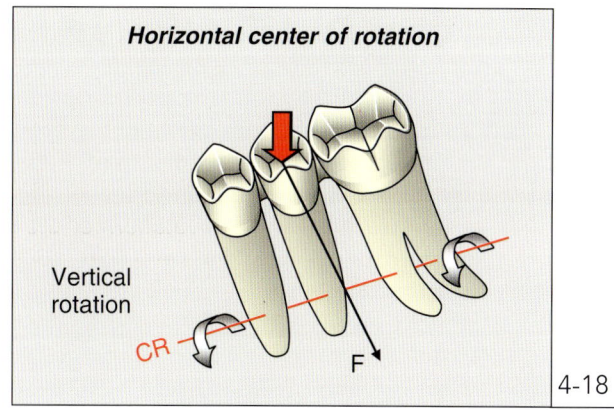

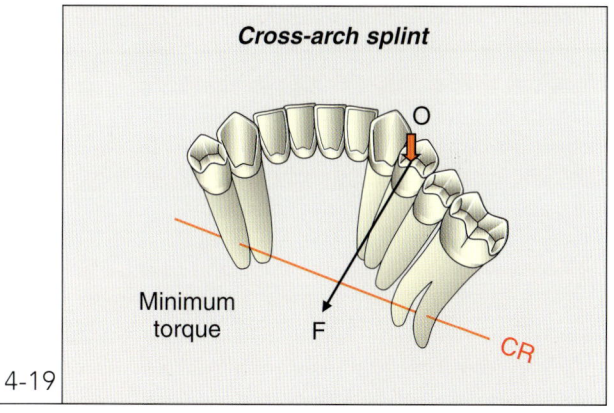

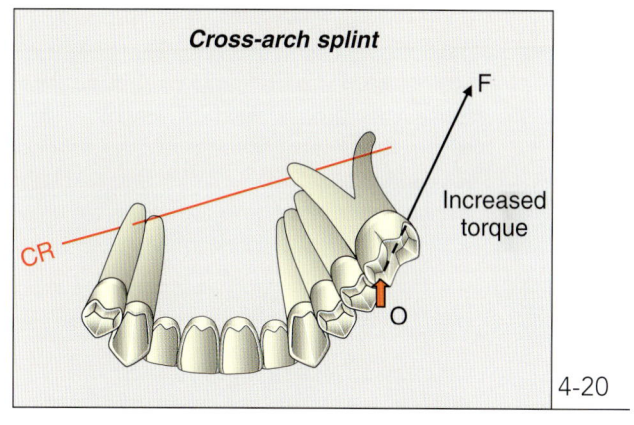

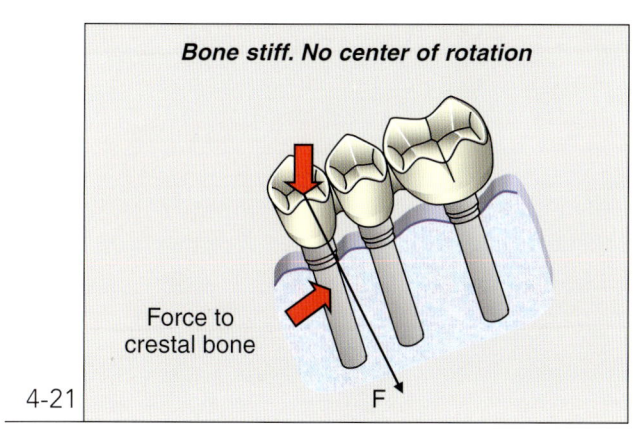

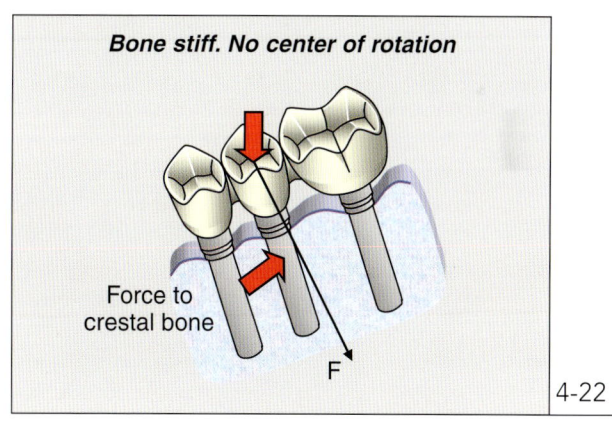

Fig 4-20 Cross-arch splint — Increased torque

Fig 4-21 Bone stiff. No center of rotation — Force to crestal bone

Fig 4-22 Bone stiff. No center of rotation — Force to crestal bone

force distribution to the supporting bone is not significantly improved by multiple splinting of implants, whereas force is distributed to all the abutments of natural teeth because of the flexion of the periodontal ligament (see Fig 4-17).

Similarly, if loading is applied to the middle restoration, the distribution of force is concentrated at the crestal bone of that restoration rather than distributed to adjacent implants (Fig 4-22). In the same configuration supported by natural teeth, the force distribution is shared by all the teeth because of the flexion of the periodontal ligament. If the loading was distributed evenly on the implant-supported prosthesis, each implant would receive similar loading *only at the crestal bone* and not along the whole length of the implant.[5,6]

55

Force Distribution in Combined Prostheses

A combined prosthesis is one supported by both natural teeth and implants. The method of attachment between the segments can be flexible, as with internal attachments (Fig 4-23), or stiff, such as when the terminal abutments are implants (Fig 4-24). The type of attachment and the location of the implants relative to the natural teeth will significantly alter the force distribution. If the osseointegrated prosthesis is freestanding or if natural teeth are included in the prosthesis, the implants will bear almost all of the load.[12,13]

Flexible attachment

An internal attachment that combines implant-supported and tooth-supported prostheses is primarily used so that the tooth-bearing prosthesis (containing the female attachment) can be finally cemented (see Fig 4-23), while the implant-supported prosthesis can remain fixed-retrievable if desired. The flexion is the result of vertical and lateral movement; even a factory-made, so-called precision attachment will develop horizontal play between the two restorations. As will be discussed shortly, this flexion between the male and female attachments is not deleterious but rather desirable.

Stiff attachment

When natural teeth are included within an implant-supported prosthesis, substructure telescope copings are permanently cemented to the natural teeth, and the osseointegrated prosthesis is temporarily cemented over the copings on the natural teeth (see Fig 4-24). In this way the osseointegrated prosthesis can maintain fixed retrievability through the access channels when desired. It should be noted that the temporary cement between the toothborne, permanently cemented substructure coping and the osseointegrated prosthesis can loosen, and in some situations the natural tooth can move apically from the osseointegrated prosthesis. A lingual retaining screw can be used between these two interfaces without penetration into the tooth structure. Choosing final cementation of the osseointegrated prosthesis rather than the maintenance of fixed-retrievability eliminates this problem. The biomechanics of combined prostheses is discussed in chapter 5.

Differential mobility

In addition to the foregoing diagnostic principles that are useful in the clinical treatment of combined prostheses, a new concept can be introduced. *Differential mobility* is based on the qualitative difference between the flexion of the periodontal ligament and the stiffness of osseointegration. Remember that inclined force on an implant is distributed only to the crestal bone and not to the apical remainder of the implant (Fig 4-25, *left*).[5,6] The same oblique force exerted on a natural tooth, however, results in force distribution throughout the periodontal ligament (Fig 4-25, *right*).

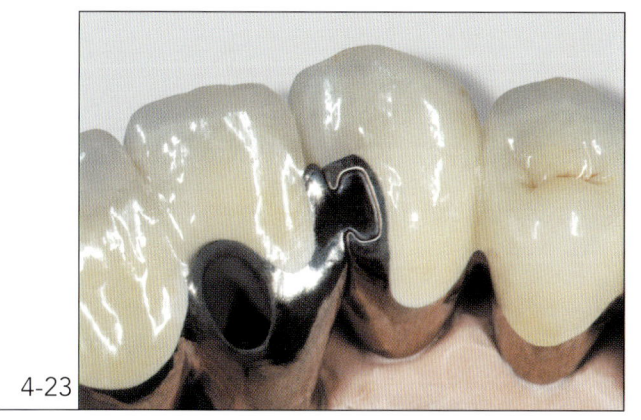

Force Distribution in Combined Prostheses

4-23

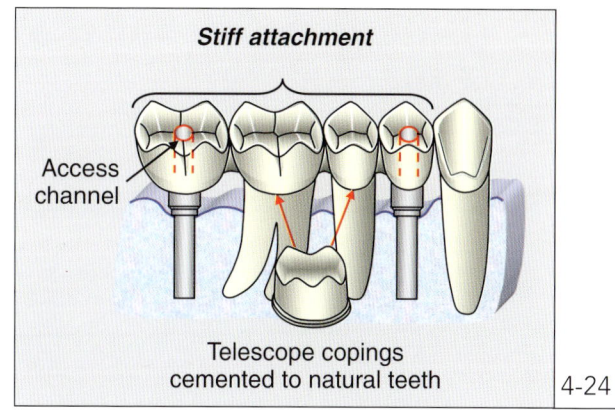

4-24 Stiff attachment — Access channel — Telescope copings cemented to natural teeth

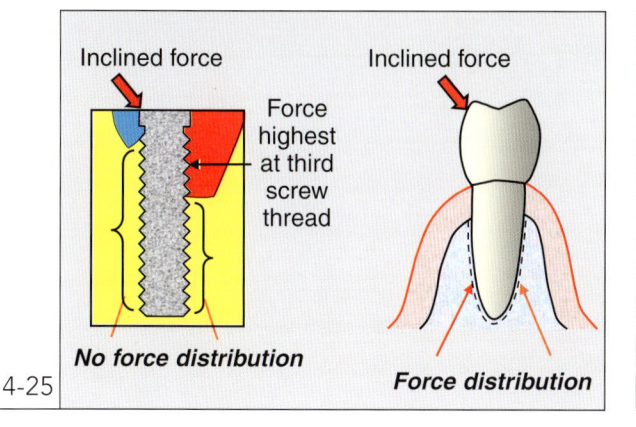

4-25 Inclined force — Force highest at third screw thread — No force distribution | Inclined force — Force distribution

4-26 Micromovement (0.5 mm) Periodontal ligament | Micron movement (0.1 mm) Osseointegration

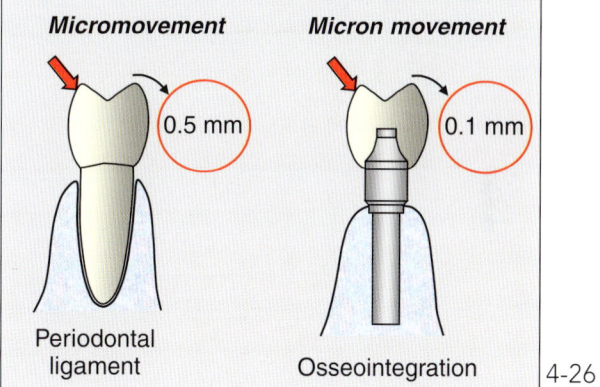

Micromovement

Quantitatively, in response to oblique force, a natural tooth with good bone will move laterally approximately 0.5 mm or less as measured at the occlusal (Fig 4-26, *left*). Movement of more than 0.5 mm is considered macromovement and is associated with bone loss and/or a thickened periodontal ligament related to occlusal trauma.

Micron movement

In response to the same oblique force, an implant-supported restoration can move laterally approximately 0.1 mm or less as measured at the occlusal (Fig 4-26, *right*).[14] This will be referred to here as *micron movement*.[13] In an in vitro experiment, Rangert et al[14] attributed this degree of movement to the gold and abutment screws used in the restoration.

Differential Mobility: A Significant Diagnostic Criterion

Natural teeth

If a tooth with good bone and with micromobility of less than 0.5 mm is splinted to a tooth with poor bone support and macromobility of approximately 1.0 mm, then a lateral force exerted on the mobile tooth will be distributed entirely to the less mobile tooth (Fig 4-27).[13] This can be explained by physical dynamics as follows: *(a)* The more mobile tooth will move as much as 1 mm before its periodontal fibers will begin to resist further movement and share the load; *(b)* the less mobile tooth will permit movement of less than 0.5 mm before its periodontal fibers will resist; *(c)* therefore, the maximum range of movement of the firm tooth will prevail, and all the force will be distributed to its bone support. When the differential mobility is in the range of 2:1, the less mobile tooth will receive all of the force distribution.

Implant and tooth splint

When a firm tooth of less than 0.5 mm micromovement is splinted to an implant with micron movement of less than 0.1 mm, the differential mobility is 5:1 (Fig 4-28).[13] In this case, a lateral force on the natural tooth would be borne *entirely* by the implant since its osseointegrated interface will not permit movement even approximating that of the natural tooth without fracture of the osseointegrated interface bone. Therefore, the higher the disparity (ratio) of the differential mobility, the more concentrated the force distribution will be to the less mobile component.[13]

Lever arm effect

When an implant and a natural tooth are the terminal supporting units connecting a long pontic, lateral force on the natural tooth will distribute all of the force to the implant and none of the force to the tooth because of the 5:1 differential mobility (Fig 4-29). Not only does the implant take all of the loading, but the long pontic causes an extremely destructive lever arm force.

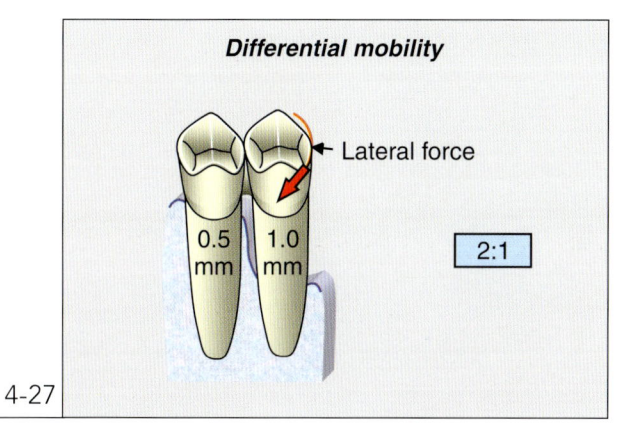

Differential Mobility: A Significant Diagnostic Criterion

4-27

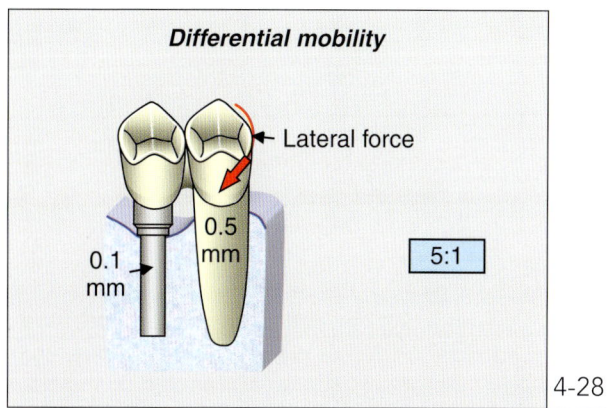

4-28

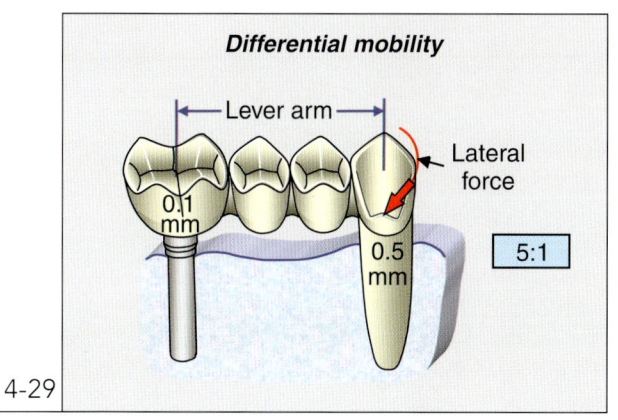

4-29

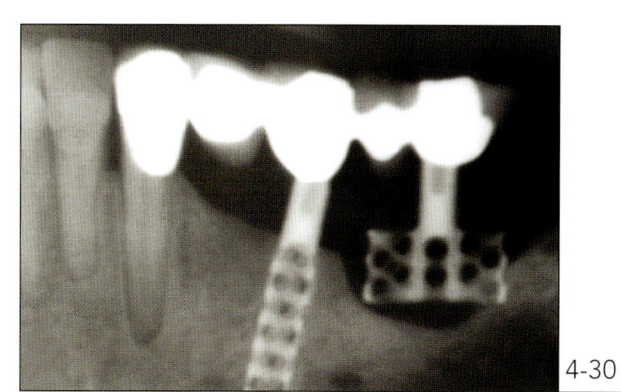

4-30

Clinical implications

There is a common misconception that implants are equivalent to natural teeth when used as abutments for prostheses. If this were so, the radiograph shown in Fig 4-30 would be diagnostically correct. However, since the flexion of the three interfaces is completely different, the reverse is true. The periodontal ligament provides the greatest degree of flexion, the osseointegrated implant the least, and the fibro-osseous integration of the blade falls somewhere in between. Equal occlusal loading would transfer three different force distributions to the supporting bone because each of them has a different level of flexion. However, the stiffest interface would bear the highest loading, and the length of the lever arm distances would also have to be taken into consideration. In Fig 4-30, the rapid breakdown of bone surrounding the posterior blade implant might indicate a loosening of the abutment screw (or another portion) of the premolar implant, which would cause an extremely long lever arm force on the blade implant.

Diagnostic Factors in Combined Prostheses

Standard prosthesis design

A standard treatment plan for a posterior osseointegrated prosthesis would combine a two-unit cantilever with an anterior splint comprising multiple natural teeth (Fig 4-31). An internal attachment in the distal of the natural tooth splint in such a design is erroneously thought to support the implant cantilever. As discussed previously (see Fig 4-29), the natural teeth cannot support the implant because of the 5:1 differential mobility, regardless of the length of the natural tooth splint. To add to the problem, the long lever arm increases the degree of mechanical leverage (see Fig 4-31). Despite the benefit of the internal attachment flexion, the implants always support the natural teeth and not vice versa.

Recommended prosthesis design

A recommended treatment plan for a posterior osseointegrated prosthesis would be to have one cantilever pontic extended from each segment of the prosthesis to safely support the respective splinted natural teeth and implants (Fig 4-32).[9] To reduce the lever arm effect, the internal attachment should not be rigid (see Fig 4-29). The purpose of the internal attachment in this design would be to prevent the drifting apart of the segments rather than lateral force transmission. (This is particularly true in the maxillary arch, where a labially inclined force is produced as a result of vertical overlap articulation [see Fig 4-5].) This design also reduces the torque on the implants without overloading the natural teeth. In the event that the pontic is too long for this approach, the author would recommend placing another implant anteriorly to create a freestanding implant-supported prosthesis (see below).

Natural teeth

Figure 4-33 shows two nonvital premolars along with a missing first molar. If the premolars can be saved, a fixed prosthesis that would include the premolars and the second molar would be biomechanically sound (Fig 4-34). Lateral force on the first premolar would be distributed to all the abutments because of the flexion in the periodontal ligament (Fig 4-35). The quantity and quality of the distribution of force depends on the location within the periodontal ligament and the site and direction of the force application. If the premolars were not salvagable, a fixed prosthesis from the canine to the second molar would create a span that is usually too long for the abutments biomechanically and would cause overload (Fig 4-36).

As stated above, implants are unlike natural teeth in their force distribution. If an attempt is made to solve the diagnostic problem of two hopeless premolars by placement of a molar implant (Fig 4-37), the combined prosthesis would overload the implant as a result of the 5:1 differential mobility and the long lever arm (Fig 4-38; see also Fig 4-29).

Diagnostic Factors in Combined Prostheses

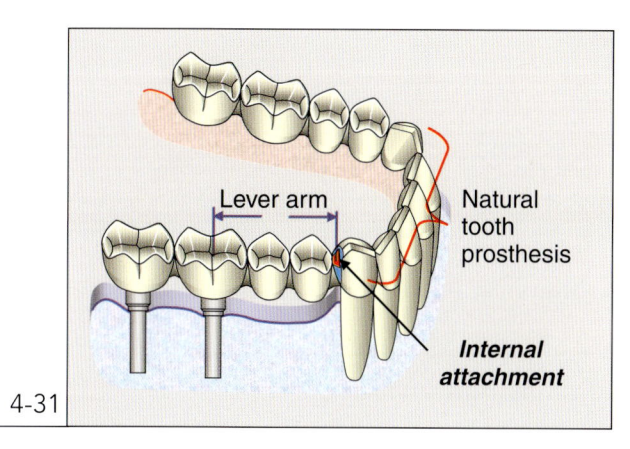

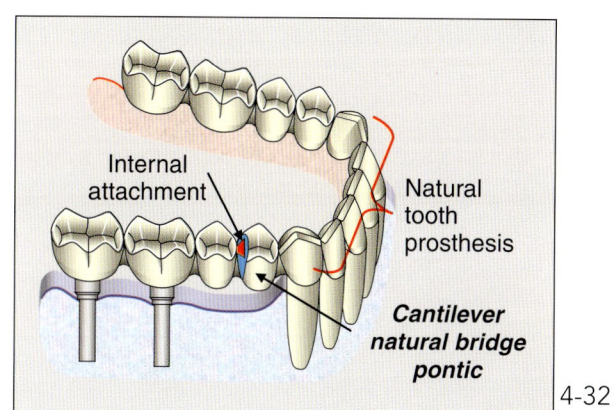

4-31 — Lever arm, Natural tooth prosthesis, **Internal attachment**

4-32 — Internal attachment, Natural tooth prosthesis, **Cantilever natural bridge pontic**

4-33 — *Diagnosis* — Nonvital teeth

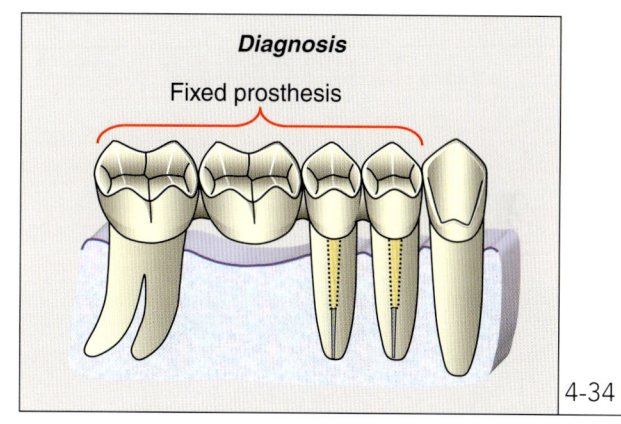

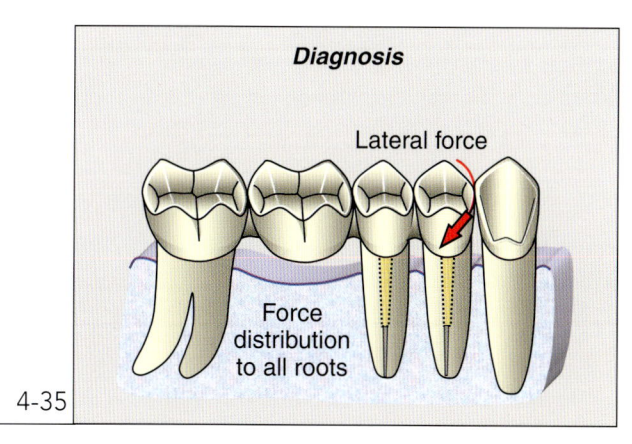

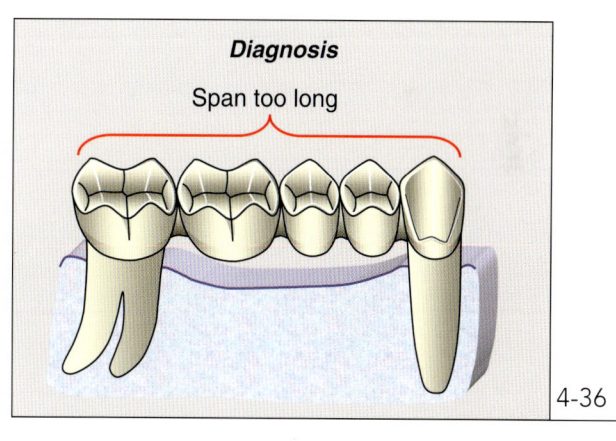

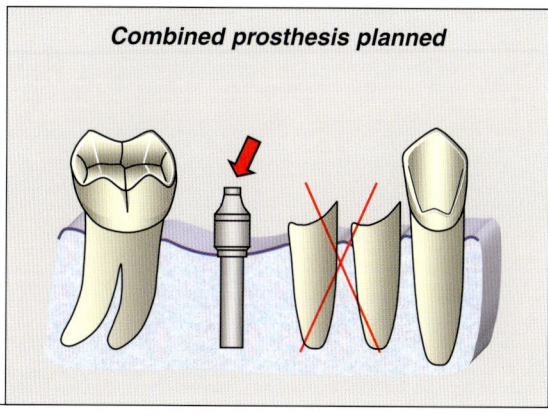

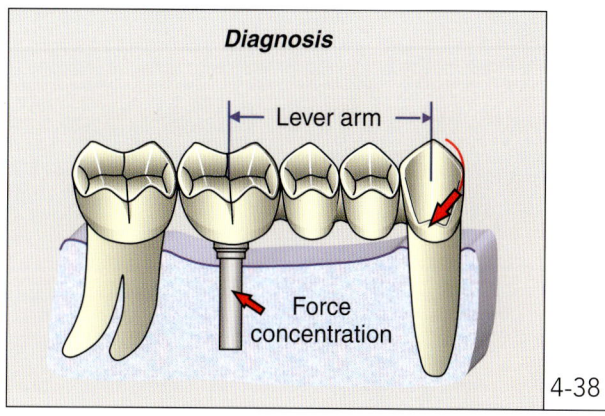

4-34 — *Diagnosis* — Fixed prosthesis

4-35 — *Diagnosis* — Lateral force, Force distribution to all roots

4-36 — *Diagnosis* — Span too long

4-37 — **Combined prosthesis planned**

4-38 — *Diagnosis* — Lever arm, Force concentration

61

Terminal implants

It should be noted that the inclusion of natural teeth within an implant-supported prosthesis does not distribute force to the natural teeth because of the differential mobility of 5:1 (Fig 4-39). From a biomechanical point of view, it would be as if the teeth were not present, and the distance between the implants would be treated as a lever arm. Lateral force on the terminal implant would concentrate the force at the loading site and could overload the implant (see Fig 4-39). Occlusal loading at the midpoint could also overload the implants because the cantilever distance from each implant would be excessive.

Most experienced clinicians recommend using a freestanding osseointegrated prosthesis provided that the distance between the implants is not excessive (Fig 4-40).

Implant Loading with Four Clinical Variants

There are four clinical variants that dramatically affect implant loading (Fig 4-41): *(1)* cusp inclination (*upper left*); *(2)* implant inclination (*upper right*); *(3)* horizontal implant offset (*lower left*); and *(4)* vertical implant offset (*lower right*).[15] Torque (moment) is measured mathematically at the gold screw, at the abutment screw, and at the level of the third screw thread of the implant.[15] The values are constant and are averaged for each variant for simplicity of presentation.[15]

Cusp inclination

For every 10-degree increase in cusp inclination, there is approximately a 30% increase in torque (Fig 4-42).[15] Cusp inclination has been found to produce the highest level of torque and represents the most significant clinical finding.

Implant inclination

For every 10-degree increase in implant inclination, there is approximately a 5% increase in torque (Fig 4-43). This represents the least significant clinical finding.

Horizontal implant offset

For every 1-mm increase in horizontal implant offset, there is approximately a 15% increase in torque (Fig 4-44). This is the second most significant clinical finding.

Apical implant offset

For every 1-mm increase in vertical implant offset, there is approximately a 5% increase in torque (Fig 4-45). This is a minimum torque-producing factor.

A summary of the clinical variants is shown in Fig 4-46. The clinical significance of these findings is extremely important because of the variation in the amount of torque produced. In treatment planning, one can reduce torque by reducing the cusp inclines and by substituting a low torque-producing factor for a high torque-producing factor. This process of reducing the total implant loading is called *therapeutic biomechanics* and is discussed in detail in chapter 5.[16]

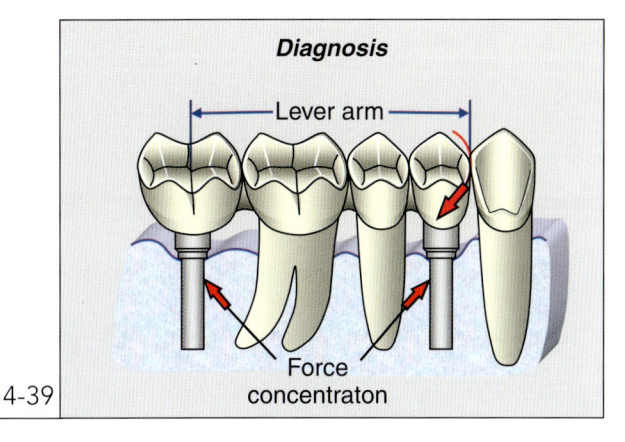

Implant Loading with Four Clinical Variants

Diagnosis

Lever arm

Force concentration

4-39

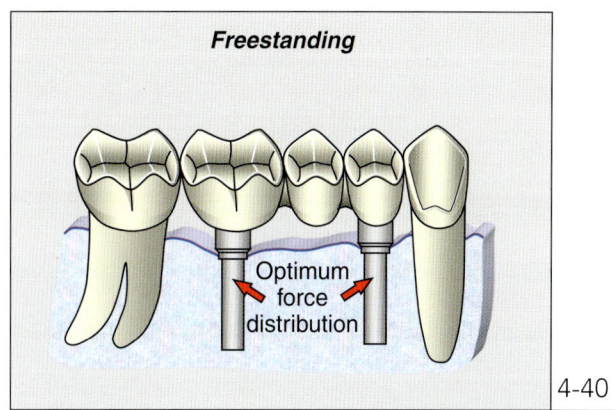

Freestanding

Optimum force distribution

4-40

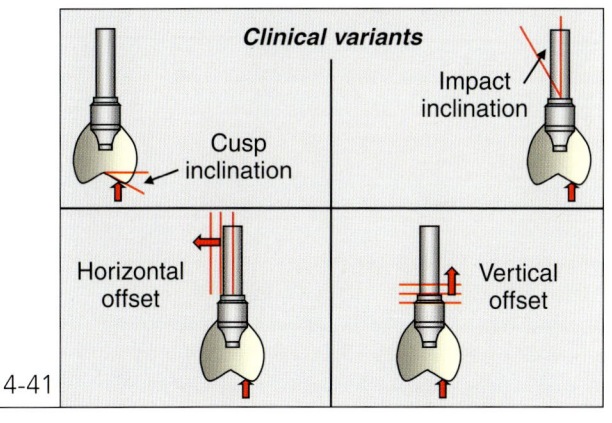

Clinical variants

Cusp inclination

Impact inclination

Horizontal offset

Vertical offset

4-41

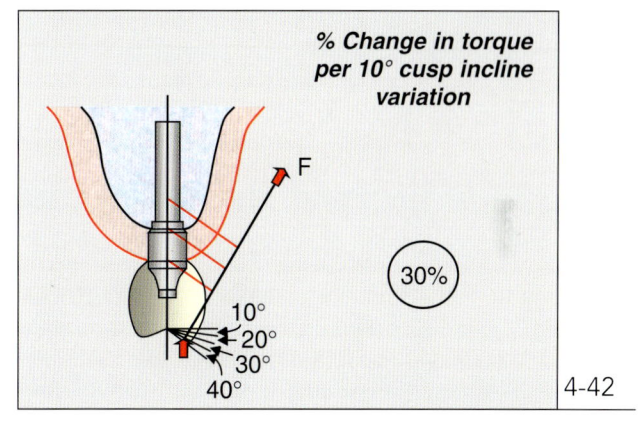

% Change in torque per 10° cusp incline variation

30%

4-42

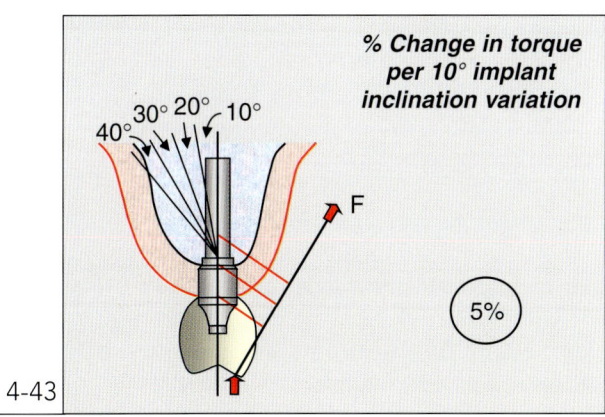

% Change in torque per 10° implant inclination variation

5%

4-43

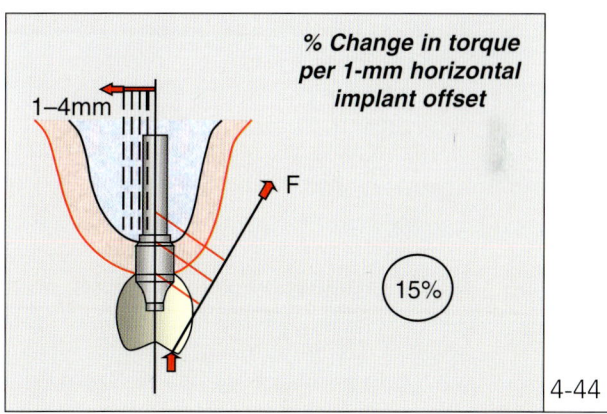

% Change in torque per 1-mm horizontal implant offset

15%

4-44

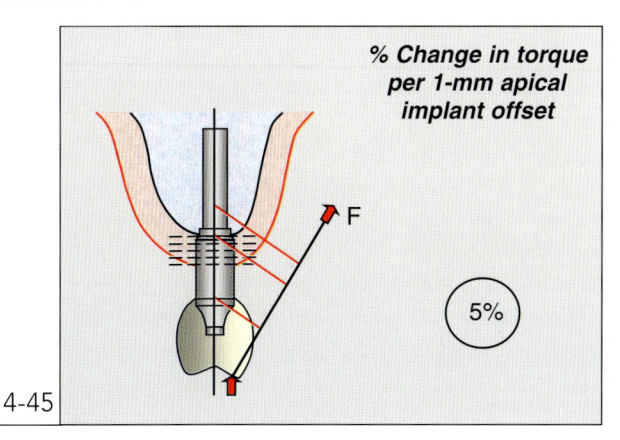

% Change in torque per 1-mm apical implant offset

5%

4-45

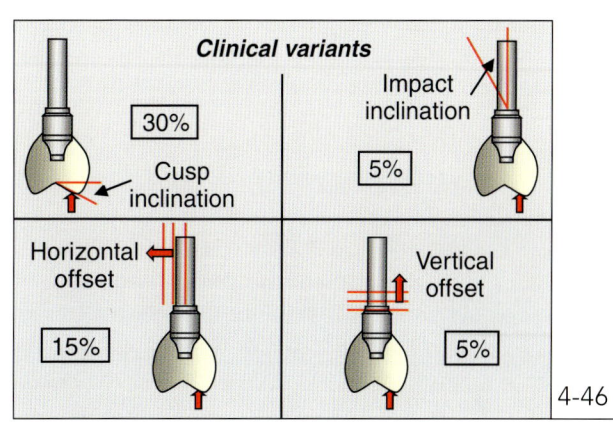

Clinical variants

Cusp inclination — 30%

Impact inclination — 5%

Horizontal offset — 15%

Vertical offset — 5%

4-46

63

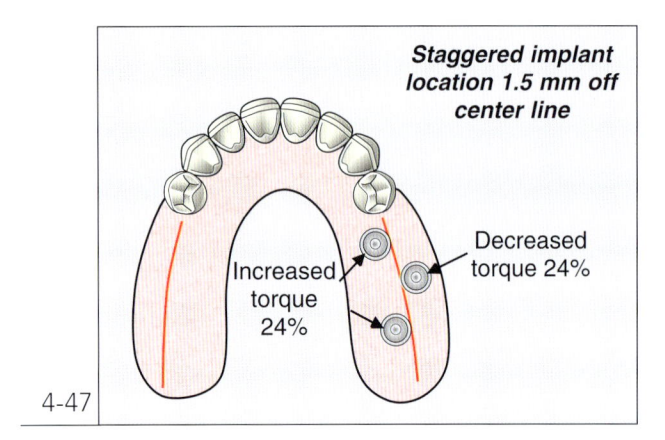

4-47 | Staggered implant location 1.5 mm off center line. Increased torque 24%. Decreased torque 24%.

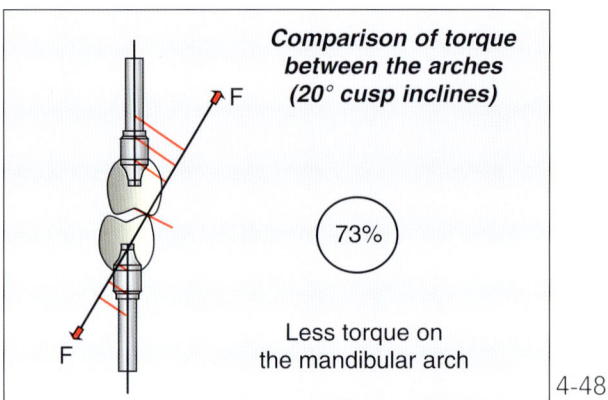

4-48 | Comparison of torque between the arches (20° cusp inclines). 73%. Less torque on the mandibular arch.

Staggered Implant Offset

Some authors have suggested placing implants in a staggered buccal and lingual offset to create a so-called tripod effect as a means of compensating for torque that is produced when occlusal forces are applied lateral to the implants, as in the maxilla shown in Fig 4-47.[17] While this concept may seem biomechanically valid, it requires evaluation mathematically. To do so, implants were staggered 1.5 mm buccal and/or lingual from the center line to achieve a tripod effect (see Fig 4-47). The torque (moment) was then evaluated mathematically with the method previously described,[15] and the maxillary arch was compared to the mandibular arch.[18] In the maxilla, the lingual offset implants created approximately 24% more torque, whereas the buccal offset implants created approximately 24% less torque. As a result of this configuration in the maxilla, evenly distributed occlusal force on the prosthesis *increased* the total torque by 24%.[18]

The posterior working-side occlusion usually produces a buccally inclined resultant line of force on the maxillary arch and a lingually inclined resultant line of force on the mandibular arch (Fig 4-48). As a result of the maxillary buccal overlap and cusp incline contact, the mandible has approximately 73% less torque than the maxilla.[18] Therefore, the concept of staggered implant offset for multiple implant-supported prostheses can be applied in the mandible with caution but is contraindicated in the maxilla.[18] In the author's opinion, it would be far better to move all of the implants as far buccally as possible in the maxilla to reduce the horizontal implant offset,[15] as described in chapter 5.

Summary

The principles of force distribution must be understood relative to the axial inclination, impact area, and location of the supporting bone. The periodontal ligament and the osseointegrated interface distribute force differently to the supporting bone. Therefore, problems develop when teeth and implants are combined in the same prosthesis. Four clinical factors have varying clinical significance relative to torque production. The clinician can apply these principles to reduce implant loading in an organized approach called *therapeutic biomechanics* (chapter 5).

References

1. Posselt U. Temporomandibular joint syndrome and occlusion: Research committee report. Am Equilib Soc Compend 1963–64;7:51.
2. Brewer AA, Hudson DC. Application of miniaturized electronic devices to the study of tooth contact in complete dentures. J Prosthet Dent 1961;11:62–72.
3. Weinberg L. Force distribution in mastication, clenching and bruxism. Dent Digest 1957;63:58–61, 116–120.
4. Misch CE. Contemporary Implant Dentistry. St. Louis: Mosby, 1993:281–282.
5. Clelland NL, Ismail YH, Zaki HS, Pipko D. Three-dimensional finite element stress analysis in and around the Screw-Vent implant. Int J Oral Maxillofac Implants 1991;6:391–398.
6. Reiger MR, Mayberry M, Brose MO. Finite element analysis of six endosseous implants. J Prosthet Dent 1990;63:671–676.
7. Weinberg L. Lateral force in relation to denture base and clasp design. J Prosthet Dent 1956;6:785–800.
8. Weinberg LA, Kruger B. Biomechanical considerations when combining tooth-supported and implant-supported prostheses. Oral Surg Oral Med Oral Pathol 1994;78:22–27.
9. Weinberg LA. Biomechanics of force distribution in implant-supported prostheses. Int J Oral Maxillofac Implants 1993;8:19–31.
10. Weinberg LA. Force distribution in splinted posterior teeth. Oral Surg Oral Med Oral Pathol 1957;10:1268–1276.
11. Weinberg LA. Force distribution in splinted anterior teeth. Oral Surg Oral Med Oral Pathol 1957;10:484–494.
12. Ericsson I, Lekholm U, Brånemark P-I, Lindhe J, Glantz P-O, Nyman S. A clinical evaluation of fixed bridge restorations supported by the combination of teeth and osseointegratedtitanium implants. J Clin Periodontol 1986;13:307–312.
13. Weinberg LA, Kruger B. Biomechanical considerations when combining tooth-supported and implant-supported prostheses. Oral Surg Oral Med Oral Pathol 1994;78:22–27.
14. Rangert B, Gunne J, Sullivan DY. Mechanical aspects of a Brånemark implant connected to a natural tooth: An in vitro study. Int J Oral Maxillofac Implants 1991;6:177–186.
15. Weinberg LA, Kruger B. A comparison of implant/prosthesis loading with four clinical variables. Int J Prosthodont 1995;8:421–433.
16. Weinberg LA. Reduction of implant loading with therapeutic biomechanics. J Implant Dent 1998;7:277–285.
17. Rangert B, Sullivan R. Preventing prosthetic overloading induced by bending. Nobelpharma News 1993;7:4–5.
18. Weinberg LA, Kruger B. An evaluation of torque (moment) on implant/prosthesis with staggered buccal and lingual offset. Int J Periodontics Restorative Dent 1996;16:253–265.

5 Reduction of Implant Loading via Therapeutic Biomechanics

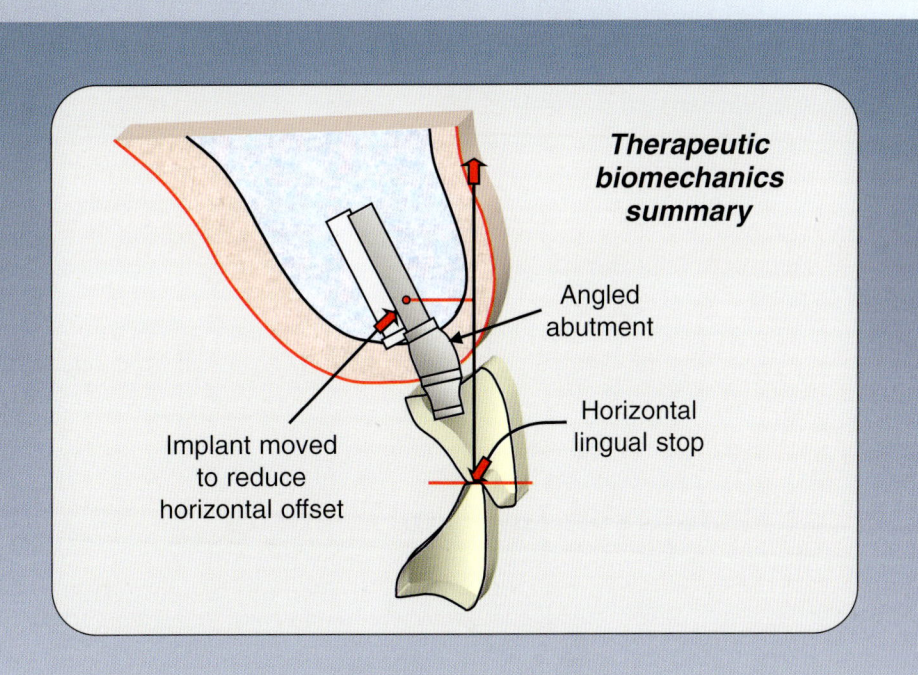

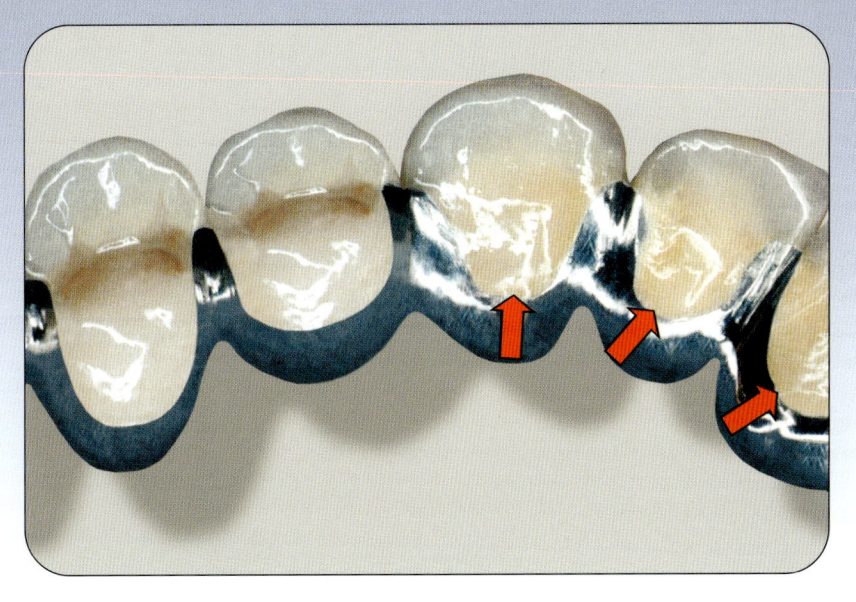

Therapeutic biomechanics summary

- Angled abutment
- Horizontal lingual stop
- Implant moved to reduce horizontal offset

The process of diagnosis and treatment planning for the osseointegrated prosthesis is influenced by long-standing successful design concepts for the tooth-supported prosthesis.[1] However, the biomechanical concept of force distribution associated with periodontal ligament flexion[2] cannot be applied to the stiff osseointegrated implant interface.[3] Biomechanical design is further complicated when natural teeth and implants support the same prosthesis.[4]

There is general consensus that implant overload is the primary cause of failure after loading[5] and that vertical force is tolerated by supporting bone more effectively than is lateral force.[6] However, in the author's opinion, corrective and remedial biomechanical designs that address these problems have not been pursued. This chapter focuses on the clinical variants that produce implant loading[7] and describes a diagnostic process known as *therapeutic biomechanics* that remediates each biomechanical factor to diminish their cumulative effect.[8]

Physiologic reactions do not take place in isolation of one another; each factor has a cumulative effect on the collective whole. Factors that contribute to implant loading are *(1)* muscle force, *(2)* cusp inclination, *(3)* location and quality of residual bone, *(4)* position of the implant, *(5)* location of the prosthesis, *(6)* physiologic variation, and *(7)* abutment design. These factors are interrelated and cumulative, and when left uncorrected they collectively increase implant loading in a process called *reactive biomechanics* (Fig 5-1).[8]

Therapeutic biomechanics is the process of remediating each biomechanical factor in the physiologic chain of events in order to diminish the cumulative result, that is, implant overload (Fig 5-2).

Clinical Variants in Implant Loading

Four clinical variants—cusp inclination, implant inclination, horizontal implant offset, and vertical implant offset—were compared mathematically in relation to torque (moment) production.[7] Variation in torque was measured at three points: the gold screw, the abutment screw, and the third screw thread of the implant. Since the values in these three areas are consistent relative to each other, the average is used for each clinical situation for the sake of simplicity of presentation (Fig 5-3).

A 10-degree increase in cusp and implant inclination produced an average 30% and 5% increase in torque production, respectively (see Fig 5-3, *top*), while every 1 mm of horizontal and vertical implant offset resulted in a respective average 15% and 5% increase in torque production (see Fig 5-3, *bottom*). Thus, cusp inclination and horizontal implant offset are shown to have the most significant effect on torque production. (See Figs 4-41 to 4-45 for a more detailed description of clinical variants affecting implant loading.)

The wide degree of variation in torque production among these four clinical variants is essential to therapeutic biomechanics. As discussed below, the clinician can not only reduce each torque-producing variant individually, but also has the option of substituting a low torque-producing variant for a high torque-producing variant in order to bring about less cumulative implant loading.

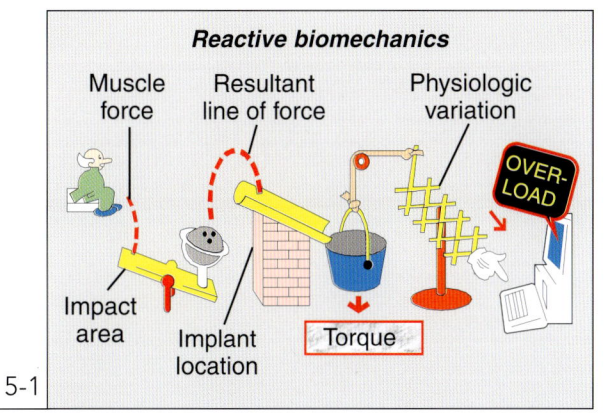

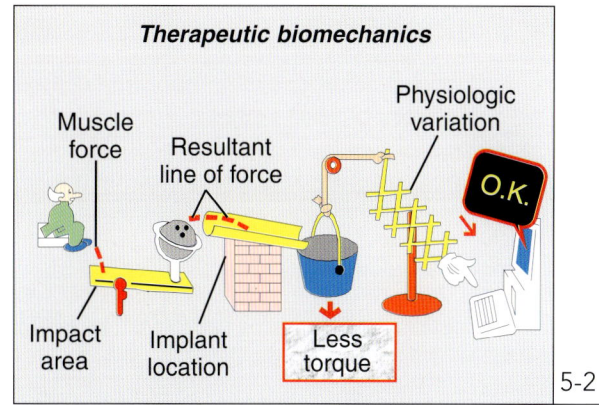

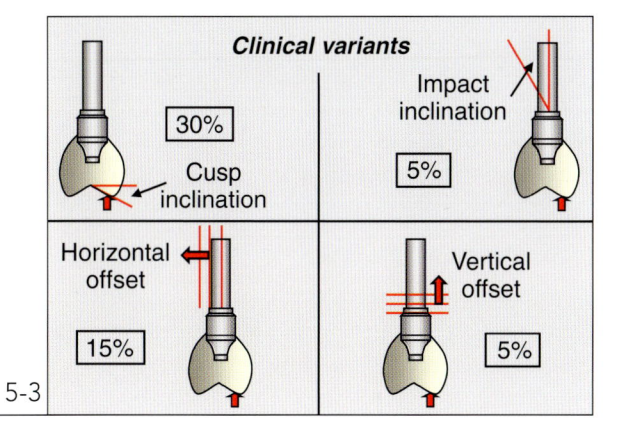

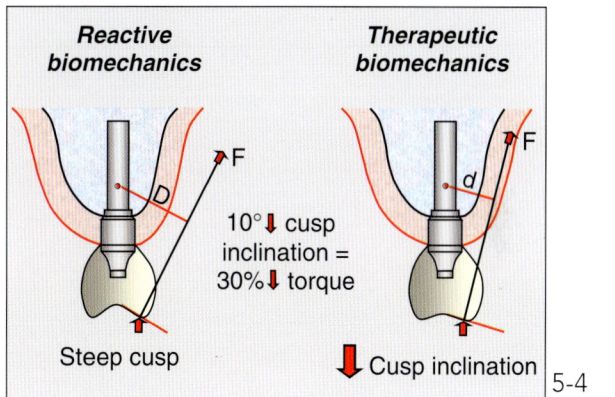

Therapeutic Biomechanics

Cusp inclination

The first step in reducing implant loading is to decrease cusp inclination. Occlusal loading on a working cusp incline produces a resultant line of force (F) that is perpendicular to the steep cusp inclination (Fig 5-4, *left*). The amount of torque produced is the force (F) times the perpendicular distance from the maximum implant loading area located approximately at the level of the third screw thread (see Fig 5-4, *left*).[9] A therapeutic biomechanical reduction in cusp inclination of 10 degrees produces an average 30% reduction in torque (see Fig 5-4, *right*). A visual means of evaluating torque is to compare the length of the distance arms (D, d) between the implant and the resultant line of force (see Fig 5-4).

5 Reduction of Implant Loading via Therapeutic Biomechanics

Altered restoration position (cross occlusion)

Figure 5-5 (*left*) shows a normal buccolingual occlusal relationship. When the restoration is repositioned in cross occlusion, the horizontal implant offset is decreased relative to the residual bone (see Fig 5-5, *right*). During function, the normal buccolingual occlusion produces exaggerated torque (Fig 5-6, *left*, D). By comparison, the cross occlusion produces less torque as measured by the shortened work arm (see Fig 5-6, *right*, d).

Esthetics and contraindications of cross occlusion

Cross occlusion may be contraindicated when an adjacent posterior natural tooth is in the normal buccolingual relationship. However, when cross occlusion is used, esthetics is usually not a problem because the first premolar is in normal buccolingual relationship, the second premolar is in cusp-to-cusp occlusion, and only the first molar is in cross occlusion. The buccolingual width of the molars can be narrowed to provide tongue space. Whenever the occlusal position is modified (ie, cross occlusion), the planned occlusion should be provided in the provisional restorations to promote patient adaptation and problem solving *prior to* the construction of final restorations.

Altered implant position

Another fundamental therapeutic biomechanical process takes advantage of the disparity in torque production among the four clinical variants discussed in Fig 5-3. The process consists of substituting a low torque-producing factor for a high torque-producing factor. For example, a standard implant-abutment-restoration design facilitates the access channel exiting the center of the restoration (Fig 5-7, *left*). However, placing the implant head as close to the center line of the restoration as possible reduces the horizontal offset. A 2-mm reduction in the horizontal implant offset *reduces* the torque by approximately 30% (see Fig 5-7, *right*). Because of the sinus, the implant must be inclined by 10 degrees, *increasing* the torque by 5%. The net result is a 25% decrease in torque. This implant inclination requires an angulated or custom-reangulated abutment in order to provide parallelism or favorable access channel location.

Favorable sinus location

Reducing the horizontal implant offset may not always require abutment reangulation. When the location of the sinus permits, the normal occlusal relationship (Fig 5-8, *left*) does not necessarily require abutment angulation when repositioned in cross occlusion (Fig 5-8, *right*). To evaluate this possibility, place the head of the implant as close to the midline of the repositioned restoration as possible; next, determine the appropriate implant inclination required by the residual bone topography. The abutment design is selected last to allow for the required parallelism and/or access.

Physiologic variation

The standard occlusal anatomy, wherein cusp inclines meet in a central groove, is shown in Fig 5-9 (*left*). In theory, the mandibular cusp causes buccal and lingual lines of force, which in turn produces a vertical resultant line of force. However, clinical

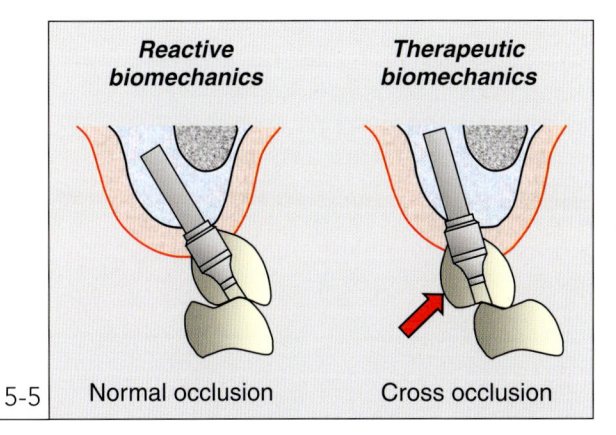

Therapeutic Biomechanics

Fig 5-5 Reactive biomechanics — Normal occlusion. Therapeutic biomechanics — Cross occlusion.

Fig 5-6 Reactive biomechanics — Working side. Therapeutic biomechanics — Reduced torque.

Fig 5-7 Therapeutic torque reduction. 2-mm reduction in horizontal offset = ↓30% torque. 10°↑ in implant inclination = ↑5% torque. Net decrease 25%.

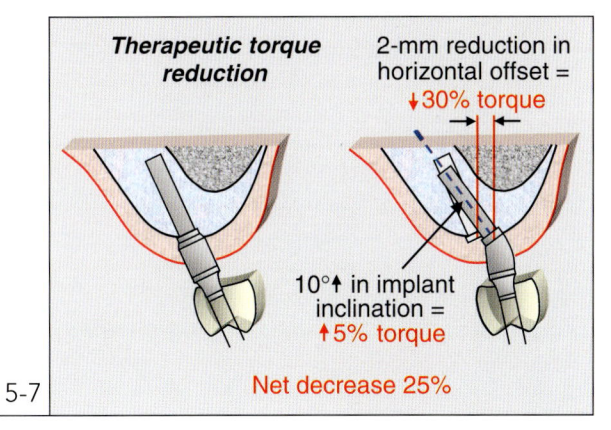

Fig 5-8 Reactive biomechanics — Lingual, Normal occlusion. Therapeutic biomechanics — Reduced horizontal offset, Cross occlusion.

Fig 5-9 Vertical resultant force — Centric occlusion. Inclined resultant force — Physiologic shift in centric occlusion.

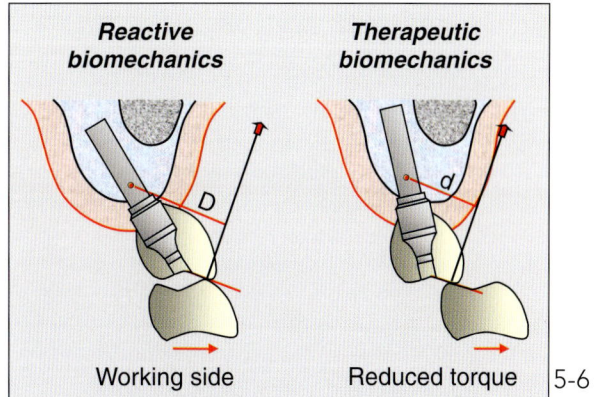

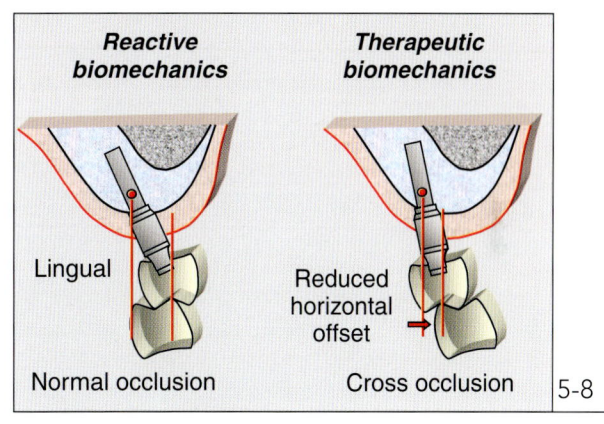

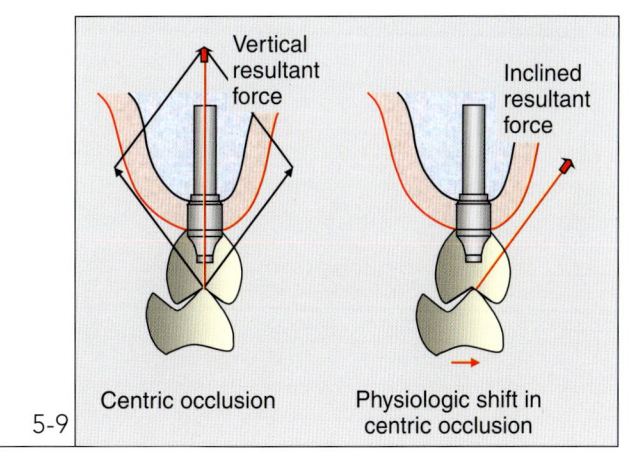

experiments based on the replication of centric relation records have all indicated a physiologic variation of approximately ± 0.4 mm with regard to time,[10] recording methods,[11] muscular de-conditioning,[12] and muscle tone.[13] As a result of this constant physiologic variation, the lateral shift in centric occlusion will result in buccally or lingually inclined resultant lines of force distributed to the supporting bone (Fig 5-9, right).

71

Modified occlusal anatomy

A posterior horizontal fossa of 1.5 mm has been proposed to compensate for physiologic variation.[14] Described as a "long centric" by Mann and Pankey,[15] the concept of a horizontal fossa is not new. Originally, the technique for creating a horizontal fossa relied on functionally generated intraoral records, which have fallen out of favor. The simple laboratory technique described in chapter 2 is designed to produce a modified occlusal anatomy containing a 1.5-mm horizontal fossa (Fig 5-10, *right*). With this configuration, a mandibular cusp will produce a vertical resultant line of force within the expected range of physiologic variation (see Fig 5-10, *left*).

Pattern of Bone Loss

Posterior mandibular bone loss

When teeth are lost, the bone atrophies along the root inclination toward the basal bone. The pattern of posterior bone loss has a significant biomechanical impact. The normal lingual axial inclination of the posteriormost molars is in the range of 33 to 35 degrees (Fig 5-11, *left*). The inclination gradually decreases as the location moves anteriorly and becomes nearly vertical at the premolars (see Fig 5-11, *right*). At the canine, the axial inclination is buccal in direction (Fig 5-12, *left*) and increases in severity toward the midline. The incline of the incisors is markedly labial (see Fig 5-12, *right*).

Biomechanical effect

The biomechanical effect of this pattern of bone loss is to move the implant-supporting bone lingual to the occlusal impact area. As discussed in chapter 4, the resultant torque depends on the character of the impact area and the direction of the resultant line of force relative to the implant and its supporting bone.[2–4,7] Often, the reactive biomechanics posteriorly is exaggerated by the required lingual position of the restoration relative to the residual bone (Fig 5-13). A bad situation is made worse by the combined effect of the loss of vertical bone height and the location of the mandibular nerve. This combination usually results in the buccal placement of the implant and excessive torque due to the long working arm (D) generated by the exaggerated lingual resultant line of force (F) created by the occlusion (see Fig 5-13).

Therapeutic biomechanics

The exaggerated implant torque previously described (see Fig 5-13) is contrasted with the reduced torque (shorter working arm [d]) produced as a result of a series of therapeutic biomechanical remedial procedures (Fig 5-14): *(1)* The cusp inclination is reduced, causing the resultant line of force to pass much closer to the implant and supporting bone; *(2)* the head of the implant is placed closer to the midline of the restoration, reducing the horizontal implant offset; *(3)* the angulated abutment facilitates the required parallelism and/or access. It should be emphasized that the precise location and inclination of the implant, ie, safely avoiding the mandibular canal, is a practical clinical result of a precise three-dimensional guidance system for implant insertion (see chapter 6).[16,17]

Pattern of Bone Loss

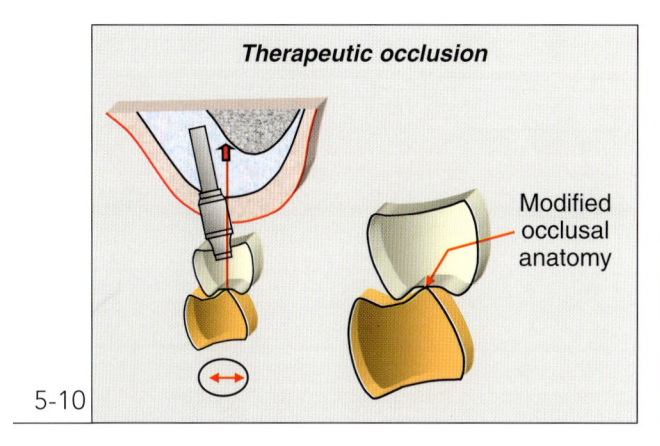

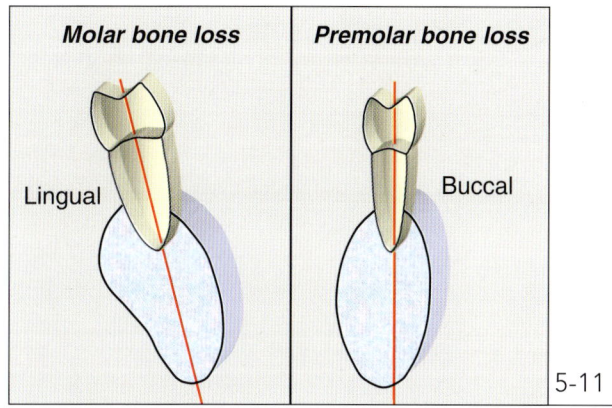

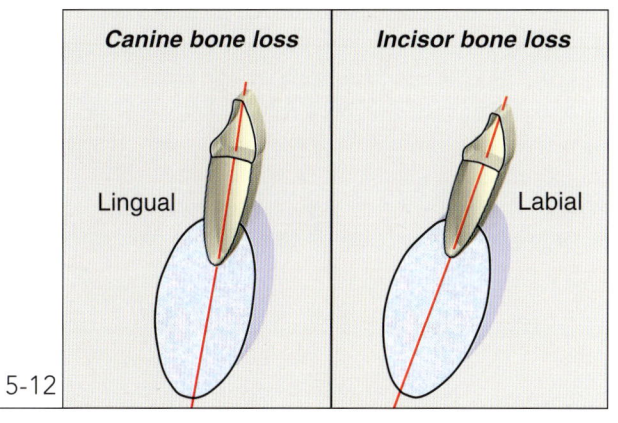

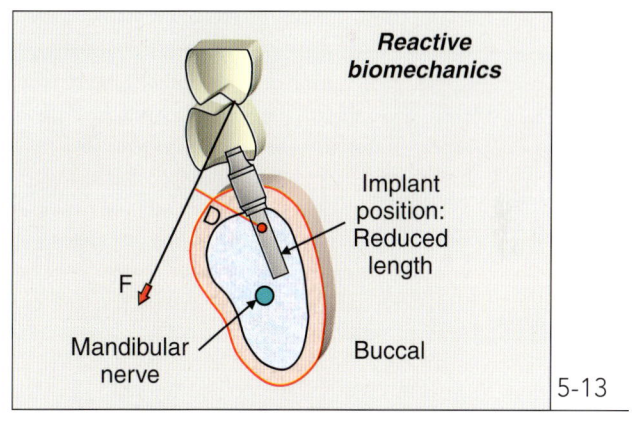

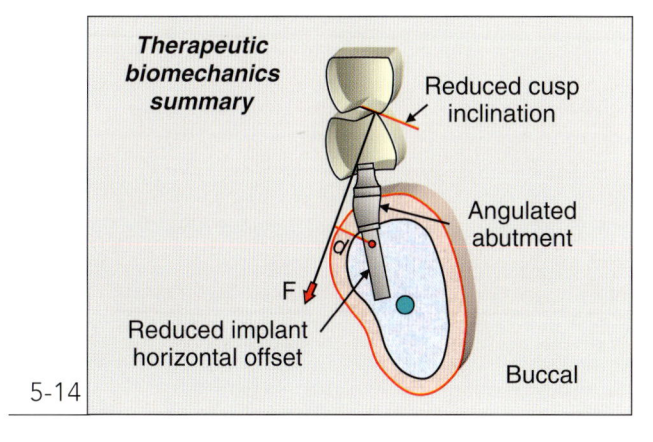

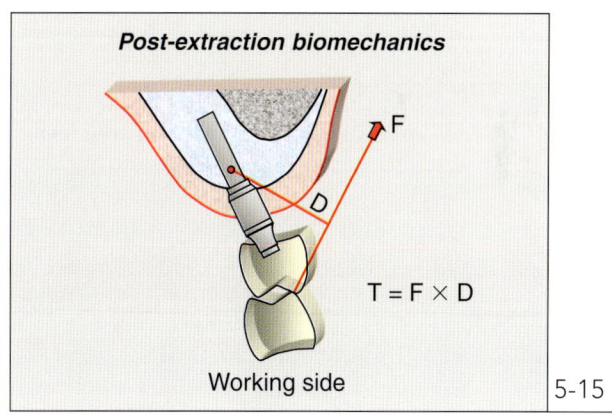

Figs 5-10 to 5-15

Posterior maxillary bone loss

Often, the posterior maxillary residual alveolar bone is more restricted than the mandibular residual bone as a result of the lingual pattern of bone loss, the location of the sinus, and frequent fracture of the buccal plate of bone during surgery. Consequently, the post-extraction biomechanics are extremely unfavorable. With a standard occlusion and implant-abutment-restorative configuration, working-side occlusion produces a resultant line of force that falls at an exaggerated distance (D) from the implant and supporting bone (Fig 5-15). This usually produces an extremely high level of torque and results in implant overload.

Therapeutic biomechanics

Assuming that the prosthesis cannot be placed in cross occlusion, several remedial therapeutic biomechanical procedures may be employed (Fig 5-16): *(1)* Marked reduction in cusp inclination will cause the resultant line of force to pass much closer to the supporting bone (D); *(2)* the head of the implant can be aligned with the midline of the restoration, reducing the horizontal implant offset; and *(3)* an angled or custom-reangulated abutment will provide parallelism and/or access. The therapeutic biomechanical process reduces the distance (D) of the work arm (see Fig 5-16) and can reverse a completely untenable implant-overloaded system (see Fig 5-15).

Cross occlusion

For comparison purposes, Fig 5-17 (*left*) shows the original reactive working-side occlusion, with the exaggerated torque-producing long working arm (D). In addition to the many therapeutic remedial changes shown in Fig 5-16, a cross occlusion further reduces the working arm (d) and resulting torque (Fig 5-17, *right*).

As many as five therapeutic biomechanical procedures can be used in conjunction with each other to reduce torque in the maxillary posterior area (Fig 5-18): *(1)* cross occlusion (reduction of horizontal implant offset); *(2)* placement of the implant head as close to the midline of the restoration as possible; *(3)* use of an angled abutment; *(4)* creation of shallow cusp inclines; and *(5)* modification of the centric occlusion anatomy (1.5-mm horizontal fossae). It may not be practical to use all five in some clinical cases. While these procedures do not necessarily rule out sinus lifts, they are valuable alternatives and/or additions.

Anterior maxillary bone loss

Reactive biomechanics

Figure 5-19 shows an example of pre-extraction bone level (*left*) and post-extraction bone loss superiorly and lingually (*right*). In this case, esthetic demands require the restoration to remain in the original position, considerably labial to the residual supporting bone (see Fig 5-19, *right*). To compound the problem, a steep vertical overlap produces a resultant line of force (F) that has exaggerated labial inclination (see Fig 5-19, *right*). The distance arm (D) is extremely long, producing an unacceptable overload on the retaining screws, implant, and supporting bone (see Fig 5-19, *right*).

Therapeutic biomechanics

When standard alignment of the implant-abutment-restoration is used to facilitate access channel placement, the lingual horizontal implant offset increases by 2 mm, resulting in a 30% increase in torque (Fig 5-20). However, by positioning the implant anteriorly 2 mm, the implant head may be placed closer to the midline of the restoration. An angled or custom-reangulated abutment provides the access channel without an increase in torque (Fig 5-21).

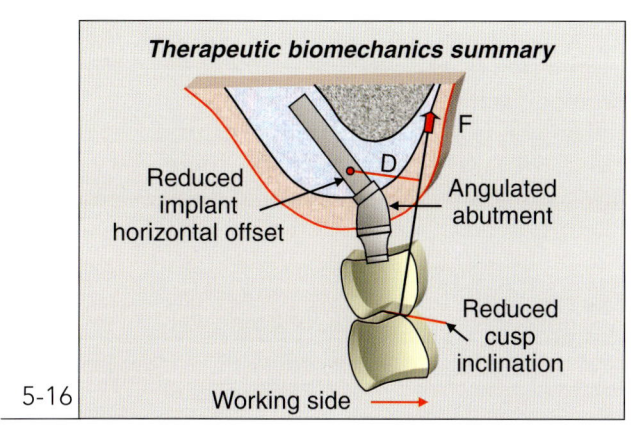

Pattern of Bone Loss

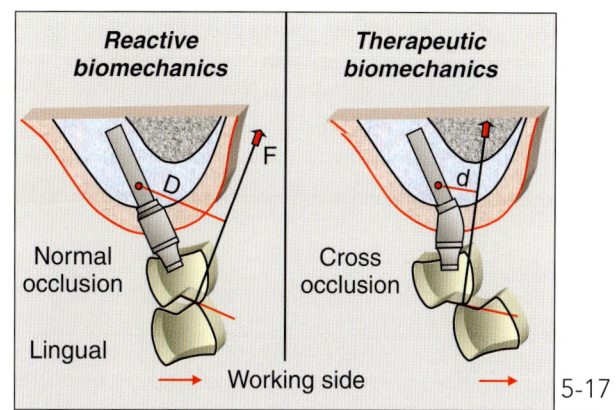

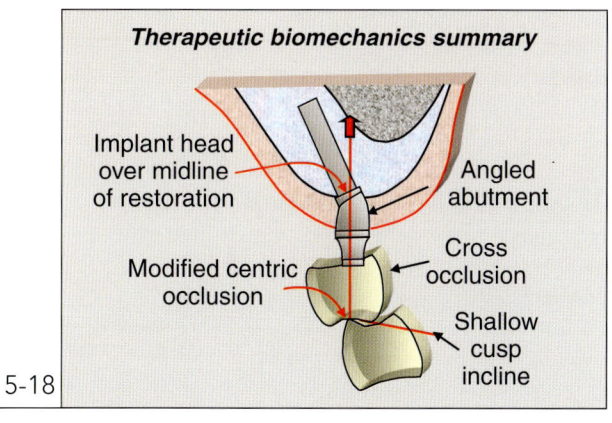

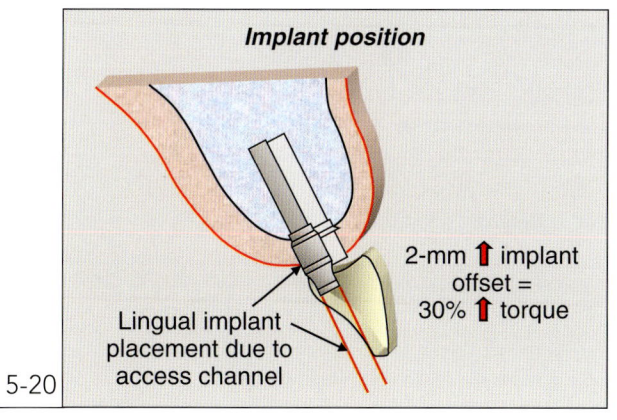

5-16 **Therapeutic biomechanics summary** — Reduced implant horizontal offset, Angulated abutment, Reduced cusp inclination, Working side →

5-17 **Reactive biomechanics** / **Therapeutic biomechanics** — Normal occlusion, Lingual, Cross occlusion, Working side →

5-18 **Therapeutic biomechanics summary** — Implant head over midline of restoration, Angled abutment, Cross occlusion, Modified centric occlusion, Shallow cusp incline

5-19 **Pre-extraction bone** / **Reactive biomechanics**

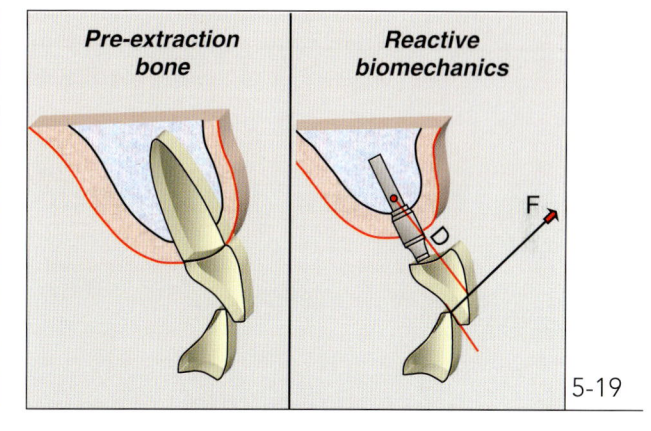

5-20 **Implant position** — Lingual implant placement due to access channel, 2-mm ↑ implant offset = 30% ↑ torque

5-21 **Abutment design** — Angulated abutment, Access channel without increase in torque

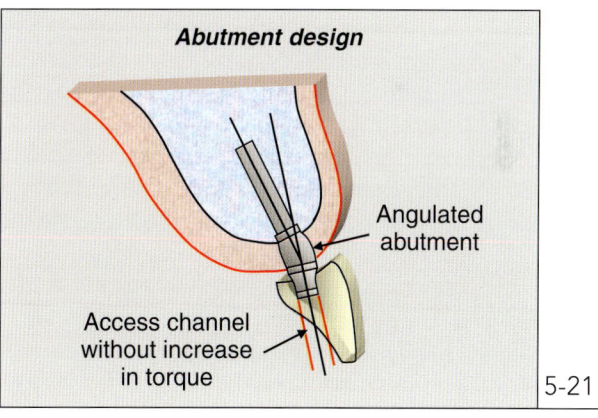

75

Regardless of the placement of the implant labially, lingual incline contact with a deep vertical overlap (O) produces a severely inclined resultant line of force (F), which induces excessive torque from the extremely long working arm (D) (Fig 5-22). This can be reduced by providing a horizontal lingual stop on the maxillary restoration, which will redirect the resultant line of force (F) as vertically as possible, thereby reducing the working arm (d) and effectively diminishing the torque (Fig 5-23). Horizontal lingual stops may also be used with tooth-supported fixed prostheses (Fig 5-24, *arrows*).

Because of esthetic demands, there are three possible therapeutic procedures that can be used alone or in combination to reduce torque in the anterior maxillary area: *(1)* placing the implant head as close to the midline of the restoration as possible; *(2)* using an angled abutment; and *(3)* providing a maxillary horizontal lingual stop (see Fig 5-23). It may not be practical in some clinical cases to use all three of these procedures. However, to gain maximum benefit from therapeutic biomechanics, optimum implant placement using a three-dimensional guidance system for implant insertion is recommended (see chapter 6).[16,17]

Occlusion: Therapeutic Differential Loading

A new concept called *therapeutic differential loading* improves long-term prognosis when implants and natural teeth support separate prostheses in the same arch.

Differential occlusal adjustment

Two new dynamic biomechanical factors are introduced, requiring differential occlusal adjustment procedures in addition to the standard methods. When separate implant-supported and tooth-supported prostheses co-exist in the same arch,[4] the new biomechanical factors have entirely different characteristics from each other: One concerns the constant differential mobility between the natural teeth and implants, while the other deals with the dynamic changes in biomechanics brought about over time. Differential occlusal adjustment techniques are therefore used to provide *therapeutic differential loading*.

Differential mobility

The periodontal ligament provides a degree of flexion in the range of 0.1 mm, whereas the osseointegrated implant interface is stiff.[3,4,8,9] Because of this differential mobility, occlusal loading between the implant- and tooth-supported prostheses, which is thought to be equal on light occlusal contact (Fig 5-25, *left*), is not equal *upon forceful closure* (see Fig 5-25, *right*). Instead, the flexion of the periodontal membrane shifts the loading to the implants and their supporting bone.[4]

Long-term natural tooth intrusion

This clinical problem becomes even more complicated over a period of time. Regardless of the status of occlusal contact upon completion of the tooth-supported and implant-supported prostheses (Fig 5-26, *left*), over time individual teeth or a tooth-supported prosthesis can be intruded apically (see Fig 5-26, *right*).[18] Because natural

Occlusion: Therapeutic Differential Loading

5-22 Reactive biomechanics — Torque produced, F, Lingual incline contact, O

5-23 Therapeutic biomechanics summary — Angled abutment, Implant moved to reduce horizontal offset, Horizontal lingual stop

5-24

5-25 Light occlusal contact / Heavy occlusal contact — 0.1-mm flexion, Hyperocclusion

5-26 Even contact on loading / Time: Tooth intrusion — Hyperocclusion

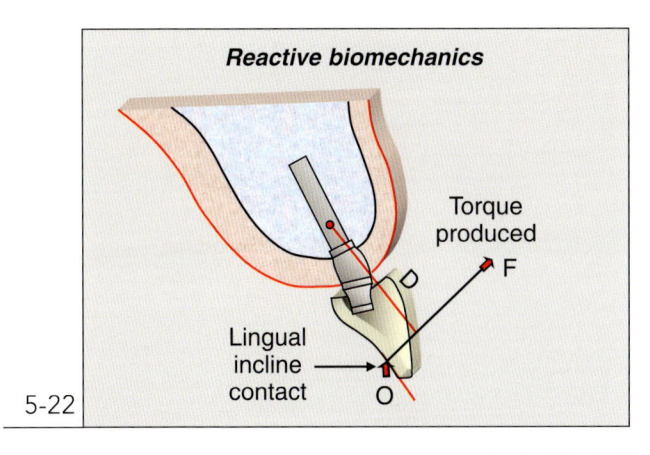

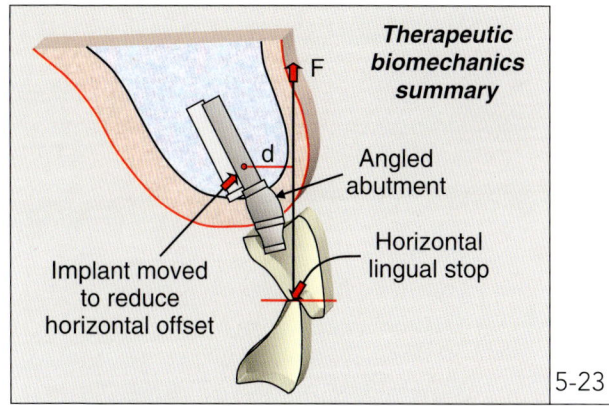

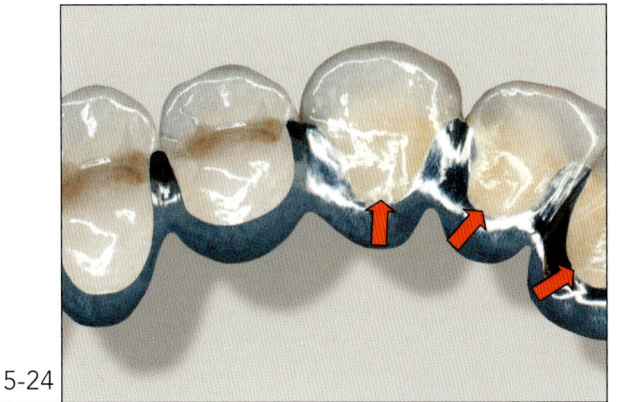

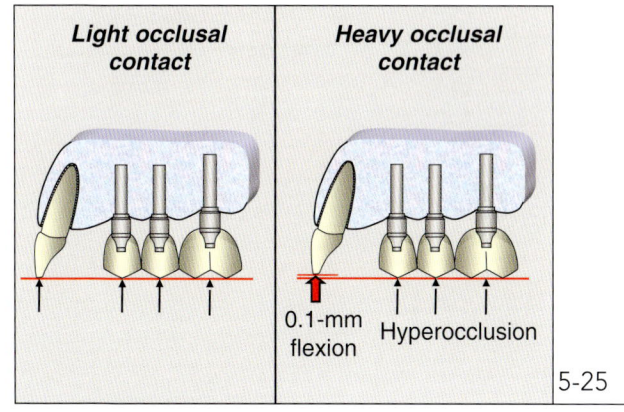

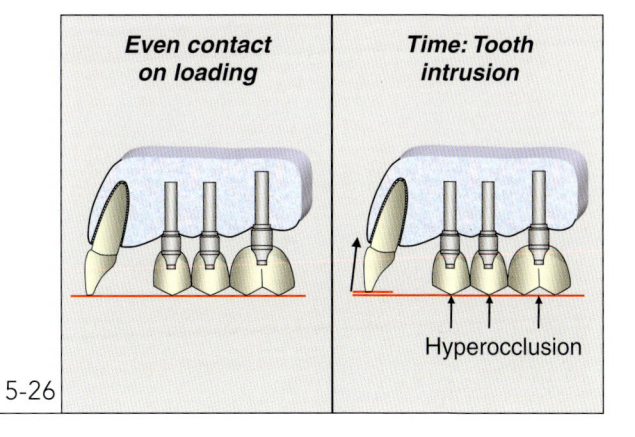

tooth loading is reduced, the burden of force distribution shifts to the implants, causing hyperocclusion. Because two new dynamic factors have been introduced—ie, differential mobility of the supporting interfaces and long-term natural tooth intrusion relative to the implants—differential occlusal adjustment procedures are needed in addition to the standard methods.

Standard and Differential Occlusal Adjustment

The clinical objective of differential occlusal adjustment is to provide *therapeutic differential loading* when individual tooth-supported and implant-supported prostheses are present in the same arch. The flexion of the periodontal ligament requires a two-step corrective procedure. First, the standard intraoral occlusal adjustment should be carried out as usual on all the prostheses regardless of the nature of the supporting structures.[19,20] This is followed by a new procedure known as *differential occlusal adjustment*, which is described below.

Standard occlusal adjustment

Centric occlusion is adjusted[19,20] to obtain simultaneous contact on *all the occlusal surfaces* (*arrows*), as evidenced by tight occlusal contact on 0.0005-inch-thick Mylar occlusal registration strips (Artus, Englewood, NJ) held in a hemostat (Fig 5-27). To eliminate false negatives, the patient should be instructed to keep the teeth together (in centric occlusion) and to try to resist lateral movement of the Mylar registration strip. To facilitate the occlusal-correction process, pressure-sensitive Mylar ribbon (Bausch 40μ Micro-Thin; Bausch Articulating Papers, Nashua, NH) used with repeated forceful occlusal contact is recommended to mark the areas requiring occlusal adjustment.

To obtain an effective marking, the teeth must be completely dry. Centric occlusal contact areas are very small and fully delineated (*arrows*) when recorded with the pressure-indicating strips, while those obtained with standard articulating paper result in broad smudges (*circles*) (Fig 5-28) and are therefore unreliable for determining hyperocclusal contact. Preliminary standard centric occlusal adjustment is complete when *all* the occlusal surfaces have at least one discrete occlusal marking as indicated by the *arrows* in Fig 5-28 and when the Mylar strips cannot pass through them occlusally.

Differential occlusal adjustment

Differential occlusal adjustment is designed to selectively reduce occlusal loading on the implant-supported prosthesis relative to the natural teeth and/or tooth-supported prosthesis in the same arch by means of a two-step process. Occlusal adjustment is performed on one restoration at a time using the discrete pressure markings on the implant-supported prosthesis (see Fig 5-28, *arrows*). This is followed immediately by checking the degree of pull on the Mylar strips between that corrected surface and the opposing arch (Fig 5-29). The author was introduced to the concept of pulling a thin strip of tissue paper through corrected occlusal surfaces by Dr C. Schuyler in 1952. If the Mylar strip cannot be pulled through, then more adjustment is necessary. If, on the other hand, the Mylar strip passes freely through the occluded surfaces, then the restoration was overcorrected. The Mylar strip should pass through with a clear "tugging" resistance, indicating that the correction was less then 0.0005 inches and more in the range of 0.00025 inches. This technique enables a much higher degree of accuracy and control than that attainable with the wax penetration technique of the past. The tight occlusal contact of the Mylar strip on the adjacent tooth-supported prosthesis serves as a constant point of reference (see Fig 5-29, *arrow*).

For accurate results it is essential that the patient maintain constant pressure during the Mylar testing procedure. This procedure is designed to adjust for the difference in flexion of the periodontal ligament compared to the stiffness of the adjacent osseointegrated interface. The osseointegrated prosthesis is then glazed and repositioned, and the occlusion is confirmed (Fig 5-30).

5-27

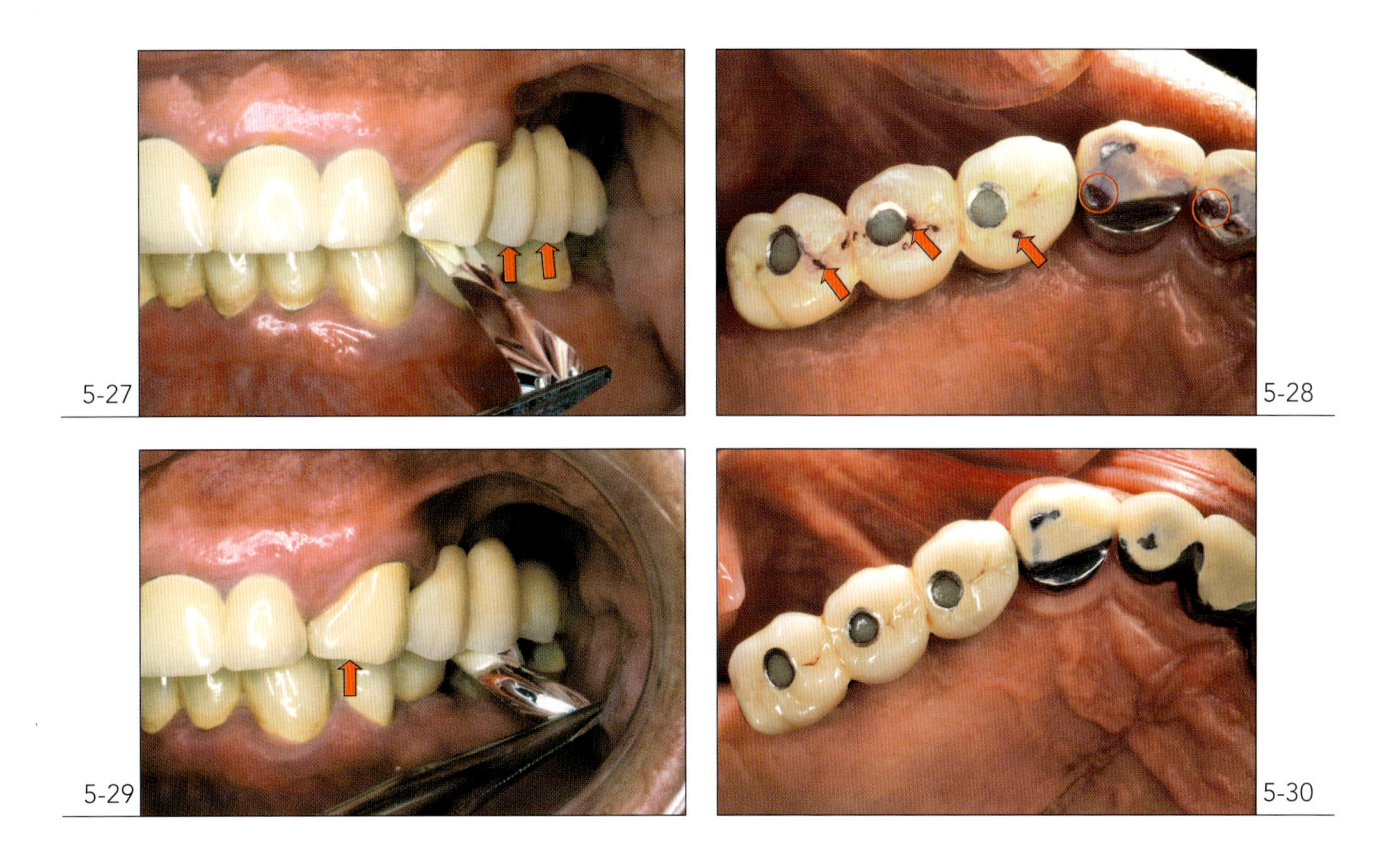

5-28

5-29

5-30

Long-Term Therapeutic Differential Loading

The process of therapeutic differential loading should be performed annually to accommodate for the ongoing intrusion of natural teeth relative to that of the adjacent implant-supported prostheses.[18] The rate of natural tooth intrusion has a mixed etiology, but an increased rate is found in patients who have habitual or nocturnal clenching. These severe cases can be identified by exaggerated crestal bone loss around implants. The author recommends a disocclusion night guard with anterior contact and 1 mm of posterior clearance.[21] In the author's opinion, the use of occlusal onlay night guards to decrease posterior implant loading is counterproductive and contraindicated.[21] The problem of natural tooth intrusion in such patients is inescapable; however, long-term prognosis is dramatically improved when these patientis are periodically observed and undergo therapeutic differential loading as needed.

Long-term supervision

Figure 5-37 shows the radiographic view upon loading. The 9-year postoperative radiograph shows minimal bone loss (Fig 5-38). During the observational period, bone loss around the natural canine anterior to the implant-supported prosthesis required extraction and replacement by an implant-supported restoration (see Fig 5-38). Figure 5-39 shows the radiographic view of the contralateral osseointegrated prosthesis upon loading; the 9-year postoperative radiograph also demonstrates minimal bone loss (Fig 5-40).

Summary

All physiologic processes are multileveled and biomechanically interactive. Their effect is cumulative and can result in implant overload. Therapeutic biomechanics[8] uses multiple corrective procedures to reduce implant loading. Previous mathematical data on clinical variables[7] suggested five possible corrective procedures to reduce torque and implant loading: *(1)* The head of the implant is placed as close as possible to the midline of the restoration. This may require implant inclination, which produces much less torque than horizontal implant offset.[7] *(2)* Wherever possible, cross occlusion is advocated posteriorly to reduce the horizontal implant offset.[8] *(3)* Angulated or custom-reangulated abutments provide parallelism and/or access. *(4)* Posterior cusp inclination produces maximum torque[7] and therefore should be substantially reduced. *(5)* Because of physiologic variability, a modified centric occlusal anatomy containing 1.5-mm horizontal fossae is recommended to maintain vertical resultant forces[14] within the range of physiologic variation (± 0.4 mm).[10–13]

Vertical overlap in the anterior maxilla produces a sharply inclined resultant line of force perpendicular to the impact surface. A lingual horizontal stop on the maxillary restoration (an *anterior* modified centric occlusion) redirects the resultant line of force in a vertical direction, much closer to the implant and supporting bone.[8] While it is not always possible to employ all therapeutic biomechanic corrective procedures clinically because of limitations of space, esthetics, and occlusal demands, maximum effectiveness is obtained in conjunction with a three-dimensional guidance system for implant insertion[16,17] (see chapter 6).

When tooth-supported and implant-supported prostheses are in the same arch, therapeutic differential loading can be introduced. The technique of differential occlusal adjustment prevents overloading of the implant-supported prosthesis caused by the differences in force distribution between the stiff osseointegrated interface and the flexion of the periodontal ligament. Long-term postoperative radiographs reveal minimum bone loss in response to the remedial therapeutic biomechanic procedures described.

Acknowledgments

Portions of this chapter were reprinted from articles appearing in the *Journal of Oral Implantology* by Weinberg[22,23] with permission from Alliance Communications Group and adapted from an article appearing in *Implant Dentistry* by Weinberg[8] with permission from Lippincott Williams & Wilkins.

5-37

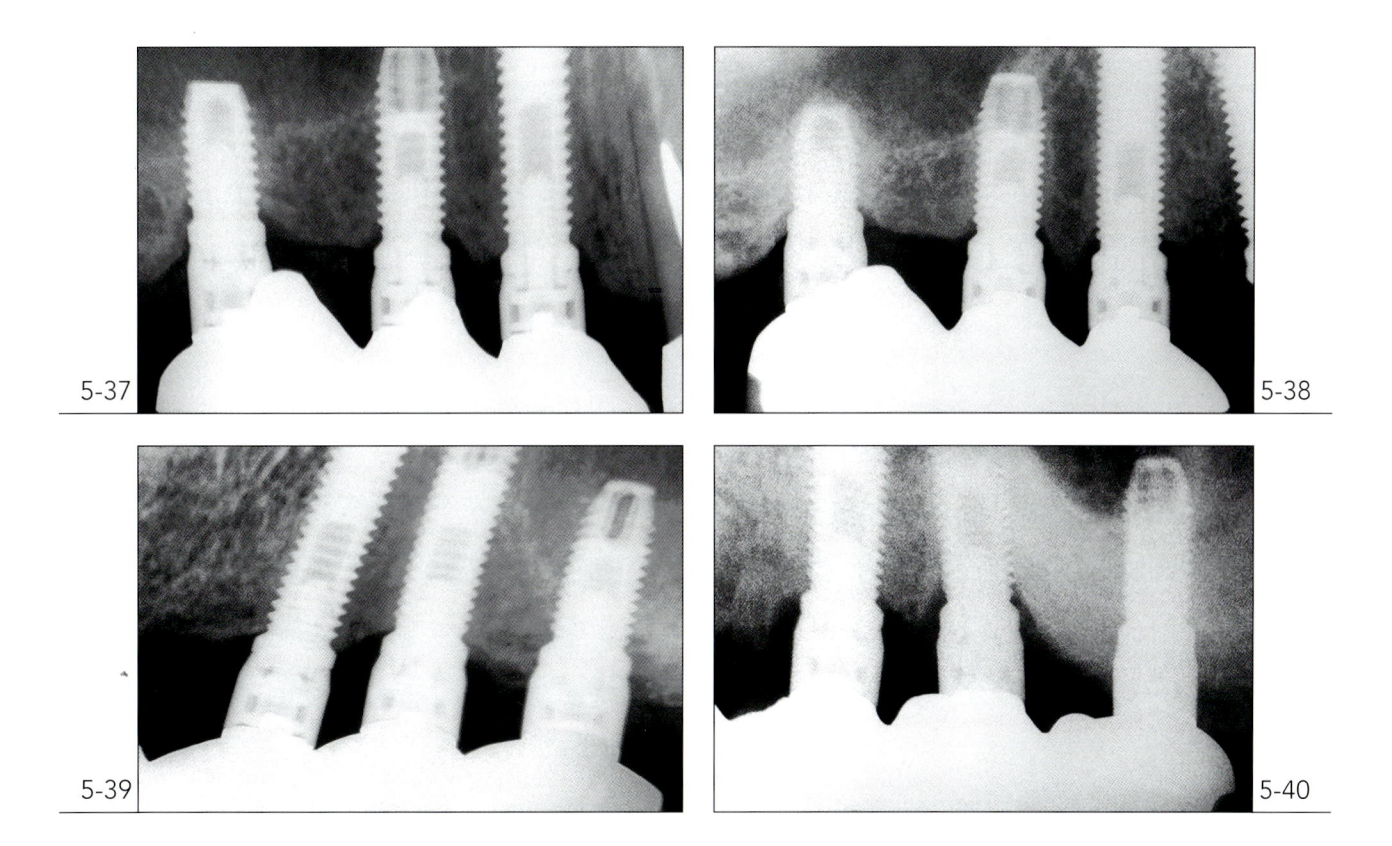

5-38

5-39

5-40

References

1. Lundeen D, Laurell L. Occlusal forces in prosthetically restored dentitions: A methodological study. J Oral Rehabil 1984;11:29–37.
2. Weinberg LA. Axial inclination and cuspal articulation in relation to force distribution. J Prosthet Dent 1957;7:804–813.
3. Weinberg LA. Biomechanics of force distribution in implant-supported prostheses. Int J Oral Maxillofac Implants 1993;8:19–31.
4. Weinberg LA, Kruger B. Biomechanical considerations when combining tooth-supported and implant-supported prostheses. Oral Surg Oral Med Oral Pathol 1994;78:22–27.
5. Smith DC. Dental implants: Materials and design considerations. Int J Prosthodont 1993;6:106–117.
6. Misch CE. Contemporary Implant Dentistry. St Louis: Mosby, 1993:281–282.
7. Weinberg LA, Kruger B. A comparison of implant/prosthesis loading with four clinical variables. Int J Prosthodont 1995;8:421–433.
8. Weinberg LA. Reduction of implant loading with therapeutic biomechanics. Implant Dent 1998;7:277–285.
9. Clelland NL, Ismail YH, Zaki HS, Pipko D. Three-dimensional finite element stress analysis in and around the Screw-Vent implant. Int J Oral Maxillofac Implants 1991;6:391–398.
10. Grasso J, Sharry J. The duplicability of arrow-point tracing in dentulous subjects. J Prosthet Dent 1968;20:106–115.
11. Kantor M, Silverman S, Garfinkel L. Centric relation recording techniques: A comparative investigation. J Prosthet Dent 1972;28:593–600.
12. Calagna L, Silverman S, Garfinkel L. Influence of neuromuscular conditioning on centric relation registrations. J Prosthet Dent 1973;30:598–604.
13. Celenza FV. The centric position: Replacement and character. J Prosthet Dent 1973;30:591–598.
14. Weinberg LA. Reduction of implant loading using a modified centric occlusal anatomy. Int J Prosthodont 1998;11:55–69.

15. Mann A, Pankey K. Oral rehabilitation. II. Reconstruction of the upper teeth using functionally generated path technique. J Prosthet Dent 1960;10:151–162.
16. Weinberg LA, Kruger B. Three-dimensional guidance system for implant insertion: Part I. Implant Dent 1998;7:81–91.
17. Weinberg LA, Kruger B. Three-dimensional guidance system for implant insertion: Part II. Dual axes table. Problem solving. Implant Dent 1999;8:225–264.
18. Ericsson I, Lekholm U, Brånemark P-I, Lindhe J, Glantz P-O, Nyman S. A clinical evaluation of fixed bridge restorations supported by the combination of teeth and osseointegrated titanium implants. J Clin Periodontol 1986;13:307–312.
19. Schuyler CH. Correction of occlusal disharmony of the natural dentition. N Y State Dent J 1947;13:445–462.
20. Weinberg LA. Rationale and technique for occlusal equilibration. J Prosthet Dent 1964;14:74–86.
21. Weinberg LA. Vertical dimension: A research and clinical analysis. J Prosthet Dent 1982;47:290–302.
22. Weinberg LA. Therapeutic biomechanics concepts and clinical procedures to reduce implant loading. Part I. J Oral Implantol 2001;27:293–301.
23. Weinberg LA. Therapeutic biomechanics concepts and clinical procedures to reduce implant loading. Part II: Therapeutic differential loading. J Oral Implantol 2001;27:302–310.

6 Three-dimensional Guidance System for Implant Placement

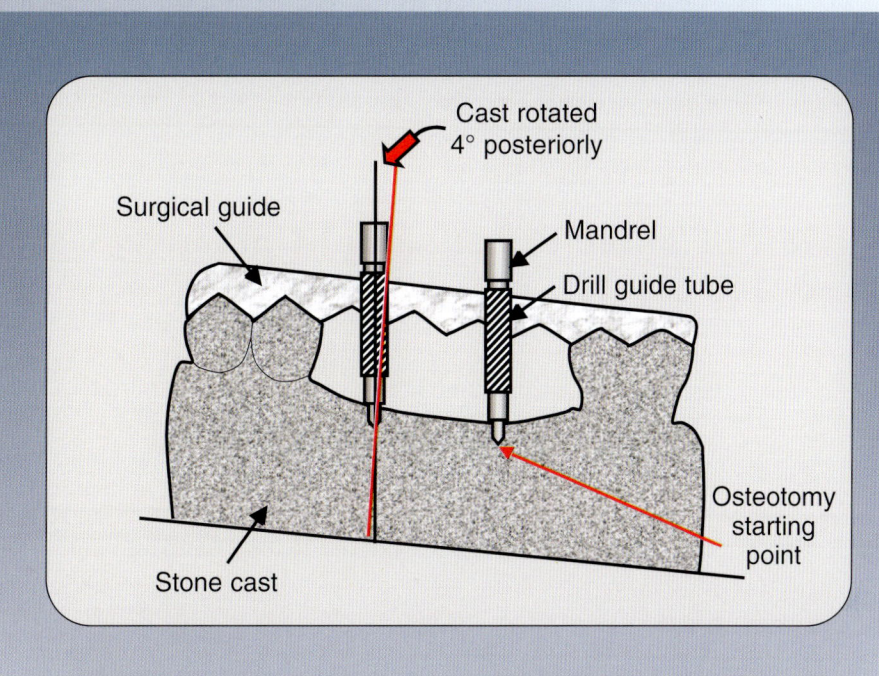

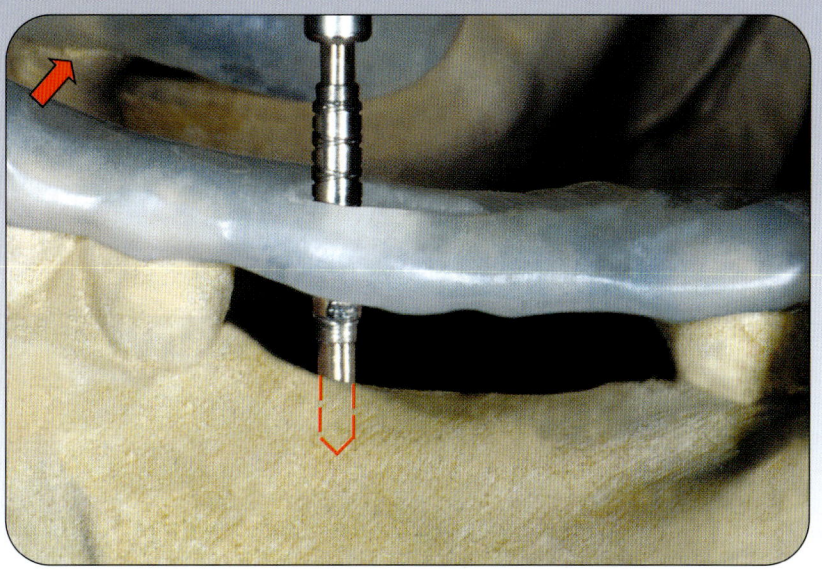

Despite the availability of radiographic guides for outlining the occlusion,[1] there currently is no procedure for planning optimal implant orientation correlated with a three-dimensional surgical guide. In the end, the surgery remains based on clinical judgment and the three-dimensional perception of the clinician.

In a standard surgical guide procedure, a setup is completed on the study cast (Fig 6-1). A surgical guide containing a long mesiodistal occlusal slot, which delineates the buccolingual parameters for implant placement, is constructed (Fig 6-2). The surgical procedures are accomplished with the surgical guide in position to help establish the orientation of the osteotomy (Fig 6-3). However, there are no mesiodistal guidelines other than clinical judgment. Therefore, in order to create a margin of safety and avoid the distal curvature of the maxillary canine, the first premolar implant is placed too far distally (Fig 6-4, *arrows*). In turn, the distal placement of the first premolar implant requires that the second premolar be displaced distally to provide sufficient bone between them. Implants that are not centrally located can cause unwanted esthetic and hygiene problems.

Overview of Three-dimensional Guidance System Procedure

A three-dimensional guidance system for implant placement is advantageous not only because it maximizes the use of compact bone and avoids anatomic hazards, but also because it places the implant in the optimum position and orientation to decrease implant loading[2] through the use of computerized tomography (CT) scans and surgical guides.[1,3–7] For this procedure, a radiographic guide is constructed with a radiopaque vertical orientation pin in the center of each restoration. This identifies the exact location of the planned implant site in the cross-sectional and panoramic reformatted CT images. Polaroid or 35-mm prints reproduce these images of each implant site. The true vertical orientation pin images facilitate the graphic planning and measurement of the specific angulation of the implant in each cross-sectional and panoramic image. The angulations for each implant are then transferred to a surgical guide with a special dual-axis table developed for this purpose. Surgical drill guide tubes are positioned in the surgical guide to reproduce the exact starting point and planned three-dimensional orientation for each implant. Pilot osteotomies are prepared with the three-dimensional guidance of the surgical guide. Special instruments have been developed to control the exact depth and tracking of the full-length osteotomies.

Necessity of CT Scan

The cross-sectional reformatted images shown in Fig 6-5 illustrate the profound differences in residual alveolar bone every 3 mm. The shape of the residual alveolar bone varies, as does the specific location of compact bone. Unless radiographic guides are constructed with radiopaque markers placed in the center of the planned restoration, the selection of a specific cross-sectional image that represents the implant location must be determined by clinical judgment. Mistakes do happen; Fig 6-6 illustrates an implant that was erroneously placed into the mandibular canal (*arrows*), causing total lifelong paresthesia.

Necessity of CT Scan

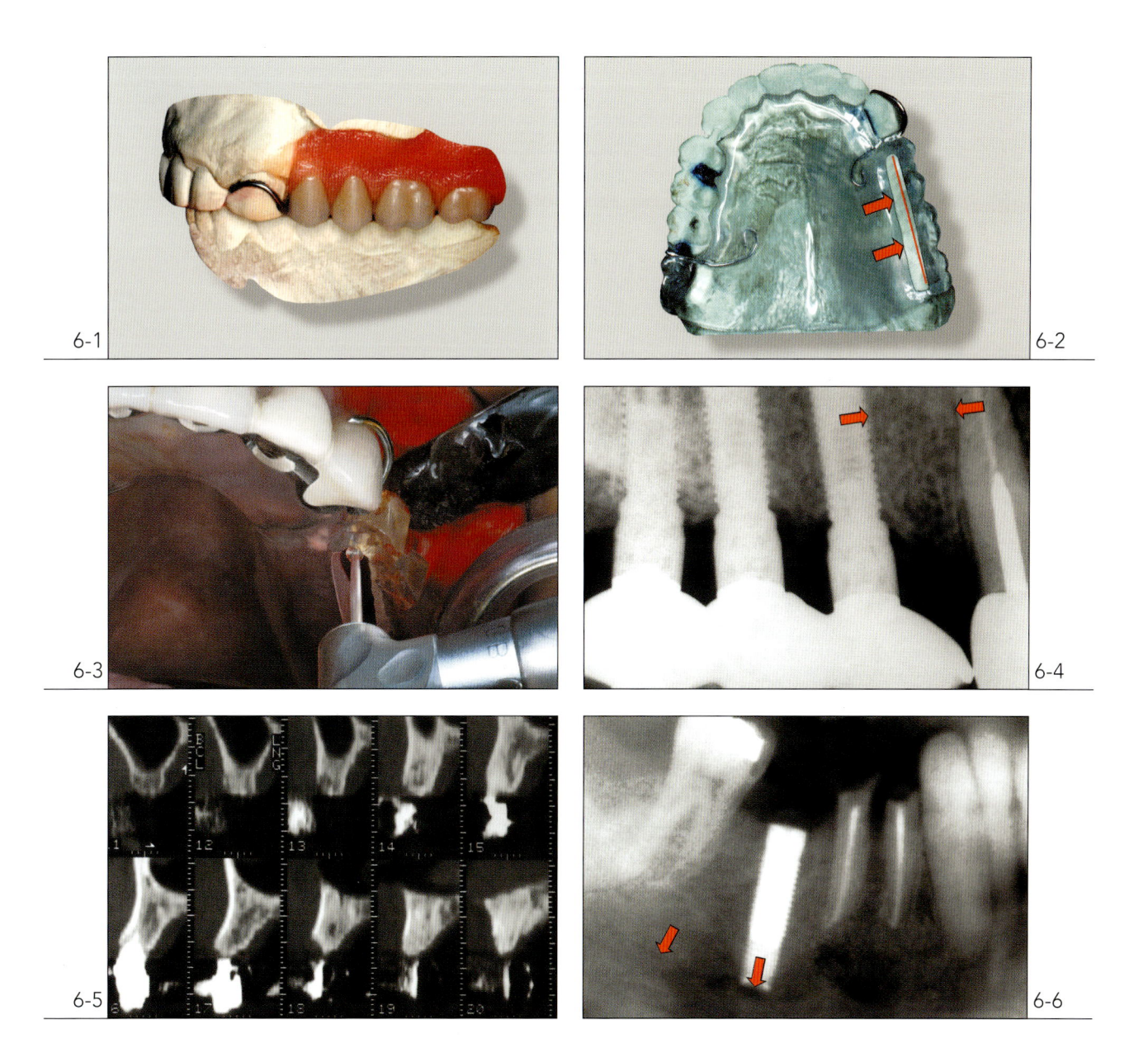

6-1

6-2

6-3

6-4

6-5

6-6

87

Radiographic Guide

The prosthetic teeth (*arrows*) are set up on mounted study casts (Fig 6-7), and an acrylic onlay radiographic guide is constructed over them. Occlusal indications are created in the radiographic guide by closing the casts while the acrylic is still soft. The occlusal imprint (Fig 6-8, *arrows*) will help ensure proper seating during the CT scan procedure. The bottom of the cast is then trimmed until the occlusal plane is parallel with the horizontal plane (Fig 6-9, *arrows*).

Vertical Orientation Pins

The restorative possibilities are at the crest of the residual alveolar ridge or buccal or lingual to it (Fig 6-10). Regardless of the location of the restoration, a vertical orientation pin is always placed at the crest of the ridge and in contact with the stone cast (Fig 6-11). To accomplish this, an access hole is made in the acrylic onlay for each implant location. (It is important to note that the occlusal plane is automatically oriented parallel to the horizontal plane when the cast is placed on the base of the drill press; see Fig 6-9.) The vertical orientation pin is placed on a mandrel held by the drill press chuck and lowered to touch the stone cast (*arrows*) while positioned in the center of the restoration (Fig 6-12). The orientation pin is then fixed to the radiographic guide with auto-curing acrylic, and the process is repeated for each restoration. This establishes the true vertical plane of reference on the crest of the ridge at the center of each restoration in all the CT scan images.

CT Scan

To limit distortion when obtaining the CT scan, it is important to have the occlusal plane perpendicular to the horizontal plane bilaterally (Fig 6-13).[8] Correct orientation of the patient's head can be accomplished with the aid of tongue blades held between the teeth on both sides. Before the CT scan is initiated, the tongue blades are removed and the proper seating and stabilization of the radiographic guide are confirmed. A scout image helps the technician ensure that the entire radiographic guide is included in the scan (Fig 6-14).

Transaxial scan image

Depending on the software and the intended coverage of the CT scan, 35 to 40 transaxial scans are obtained (see Fig 6-14). The transaxial scan that provides the maximum information on the location of the planned implant sites and on the residual alveolar bone and its topography is selected. The transaxial scan image is viewed from below, with each cross-sectional plane numbered (Fig 6-15). The solid block of information recorded in the CT scan software can be reformatted into panoramic and cross-sectional images.[8]

CT Scan

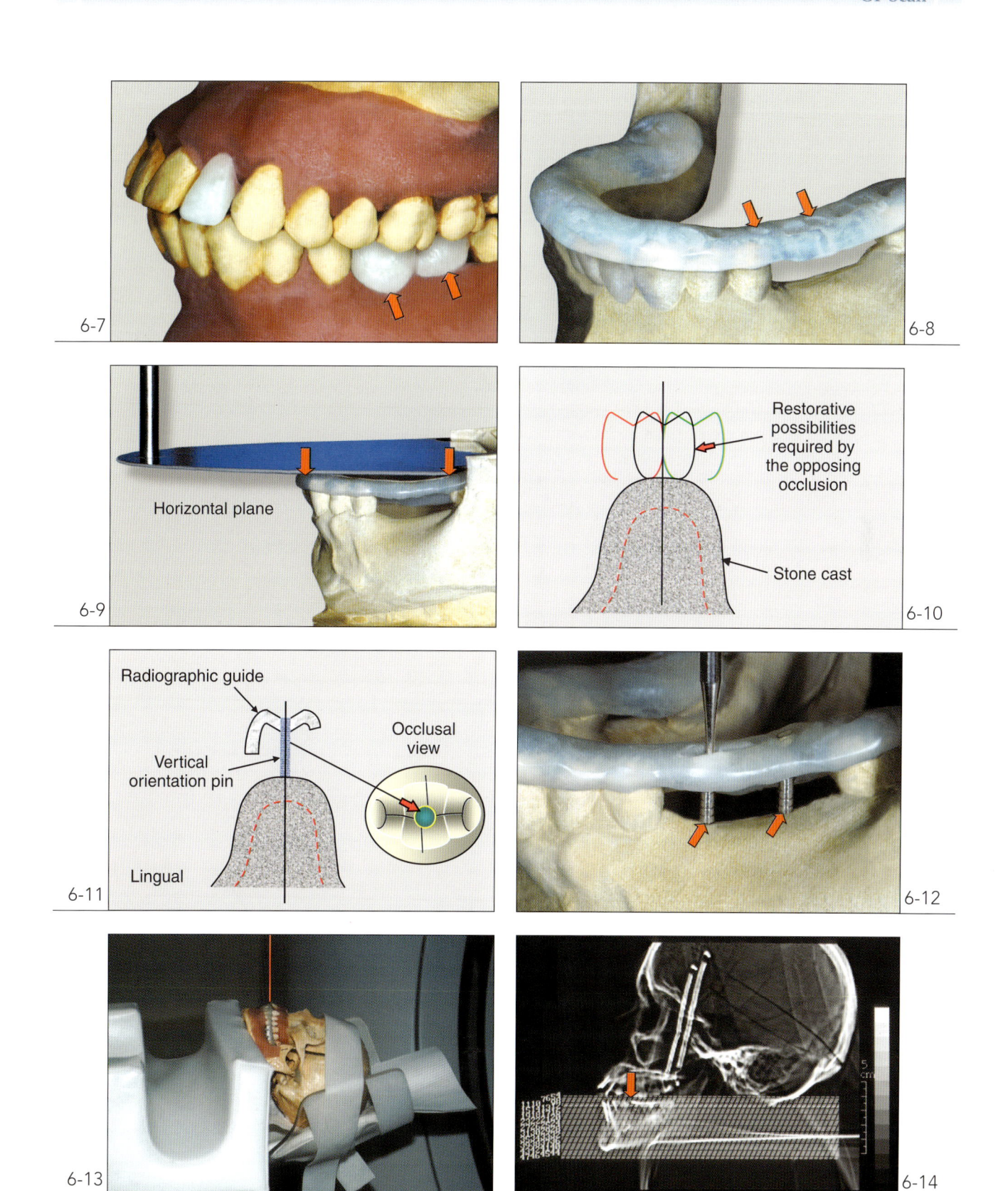

6-7

6-8

6-9 Horizontal plane

6-10 Restorative possibilities required by the opposing occlusion — Stone cast

6-11 Radiographic guide — Vertical orientation pin — Occlusal view — Lingual

6-12

6-13

6-14

89

Panoramic reformatted image

Most software programs provide three or more panoramic views: One follows the center of the mandible, and the others are buccal and lingual to it. These are reformatted into panoramic images, one of which will provide the maximum information (Fig 6-16, *bottom*). Note the vertical orientation pins (*arrow*) and the image of the radiographic guide.

Cross-sectional image

The cross-sectional drawing in Fig 6-17 illustrates the relationship of the radiographic guide, vertical orientation pin, residual bone, and soft tissue. A cross-sectional image through the left first molar area of the skull is shown in Fig 6-18. (It is important to note that with this software, the cross-sectional images are viewed from the anterior toward the posterior, so that the lingual of the left side of the mandible will be in the left corner; the reverse is true for the right side. With other software, the buccal always will appear on the lower left side, regardless of the orientation of the cross section.) The distance from the bottom of the vertical orientation pin to the residual alveolar bone represents the thickness of the gingiva (see Fig 6-18, *arrows*). The first molar area of the body of the mandible usually has a lingual inclination.

Diagnostic planning

Cross-sectional image

Figure 6-19 is an illustration of a Polaroid reproduction of the cross-sectional image shown in Fig 6-18. A line is drawn through the center of the vertical orientation pin and the residual alveolar bone. Where that line crosses the crest of the alveolar bone marks the internal starting point of the osteotomy. Based on this point, the optimum implant orientation is drawn through the residual alveolar bone. The angle between the two lines is measured and found to be 16 degrees; this represents the planned lingual inclination of the implant. The gingival thickness is the difference between the bottom of the vertical orientation pin and the crest of the alveolar bone (this measurement will be required when constructing the surgical guide). Figure 6-20 is a Polaroid reproduction of the cross-sectional image (see Fig 6-18) with the previously described planning (see Fig 6-19).

Panoramic image

Figure 6-21 is an illustration of a Polaroid reproduction of the panoramic image shown in Fig 6-16. Vertical lines are drawn in the center of the vertical orientation pins through the alveolar bone. A vertical line also is drawn parallel to the vertical orientation lines through the apex of the root of the adjacent premolar. Another line (Fig 6-21, *red*) is drawn through the center of the premolar itself, passing through the apex of the root to the center of the cusp height. The angle between this line and the vertical lines is found to be 4 degrees; this represents the mesial inclination of the implant required to ensure that the implant is parallel to the root and to avoid root perforation. Figure 6-22 is a Polaroid reproduction of the panoramic image (see Fig 6-16) with the previously described planning (see Fig 6-21).

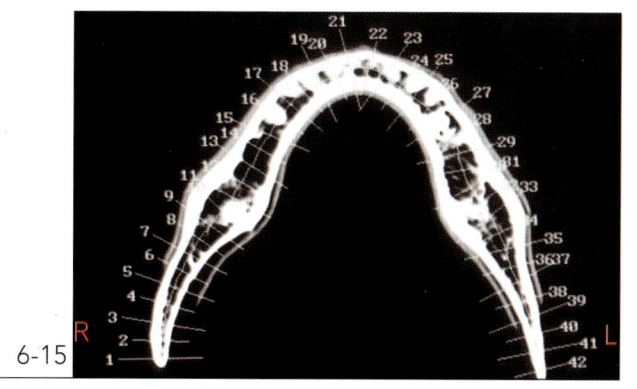

CT Scan

6-15

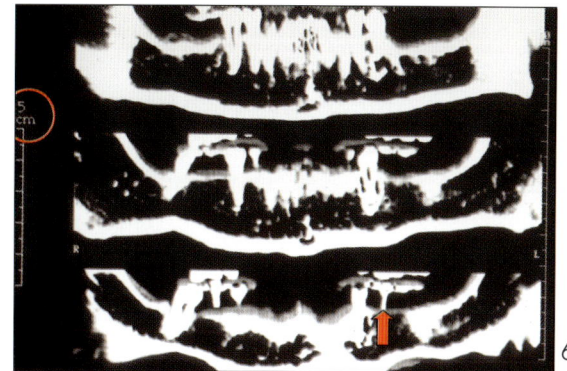

6-16

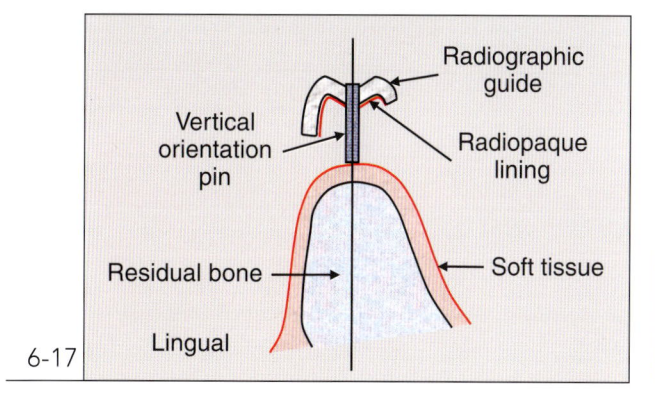

Radiographic guide
Vertical orientation pin
Radiopaque lining
Residual bone
Soft tissue
Lingual

6-17

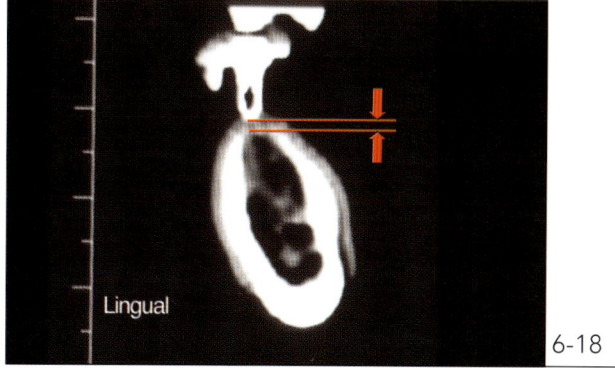

Lingual

6-18

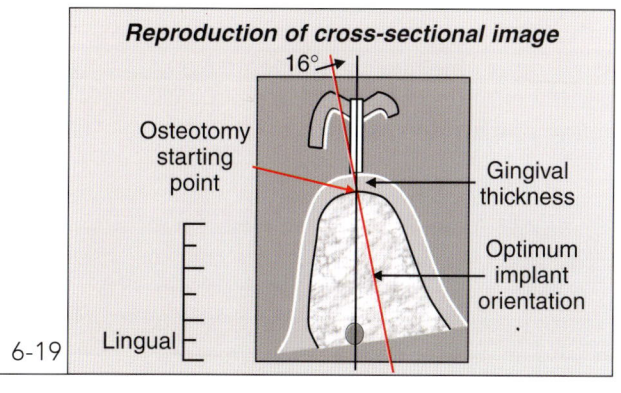

Reproduction of cross-sectional image
16°
Osteotomy starting point
Gingival thickness
Optimum implant orientation
Lingual

6-19

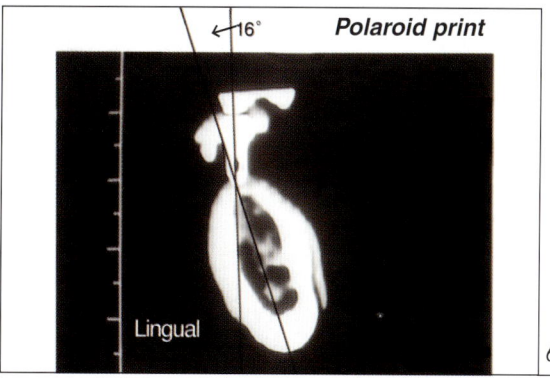

Polaroid print
16°
Lingual

6-20

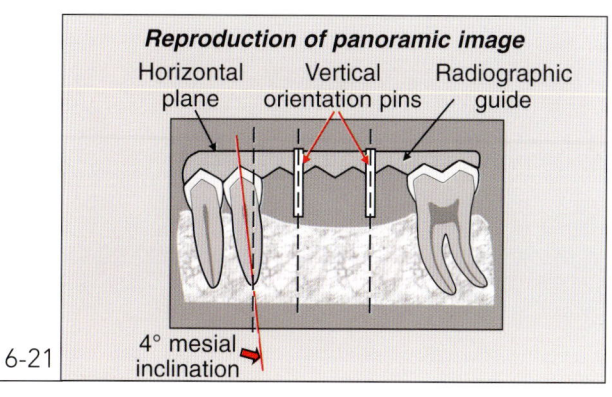

Reproduction of panoramic image
Horizontal plane
Vertical orientation pins
Radiographic guide
4° mesial inclination

6-21

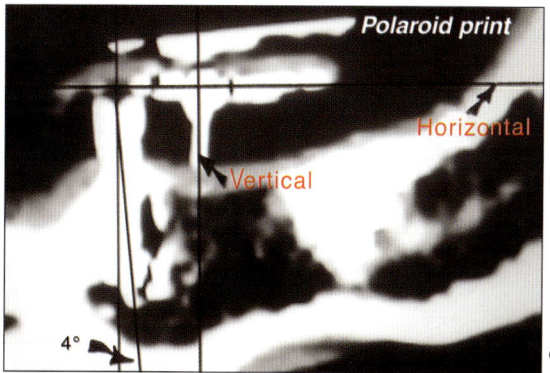

Polaroid print
Horizontal
Vertical
4°

6-22

91

6 Three-dimensional Guidance System for Implant Placement

Construction of the Surgical Guide

Transfer of internal starting point

The stone cast is placed on the drill press table (Fig 6-23), automatically positioning the radiographic guide in the horizontal plane (see Fig 6-9). The cast is moved until the mandrel can be placed into the vertical orientation pin (*arrow*), which marks the implant position on the cast (Fig 6-24). The cast is fixed to the base and the radiographic guide removed. The thickness of the gingiva (the distance between the bottom of the vertical orientation pin and the top of the alveolar bone) is obtained by caliper. This measurement must be related to the scale on the edge of the cross-sectional images (Fig 6-25), which is used to interpolate the actual gingival thickness. This procedure is necessary because there is a slight distortion factor that precludes direct measurement on any reformatted image.[8] A #701 bur in the drill press is lowered into the stone at this gingival distance to establish the internal osteotomy starting point (Fig 6-26).

Transfer of implant orientation to the cast

Once the internal starting position of the osteotomy is obtained, all that remains to be transferred to the cast are the mesiodistal and buccolingual implant inclinations. According to earlier calculations, the left first molar implant should be inclined 4 degrees mesially (see Fig 6-22) and 16 degrees lingually (see Fig 6-20). Since the upper member of the drill press can move only in the vertical plane, the cast always must be rotated in the *opposite direction* to that of the planned implant inclination. For instance, a 4-degree anterior implant inclination is obtained by a 4-degree *posterior* rotation of the stone cast (Fig 6-27). Similarly, a 16-degree *lingual* implant inclination is obtained by a 16-degree *buccal* rotation of the stone cast (Fig 6-28).

Dual-axis table

The dual-axis table was developed by Dr B. Kruger (manufactured by High Point Precision, Sussex, NJ) to provide mesiodistal and buccolingual rotation of the cast so that these inclinations can be transferred to the surgical guide. To provide this three-dimensional movement, the base has two axes of rotation that are perpendicular to each other (Fig 6-29). The axes are calibrated, and an axis-locking mechanism is provided for each on the opposite side (Fig 6-30).

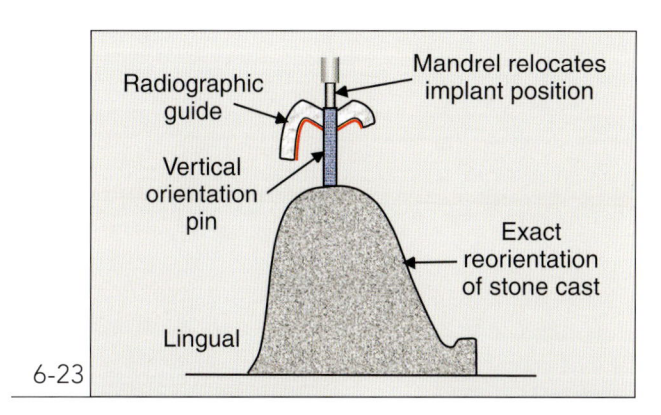

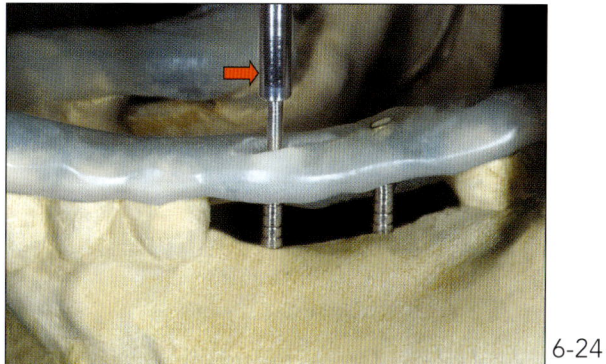

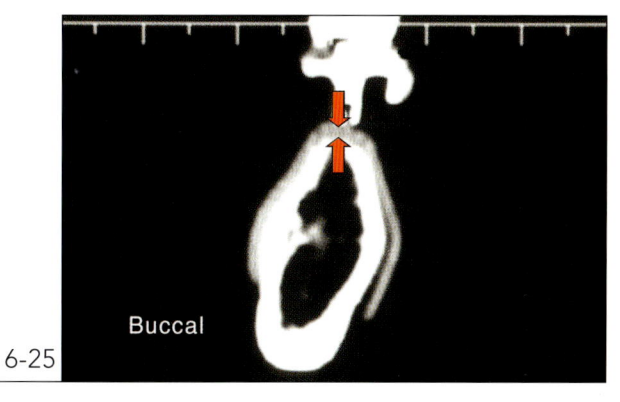

Construction of the Surgical Guide

6-23 Radiographic guide / Mandrel relocates implant position / Vertical orientation pin / Exact reorientation of stone cast / Lingual

6-24

6-25 Buccal

6-26 Osteotomy starting point / #701 in drill press to gingival depth / Stone cast / Lingual

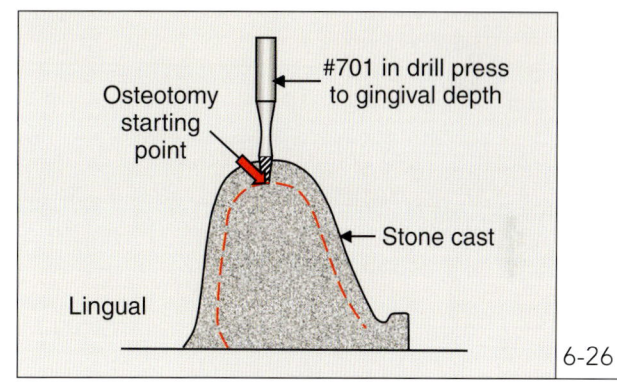

6-27 Cast rotated 4° posteriorly / Stone cast

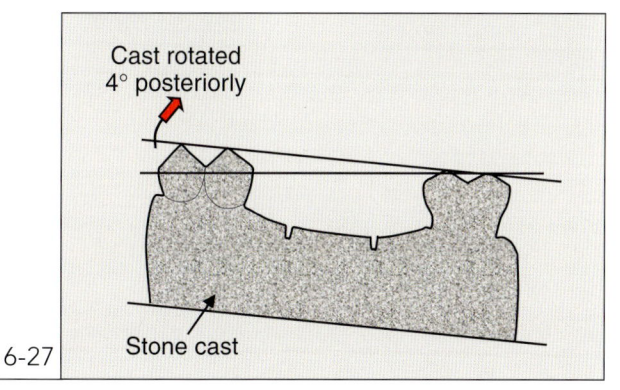

6-28 Cast rotated 16° buccally / Stone cast / Lingual

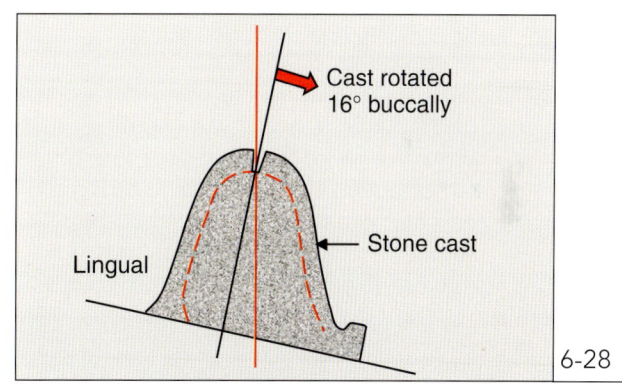

6-29 **Dual-axis base** / Buccolingual axis of rotation / Mesiodistal axis of rotation

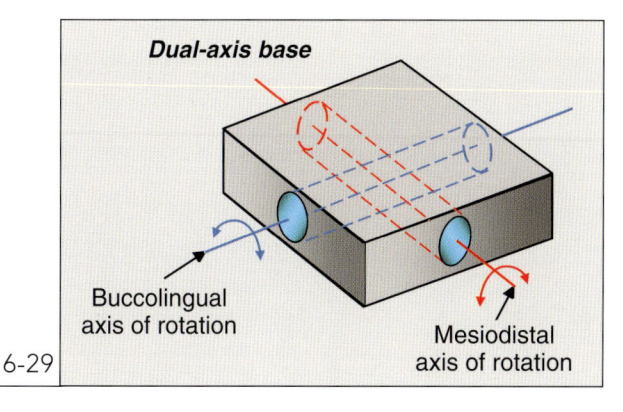

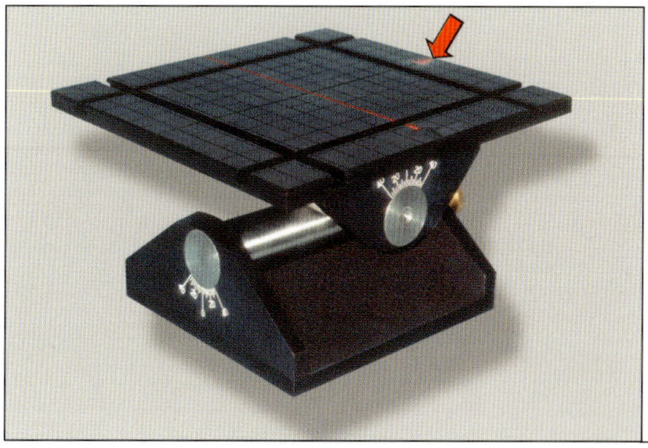

6-30

93

Cast orientation

The anterior orientation of the cast on the base is indicated by an arrow on the buccolingual axis orientation line (Fig 6-31; see Fig 6-30, *arrow*). Each implant has a buccolingual center line (Fig 6-32, *left*) that represents its cross-sectional plane; the numbered lines on the transaxial scan image represent the same cross-sectional planes (see Fig 6-15). Each implant also has an individual buccolingual and mesiodistal inclination, which must be transferred to the cast (Fig 6-32, *right*) and subsequently to the surgical guide.

To allow visualization of this process, the buccolingual center line of an implant at the right canine has been marked on the cast shown in Fig 6-33 (*arrow*). If each implant site was similarly marked and the cast was placed on the dual-axis table facing the anterior orientation arrow, none of the buccolingual center lines would align with either axis of the table (Fig 6-34). Instead, the cast must be rotated so that the buccolingual center line of each implant is placed over and parallel to the buccolingual axis of the dual-axis table (Fig 6-35). Figure 6-36 illustrates the counterclockwise rotation of the cast on the base to align the buccolingual center line of a canine implant with the buccolingual axis of the base. (For simplicity, the cast-locking mechanism has been omitted from the illustration.)

It should be emphasized that only in this position, for this one implant, do the three-dimensional relationships on the dual-axis base correspond to those shown in the reformatted cross-sectional and panoramic images of the CT scan. The cast must be manually reoriented for each implant; this is equivalent to what the CT software does in milliseconds to produce the reformatted cross-sectional and panoramic images. In other words, the dual-axis table transfers the information in the reformatted cross-sectional and panoramic images of the CT scan to reproduce the same three-dimensional relationships on the cast.

As previously discussed, in order to provide lingual implant inclination, the cast must be rotated in the opposite (ie, buccal) direction (Fig 6-37). The buccal incline of the table is adjusted, and the cast-locking mechanism tightened. Likewise, to provide mesial implant inclination, the table must be rotated in the opposite (ie, distal) direction (Fig 6-38). Since the dual-axis table, by definition, allows rotation in one axis without affecting the other axis, it makes no difference which inclination is set first. However, this is true only if the cast is oriented correctly (see Fig 6-36) and remains fixed in that position throughout the entire process for each implant.

Construction of the Surgical Guide

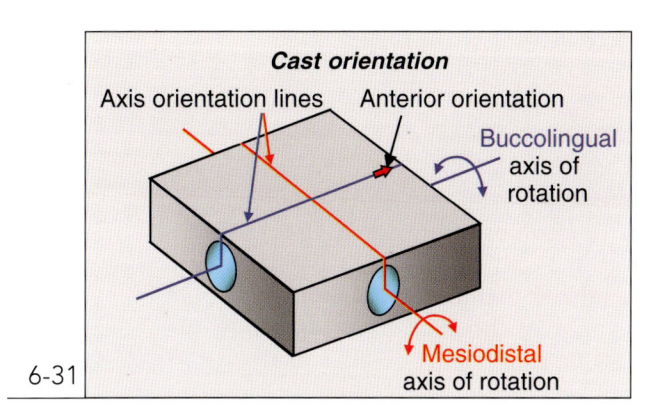

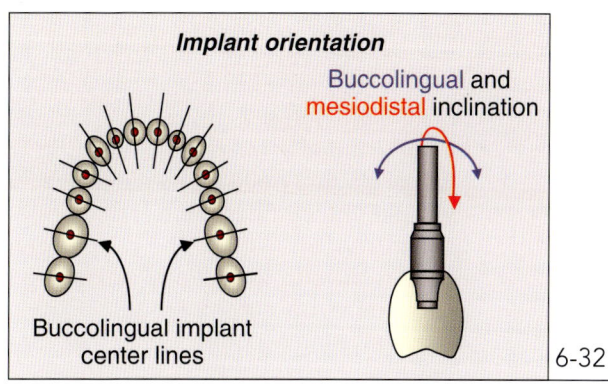

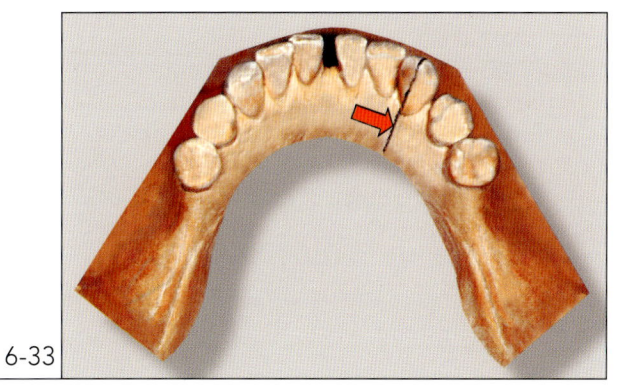

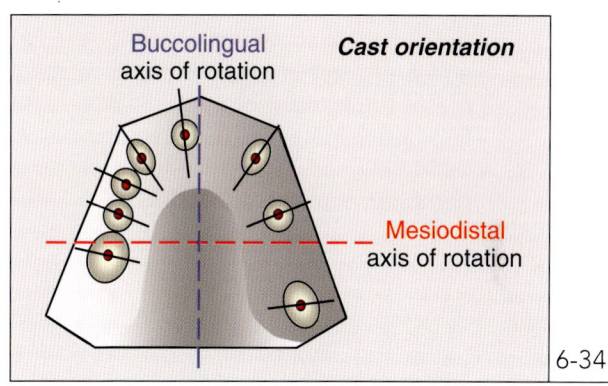

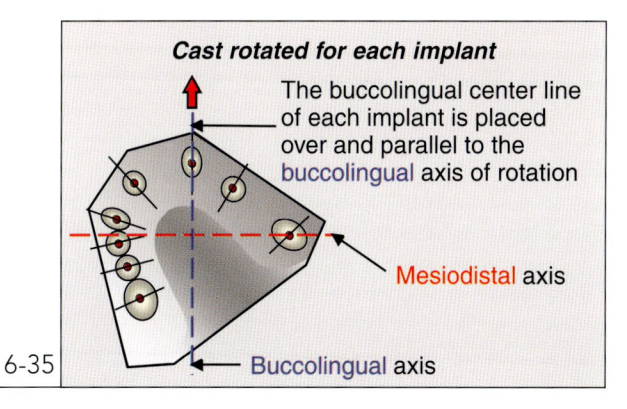

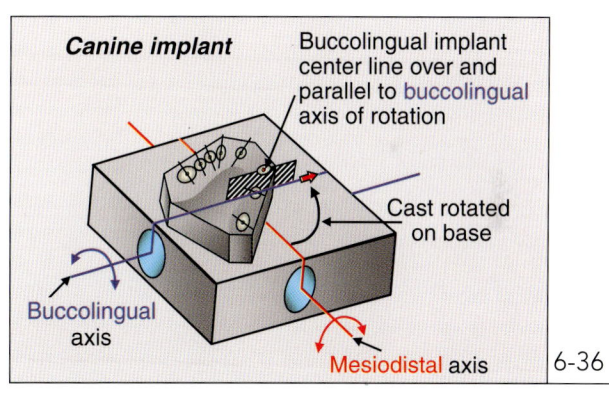

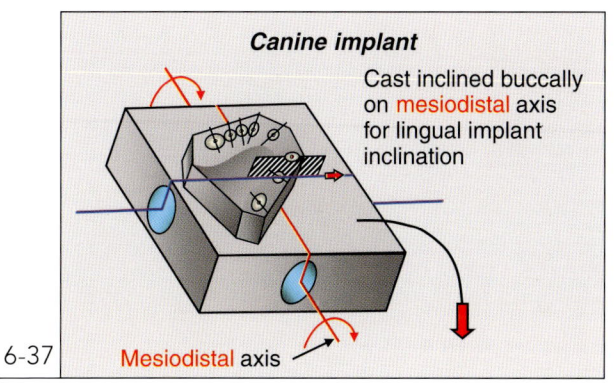

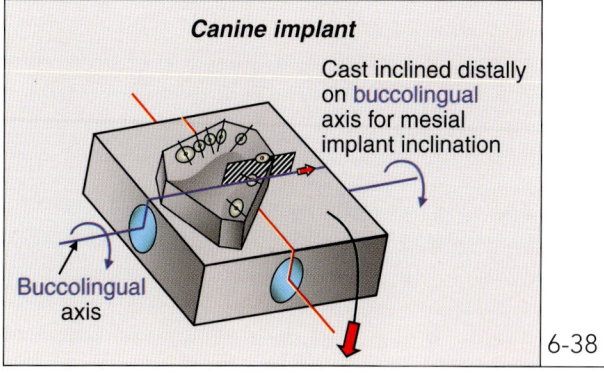

6-31 *Cast orientation* — Axis orientation lines, Anterior orientation, Buccolingual axis of rotation, Mesiodistal axis of rotation

6-32 *Implant orientation* — Buccolingual implant center lines, Buccolingual and mesiodistal inclination

6-33

6-34 *Cast orientation* — Buccolingual axis of rotation, Mesiodistal axis of rotation

6-35 *Cast rotated for each implant* — The buccolingual center line of each implant is placed over and parallel to the buccolingual axis of rotation. Mesiodistal axis, Buccolingual axis

6-36 *Canine implant* — Buccolingual implant center line over and parallel to buccolingual axis of rotation. Cast rotated on base. Buccolingual axis, Mesiodistal axis

6-37 *Canine implant* — Cast inclined buccally on mesiodistal axis for lingual implant inclination. Mesiodistal axis

6-38 *Canine implant* — Cast inclined distally on buccolingual axis for mesial implant inclination. Buccolingual axis

Transfer of implant orientation to the surgical guide

An oversized hole is made in the surgical guide corresponding to each implant location (Fig 6-39). A drill guide tube is fitted with a removable pointer (Fig 6-40) and held by the mandrel in the drill press chuck. The pointer is then placed into the osteotomy internal starting point (Fig 6-41), which was previously prepared (see Fig 6-26). In our example, the cast has been rotated buccally 16 degrees to provide a 16-degree lingual implant inclination. The buccal rotation of the cast creates lingual implant inclination relative to the surgical guide (Fig 6-42). (Note that rotation of the cast *in both planes* must be accomplished before placement of the drill guide tube into the osteotomy starting point. Either axis can be set first.)

In this case, the cast is then rotated 4 degrees posteriorly to provide 4-degree anterior (mesial) implant inclination (Fig 6-43). The mandrel positions the drill guide tube as the pointer is placed into the osteotomy internal starting point (see Fig 6-43 and 6-44, *red outline*). Fixation of the drill guide tube to the surgical guide completes the transfer of the implant orientation to the cast (see Fig 6-44). The planned lingual inclination of each implant is shown in Fig 6-45. Although the process is extremely accurate, it is nevertheless essential to have a clinical try-in to confirm complete seating of the surgical guide before surgery is scheduled (Fig 6-46).

Construction of the Surgical Guide

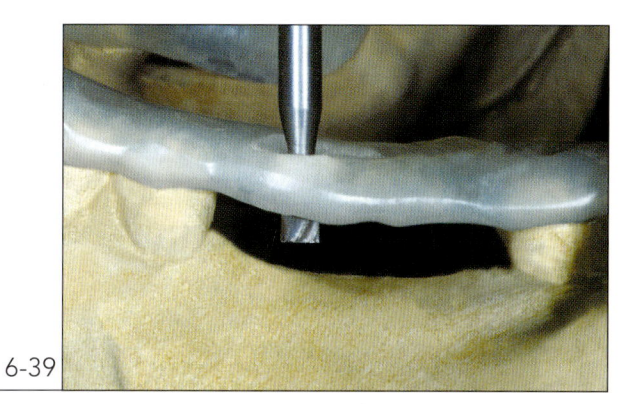

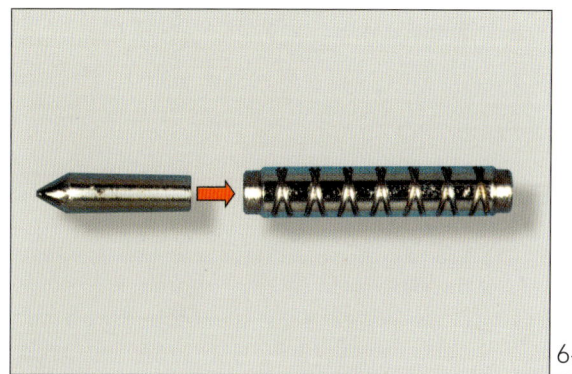

6-39

6-40

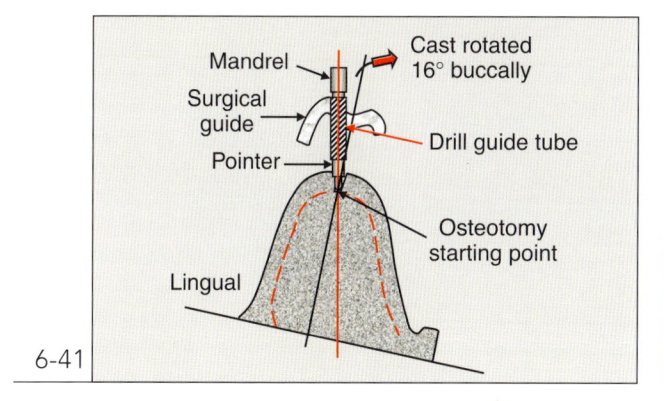

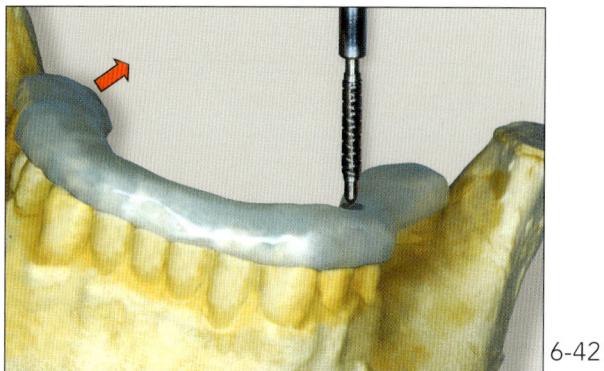

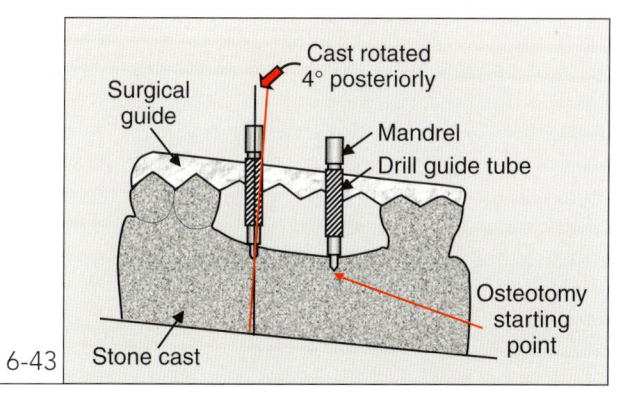

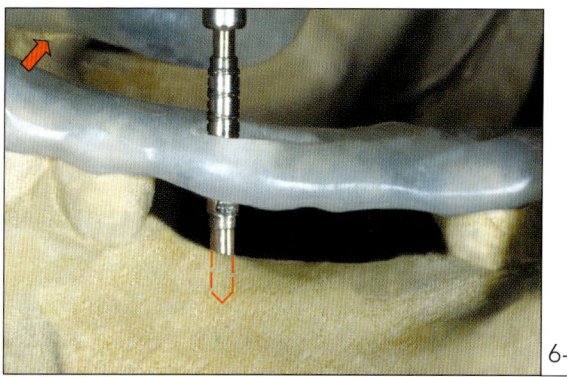

6-41

6-42

6-43

6-44

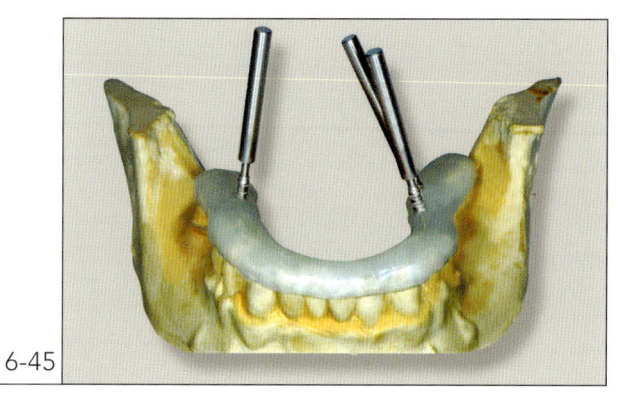

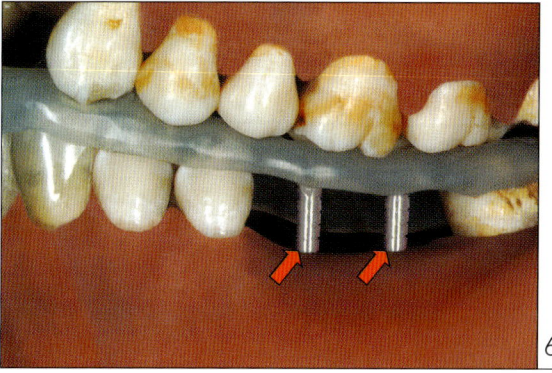

6-45

6-46

97

Surgical Procedure

Pilot osteotomy

The surgical procedure starts with a 5-mm pilot osteotomy that is prepared with the help of the surgical guide. The gingiva is retracted and the surgical guide reseated. A 1.6-mm pilot drill initiates a 5-mm preparation in alveolar bone with the guidance of the drill guide tube (Figs 6-47 and 6-48). A 1.6-mm end-cutting drill also is guided by the drill guide tube to create parallel walls in the 5-mm pilot osteotomy (Figs 6-49 and 6-50). All the pilot osteotomies are completed (with the aid of the surgical guide) before the full-length osteotomy procedure is initiated.

Full-length osteotomy

The parallel walls of the pilot osteotomy (Fig 6-51, *left*) provide guidance for extending the osteotomy to full length. In extending the osteotomy, it is important to use an end cutter that has the same diameter as the drill used to make the pilot osteotomy. This will maintain the tracking, or orientation, of the pilot osteotomy (Fig 6-51, *right*). To control the length of the osteotomy, the drill (Posi-Stop; High Point Precision) has an adjustable stop that can be set in increments of 1 mm (Fig 6-52). The instruments are color coded to facilitate efficient clinical technique.

Widening the osteotomy

During widening procedures, the walls of the pilot osteotomy must remain intact to preserve the tracking of the full-length osteotomy. For this purpose, a special tracking drill (Pilot Extension Drill; High Point Precision) has been designed with a 3-mm-long noncutting pilot extension that is attached to the 0.5-mm-wider cutting portion of the drill (Fig 6-53). The pilot extension is placed in the osteotomy to establish the correct tracking, and then the wider cutting portion widens the osteotomy as the drill advances to the full length of the osteotomy. These color-coded instruments are provided in 0.5-mm-diameter increments beginning with a 2.0-mm cutting diameter (Fig 6-54).

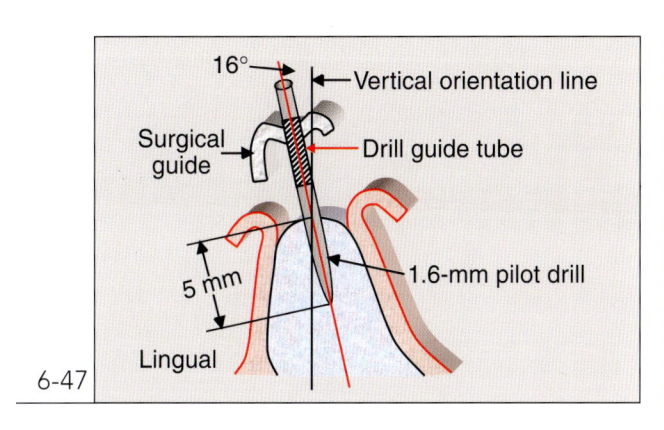

Surgical Procedure

6-47

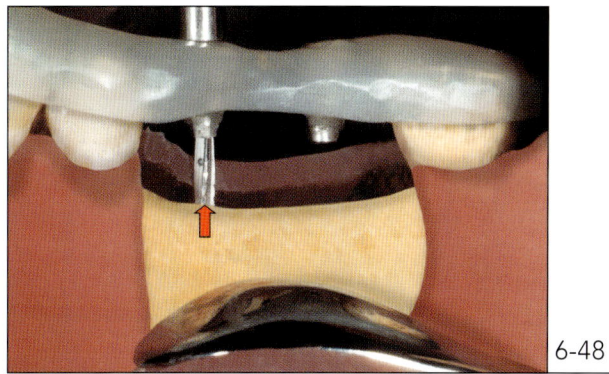

- 16°
- Vertical orientation line
- Surgical guide
- Drill guide tube
- 5 mm
- 1.6-mm pilot drill
- Lingual

6-48

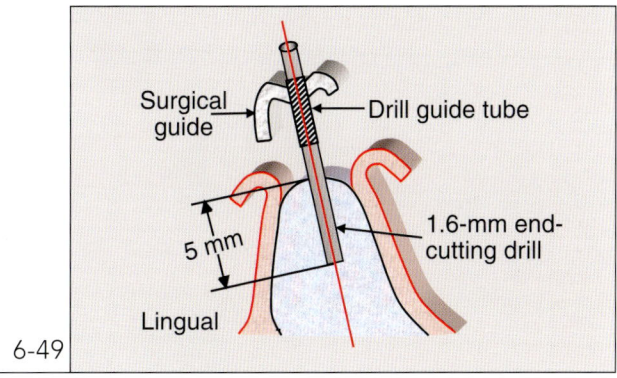

6-49

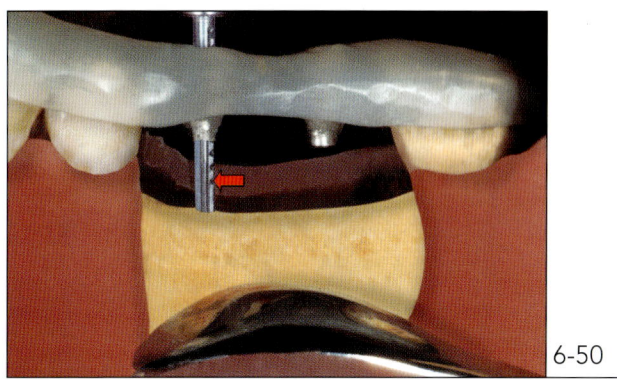

- Surgical guide
- Drill guide tube
- 5 mm
- 1.6-mm end-cutting drill
- Lingual

6-50

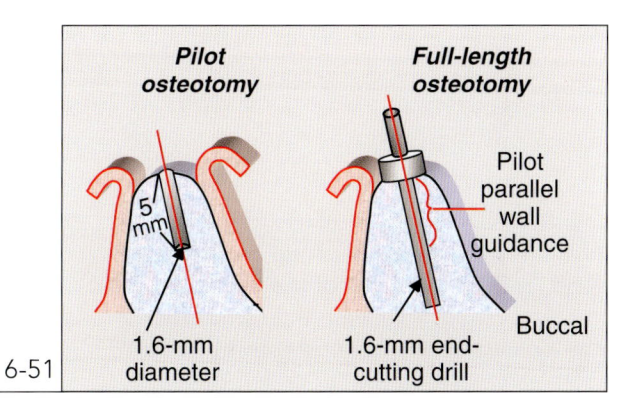

6-51

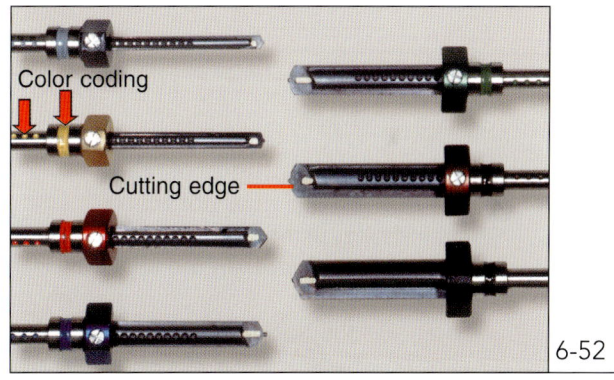

Pilot osteotomy
- 5 mm
- 1.6-mm diameter

Full-length osteotomy
- Pilot parallel wall guidance
- 1.6-mm end-cutting drill
- Buccal

6-52

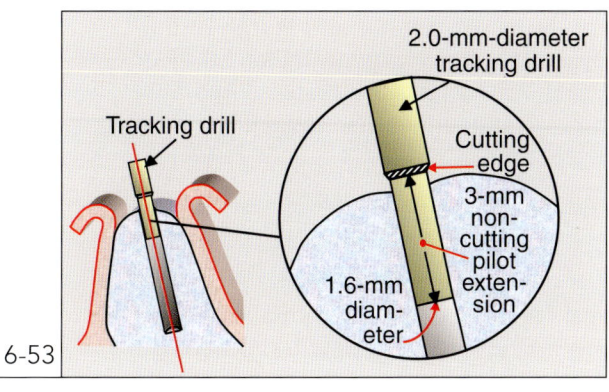

- Color coding
- Cutting edge

6-53

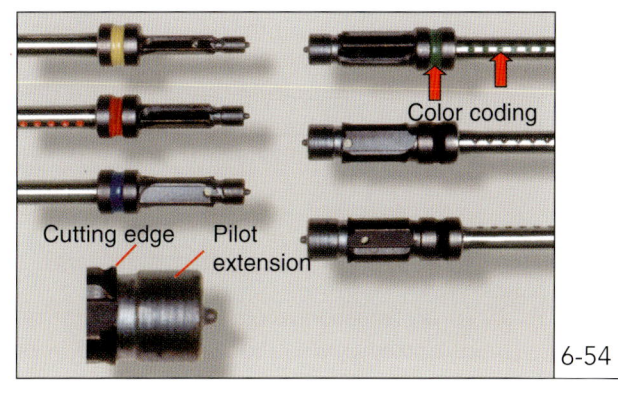

- Tracking drill
- 2.0-mm-diameter tracking drill
- Cutting edge
- 3-mm non-cutting pilot extension
- 1.6-mm diameter

6-54

- Color coding
- Cutting edge
- Pilot extension

99

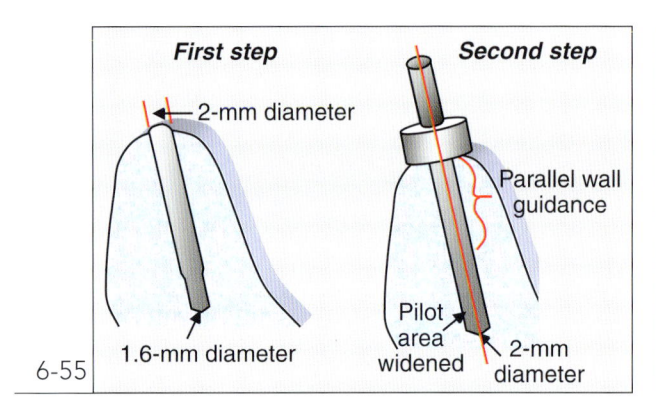

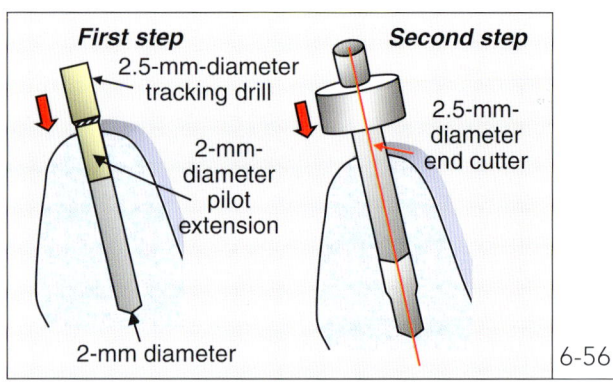

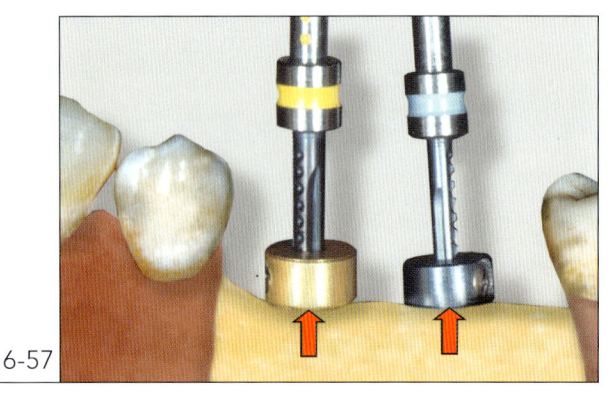

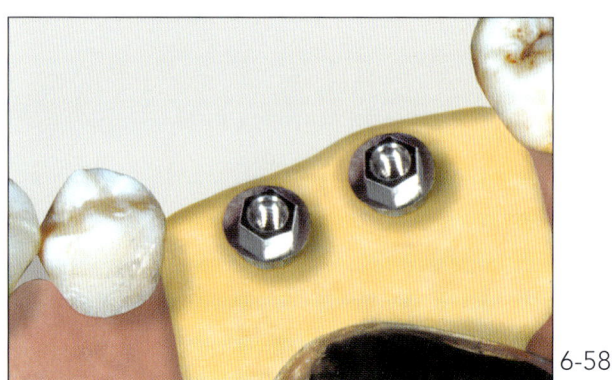

6 Three-dimensional Guidance System for Implant Placement

6-55 First step: 2-mm diameter, 1.6-mm diameter. Second step: Parallel wall guidance, Pilot area widened, 2-mm diameter.

6-56 First step: 2.5-mm-diameter tracking drill, 2-mm-diameter pilot extension, 2-mm diameter. Second step: 2.5-mm-diameter end cutter.

6-57

6-58

Two-step widening procedure

The tracking drill does not widen the osteotomy to its full length (because of the non-cutting pilot extension; see Fig 6-53); therefore, the bottom 3 mm of the osteotomy is always narrower than the top portion (Fig 6-55, *left*). The bottom of the osteotomy must therefore be widened separately using an end-cutting drill with the same color coding as the tracking drill (Fig 6-55, *right*). The parallel walls of the osteotomy serve as guidance while the end-cutting drill prepares the osteotomy to its full desired length.

This two-step procedure is continued until the final diameter and length of the osteotomy are established (Figs 6-56 and 6-57, *arrows*). The osteotomy is then beveled as needed according to the implant design, and the implants are seated (Fig 6-58). (It is advantageous to prepare the osteotomies 1.0 mm longer than required to provide clinical flexibility at the time of implant seating.)

Procedure recommendations

To prevent confusion and reduce the potential for error, preparation of all the pilot osteotomies with the surgical guide in position is recommended before proceeding. Once this is completed, the length and width should be extended in one osteotomy at a time. Proceeding in this manner has several advantages: *(1)* It is most efficient; *(2)* it prevents errors; *(3)* it reinforces hand-eye coordination through repetitive handpiece angulation; and *(4)* it simplifies the procedure, making the entire process easier for auxiliary personnel.

6-59

6-60

6-61 to 6-63 Buccal

Buccal

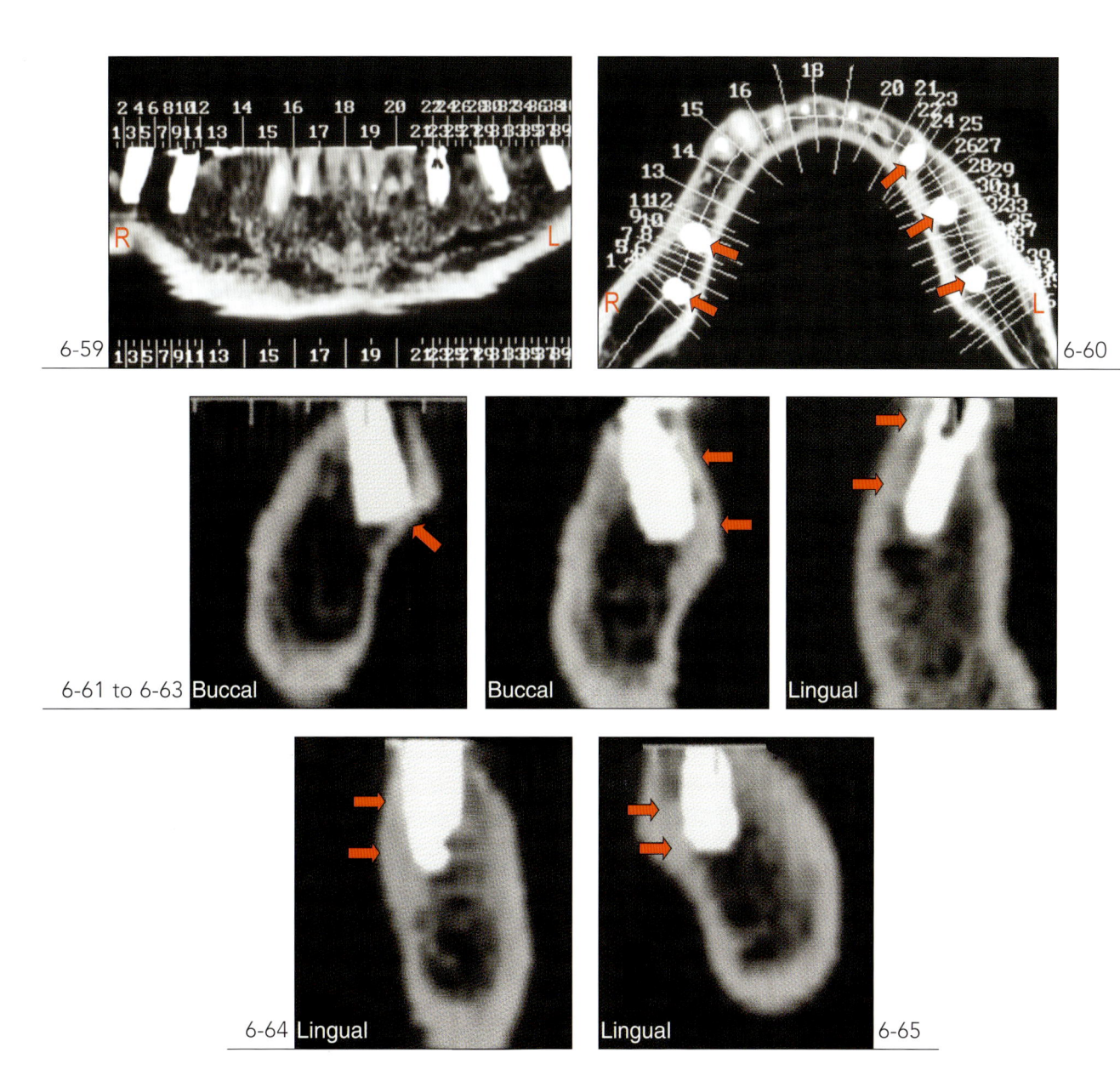

Lingual

6-64 Lingual

Lingual 6-65

In Vivo Results

Reformatted CT images

The panoramic reformatted image in Fig 6-59 reveals five implants, two on the patient's right side and three on the left. (The implants are foreshortened in the images to prevent scatter due to the prosthesis.) It should be noted that all the implants are mesially inclined approximately 4 degrees as planned. The transaxial image in Fig 6-60 indicates the position of the implants (*arrows*) relative to the remaining teeth. The patient's right second molar implant is in contact with the compact bone of the mylohyoid ridge (Fig 6-61, *arrow*), and the first molar implant on the same side is placed against lingual compact bone (Fig 6-62, *arrows*). The patient's left second premolar implant (Fig 6-63, *arrows*) and left first molar implant (Fig 6-64, *arrows*) contact lingual compact bone, while the left second molar implant is placed against lingual and mylohyoid compact bone (Fig 6-65, *arrows*).

Restorations off the Alveolar Ridge Center Line

In the case presented in this chapter, all restorations were placed at the crest of the alveolar ridge. However, restorations also may be placed lingual or buccal to the crest of the ridge depending on the requirements of the opposing occlusion (see Fig 6-10). According to therapeutic biomechanics (see chapter 5), the three-dimensional starting position and orientation of an implant are specifically designed relative to the optimal occlusal relationship and bone topography in order to reduce implant loading. The special procedural considerations associated with such cases are discussed in the following sections.

Posterior restorations

As emphasized earlier, the vertical orientation pin of the radiographic guide marks the center line of the residual alveolar ridge on the cast, and the radiopaque lining of the radiographic guide allows visualization of the center of the restoration (Figs 6-66 and 6-67). When the restoration is lingual to the crest of the ridge, lingual inclination of the implant provides proper access channel placement (Fig 6-68, *left*). When the restoration is buccal to the crest of the ridge, buccal inclination of the implant provides proper access channel placement (Fig 6-69, *left*). When the implant orientation and restoration location are not in alignment, an alternative to altering the inclination of the implant is to use an angled or custom-reangulated abutment (Figs 6-68 and 6-69, *right*).

Anterior restorations

The design of the restoration always affects the placement of the osteotomy starting point. A cemented porcelain restoration, for instance, can have the most labial osteotomy starting point, whereas a restoration of standard design requiring an access channel will have a more lingual osteotomy starting point (Fig 6-70). This lingual horizontal implant offset will increase implant loading (see chapter 5). Often, alveolar anatomy (A) dictates variations in implant inclination that require an angulated (or custom-reangulated) abutment for anatomic or esthetic considerations (Fig 6-71). Angulated or custom-reangulated abutments also permit a more labial implant placement, which reduces torque regardless of the restoration design (see chapter 5).

Radiographic guide for anterior implant placement

Anterior all-porcelain cemented maxillary restorations are usually labial to the crest of the alveolar bone, thus eliminating the need for an access channel (Fig 6-72). As always, the vertical orientation pin is placed at the crest of the alveolar ridge on the stone cast (Fig 6-73). Since, by definition, the vertical orientation pin is perpendicular to the occlusal plane, the pin is placed toward the lingual of the restoration (see Fig 6-73).

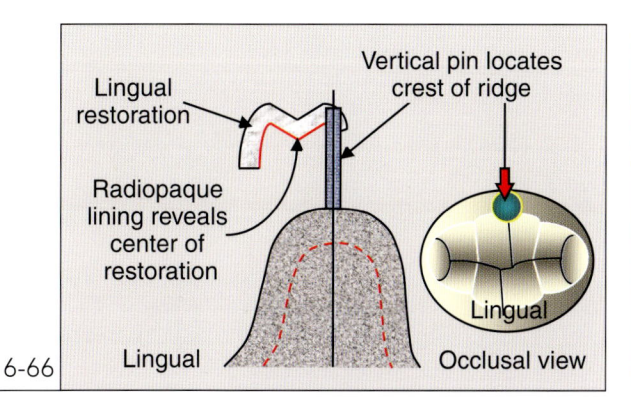

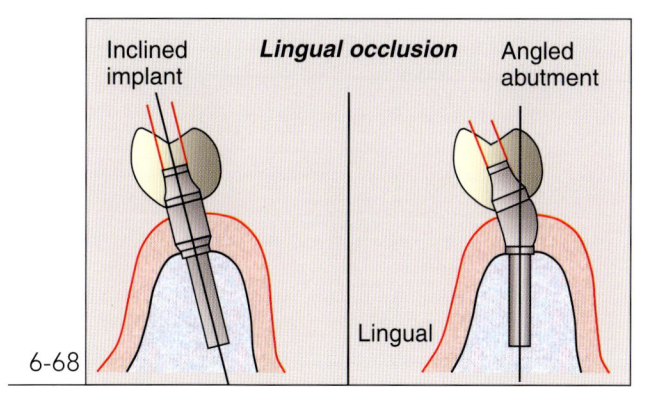

Restorations off the Alveolar Ridge Center Line

6-66
- Lingual restoration
- Vertical pin locates crest of ridge
- Radiopaque lining reveals center of restoration
- Lingual
- Occlusal view

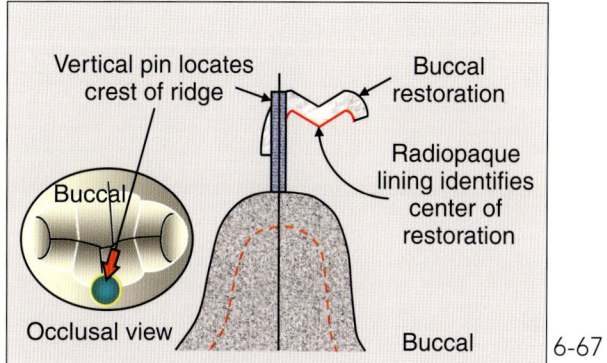

6-67
- Vertical pin locates crest of ridge
- Buccal restoration
- Radiopaque lining identifies center of restoration
- Buccal
- Occlusal view

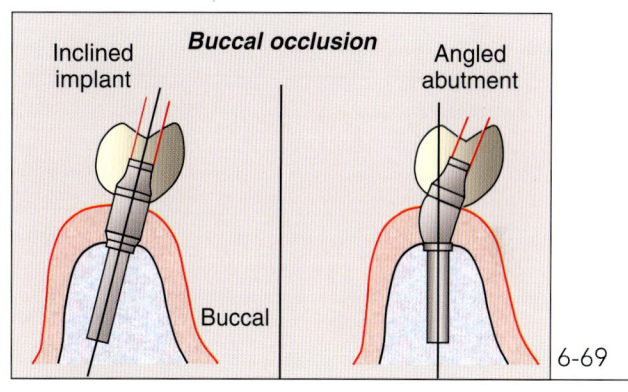

6-68 *Lingual occlusion*
- Inclined implant
- Angled abutment
- Lingual

6-69 *Buccal occlusion*
- Inclined implant
- Angled abutment
- Buccal

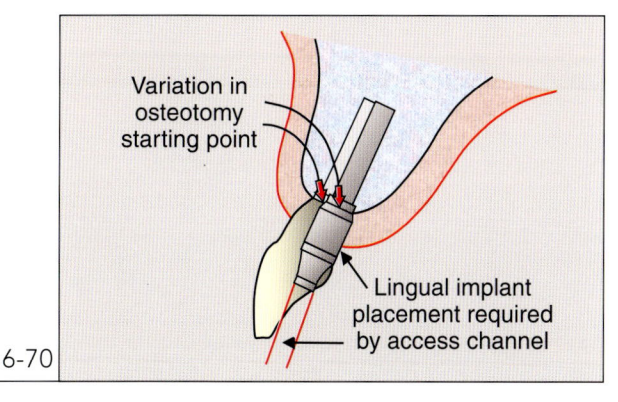

6-70
- Variation in osteotomy starting point
- Lingual implant placement required by access channel

6-71 *Variations required by alveolar anatomy*
- A
- Angulated abutment adjusts to esthetic and bone requirements

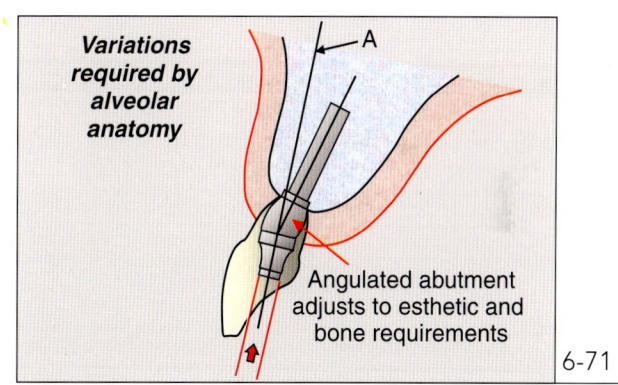

6-72 *Planning for radiographic guide*
- Stone cast
- External starting point for restoration without an access channel

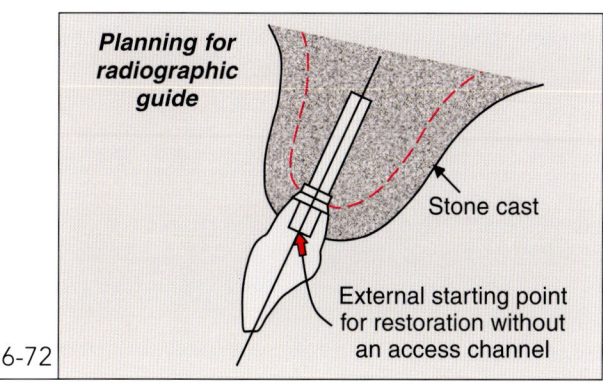

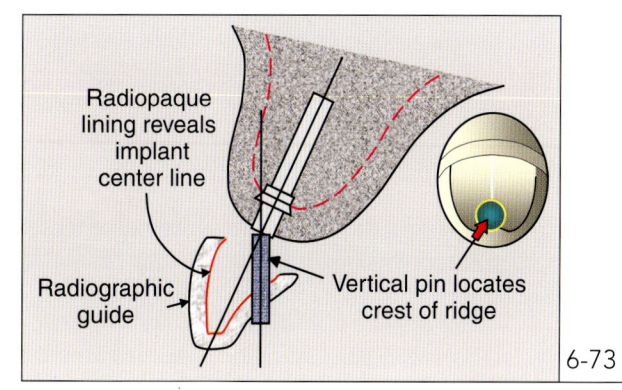

6-73
- Radiopaque lining reveals implant center line
- Radiographic guide
- Vertical pin locates crest of ridge

103

6 Three-dimensional Guidance System for Implant Placement

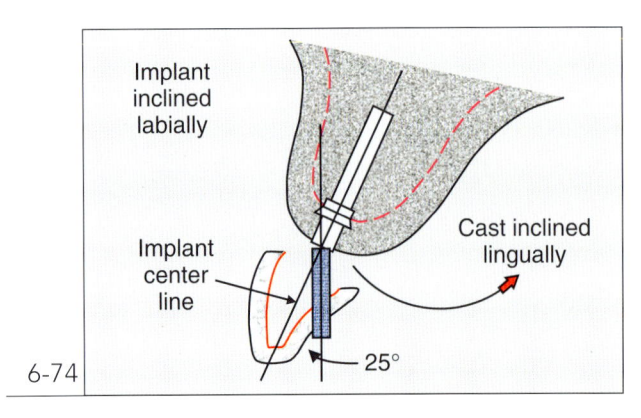

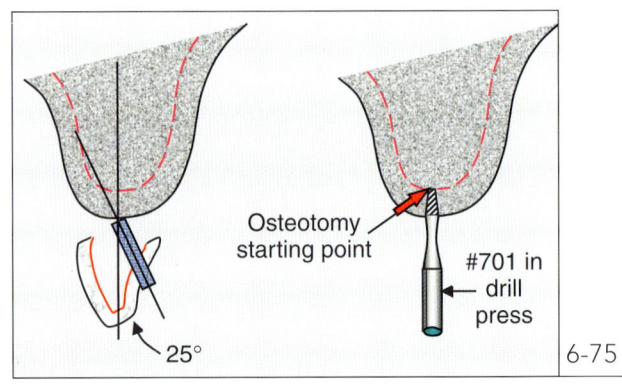

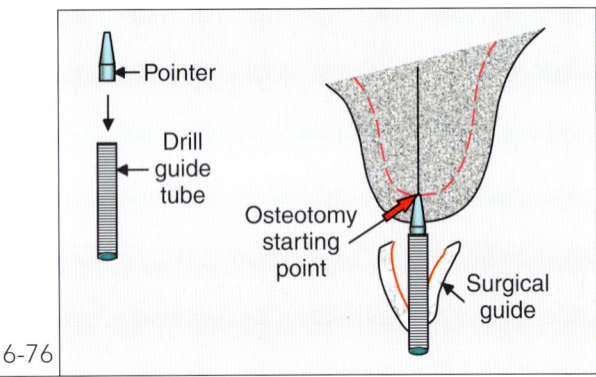

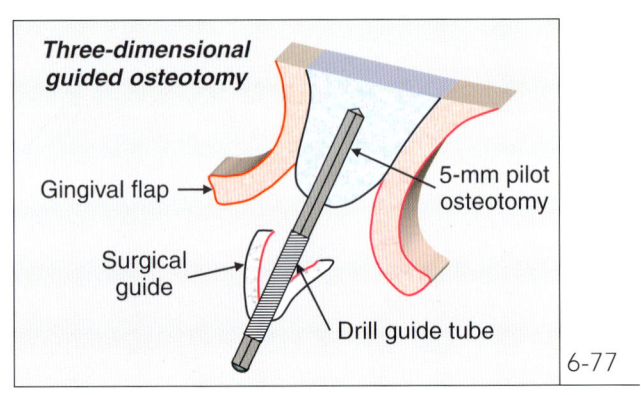

6-74 · 6-75 · 6-76 · 6-77

Surgical guide construction
When the restoration is not aligned with the planned implant orientation on the crest of the alveolar ridge, three-dimensional cast orientation is required before the internal starting point of the osteotomy can be determined (Fig 6-74). The cast is rotated *lingually* to establish the planned *labial* implant orientation. Mesiodistal correction may also be required. In Fig 6-75 (*left*), the cast has been rotated 25 degrees lingually (no mesiodistal inclination is required). The drill press prepares the internal osteotomy starting point in the stone cast to the depth of the gingiva (Fig 6-75, *right*).

Drill guide placement
A pointer is placed in a drill guide tube (Fig 6-76, *left*), which is mounted on a mandrel and guided into the internal osteotomy starting point (Fig 6-76, *right*). Fixation of the drill guide tube to the surgical guide completes the procedure.

Three-dimensional guided implant placement
After the surgical guide is seated and checked for proper placement and stability, the gingiva is resected. Pilot osteotomy procedures are initialized using drill guide tube guidance (Fig 6-77) following the step-by-step illustrations in Figs 6-47 to 6-50. The surgical guide is removed and the osteotomy is completed with the two-step procedure shown in Figs 6-51 to 6-56. (For simplicity of description, the casts in this section were described in their in vivo orientation.)

Summary

A three-dimensional guidance system for implant placment requires construction of a radiographic guide that places a true vertical radiopaque marker into the CT scan. The reformatted images are reproduced on Polaroid (or 35-mm) prints to facilitate the planned orientation and measurement of each implant mesiodistally and buccolingually. These three-dimensional inclinations are transferred to a surgical guide containing drill guide tubes that accurately reproduce each implant orientation. A newly designed dual-axis base and instruments to control depth and orientation have been developed to aid in the process.

Acknowledgments

Portions of this chapter were adapted from articles appearing in *Implant Dentistry* by Weinberg and Kruger[9,10] with permission from Lippincott Williams & Wilkins.

References

1. Edge MJ. Surgical placement guide for use with osseointegrated implants. J Prosthet Dent 1987;57:719–722.
2. Weinberg LA. Reduction of implant loading with therapeutic biomechanics. Implant Dent 1998;7:277–285.
3. Blustein R, Jackson R, Rotskoff K, Coy R, Godan D. Use of splint material in the placement of implants. Int J Oral Maxillofac Implants 1986;1:47–49.
4. Schulte JK, Peterson TA. Implants: Occlusal and prosthetic considerations. CDA J 1987;15(10):64–72.
5. Engleman MJ, Sorensen JA, Moy P. Optimum placement of osseointegrated implants. J Prosthet Dent 1988;59:467–473.
6. Chiche GJ, Block MS, Pinault A. Implant surgical template for partially edentulous patients. Int J Oral Maxillofac Implants 1989;4:289–292.
7. Langer B, Sullivan DL. Osseointegration: Its impact on the interrelationship of periodontics and restorative dentistry: Part I. Int J Periodontics Restorative Dent 1989;9:85–105.
8. Weinberg LA. CT scan as a radiologic data base for optimum implant orientation. J Prosthet Dent 1993;69:381–383.
9. Weinberg LA, Kruger B. Three-dimensional guidance system for implant insertion: Part I. Implant Dent 1998;7:81–93.
10. Weinberg LA, Kruger B. Three-dimensional guidance system for implant insertion: Part II. Dual axes table—Problem solving. Implant Dent 1999;8:225–264.

7 Clinical Procedures for Complete-Arch Osseointegrated Prostheses

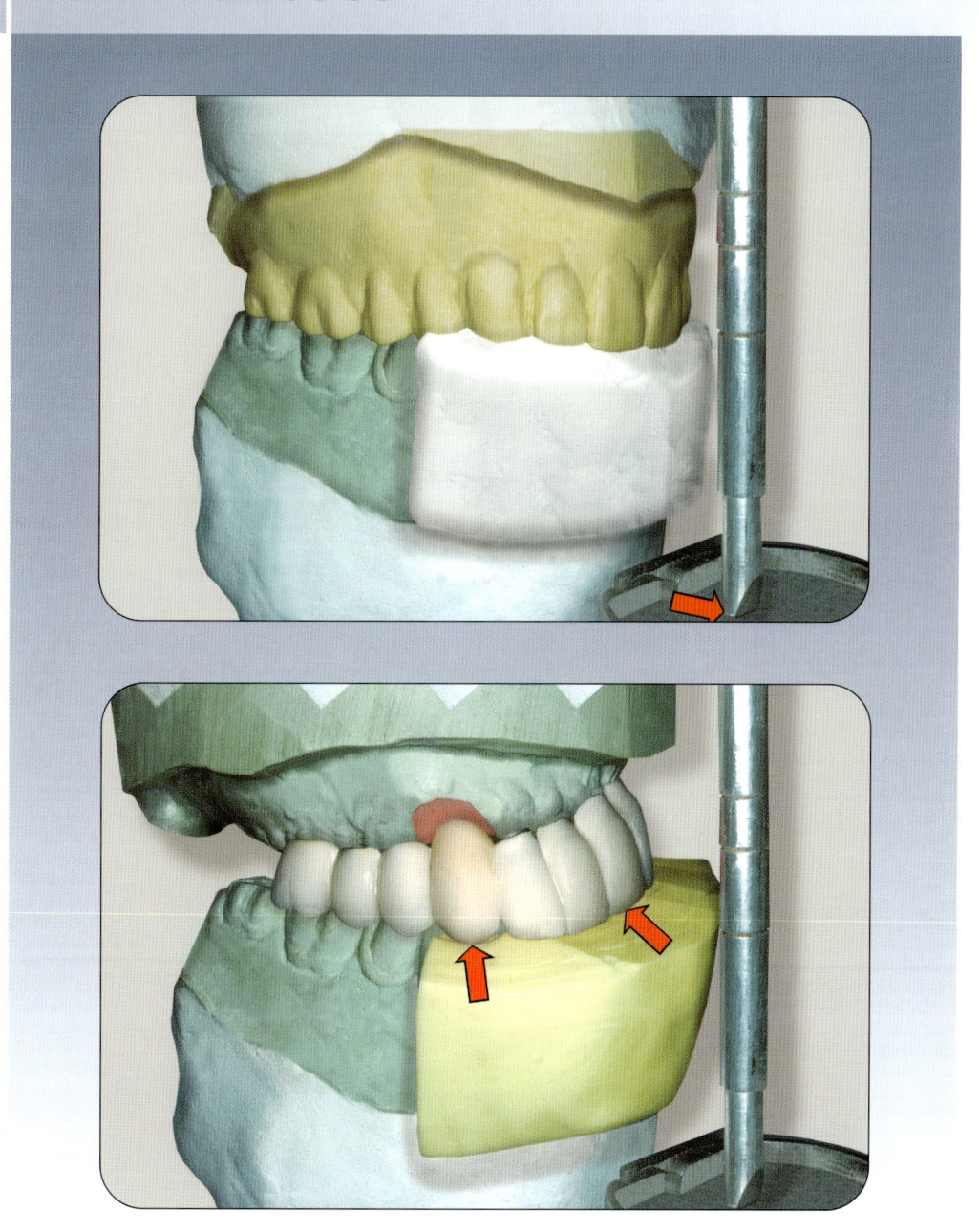

7 Clinical Procedures for Complete-Arch Osseointegrated Prostheses

This chapter presents the step-by-step clinical procedure for constructing a maxillary complete-arch osseointegrated prosthesis beginning with second-stage surgery. In the case presented, the maxillary right canine and left first molar were retained to facilitate stabilization of the surgical guide and the provisional prosthesis, which was constructed with a cast nonprecious metal framework (Fig 7-1). The mandibular arch, which held an anterior fixed prosthesis from the right first premolar to the left canine and a bilateral distal extension prosthesis, remained untreated (Fig 7-2).

First-Stage Provisional Prosthesis

A metal framework rather than an all-acrylic base design was used for the maxillary provisional prosthesis (see Fig 7-1) for several reasons: *(1)* improved patient comfort between first- and second-stage surgery; *(2)* less breakage and need for troubleshooting (ie, better cost effectiveness); and *(3)* numerous advantages provided by metal occlusal rests, including stability, better occlusion, less soft tissue impingement, and improved osseointegration prognosis.

Second-Stage Provisional Prosthesis

Optimum design requirements

The second-stage provisional prosthesis requires extensive internal soft tissue relief; however, the resultant palatal bulk limits tongue space and thus precludes its use for an extended period of time (such as that following first-stage surgery) (Figs 7-3 and 7-4, *arrows*). For this reason, the design should be simple: There should be no occlusal rests. Stainless steel bent wire clasps and acrylic teeth should be used, and the prosthesis must provide space for the abutments and healing caps (Fig 7-5) and must accommodate the extensive soft tissue edema that usually occurs. If adequate relief is not provided by the clinician before insertion, the patient may not be able to reinsert the provisional prosthesis after removal.

Progressive loading

The original technique for osseointegration, as described by Brånemark[1] and others,[2-7] required intimate and passive fit of the implant with the investing bone and a 5- to 6-month healing period during which the implant was completely isolated from the oral cavity. (Single-stage surgery and immediate loading are beyond the scope of this presentation.) When the implant was exposed after second-stage surgery, a progressive program of loading rather than the sudden application of full occlusal function was initiated using an acrylic provisional prosthesis (see Figs 7-3 and 7-4). Such a progressive loading system helped maintain successful integration of all implants. These basic concepts still hold true today.

In progressive loading, the first step is to thoroughly relieve the internal surface of the prosthesis buccally, lingually, and occlusally. The use of indicating wax is helpful for exposing impinging areas that prevent complete seating. Small holes are placed over each implant location in the acrylic base of the prosthesis. With the mandible closed in centric occlusion, the prosthesis is relined with a soft tissue treatment material. The vertical dimension is confirmed by occlusal contact of the remaining maxillary natural teeth. After the soft tissue treatment material sets, the

Second-Stage Provisional Prosthesis

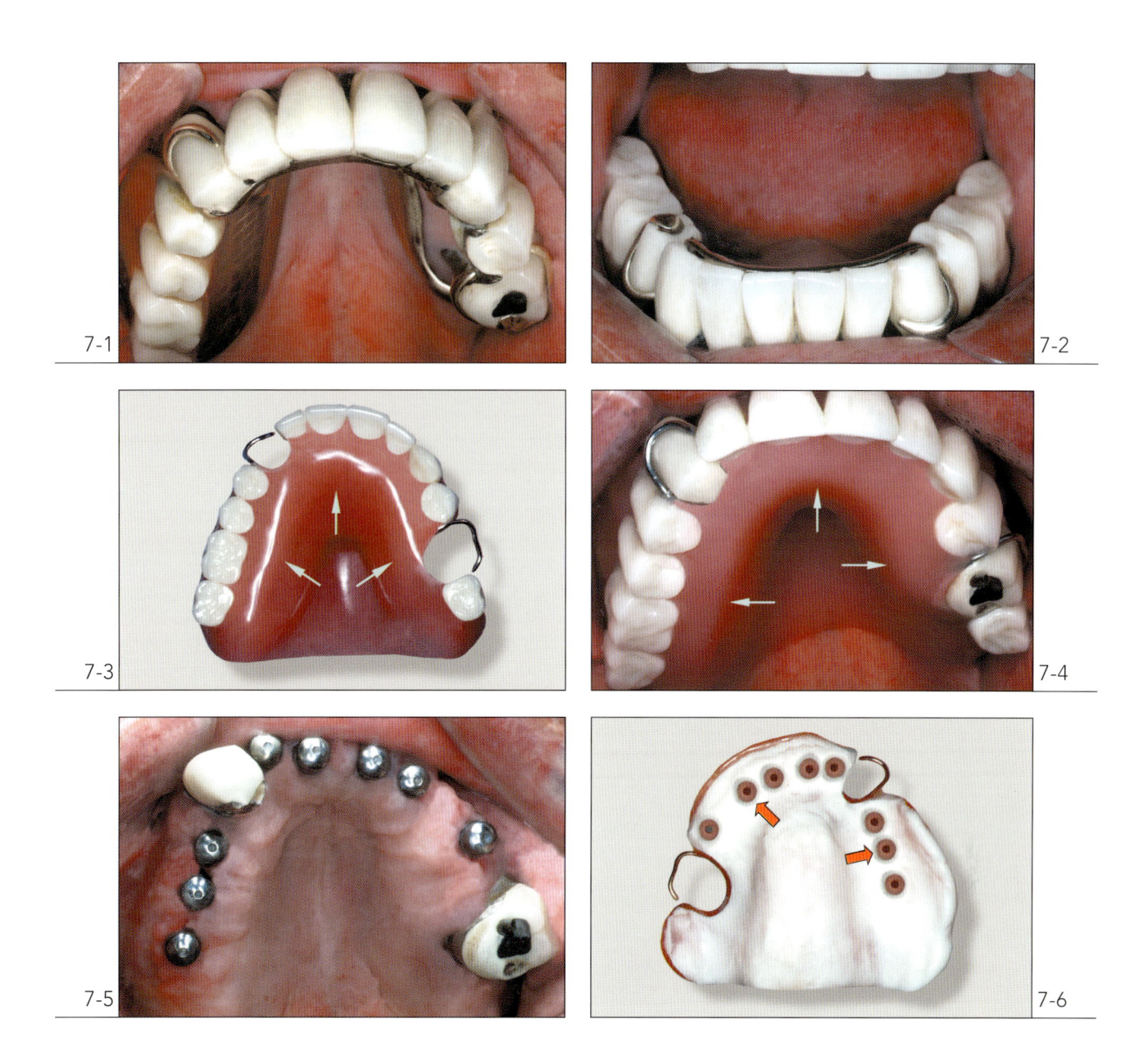

provisional prosthesis is withdrawn, and the material is removed at each implant site (Fig 7-6, *arrows*). This procedure prevents the distribution of occlusal and lateral forces on the healing cap and abutment of each implant.

The soft tissue treatment procedure can be repeated every 2 weeks until complete healing takes place. At these intervals, occlusal loading can be gradually increased by removing incrementally less soft tissue treatment material from the implant sites. The resultant increase of occlusal force on the implants is moderated by the resiliency of the material, which provides a cushioning effect. Progressive loading is further reinforced by initially placing the patient on a liquid diet and then gradually introducing soft foods to the regimen.

7 Clinical Procedures for Complete-Arch Osseointegrated Prostheses

Impression procedure

Impression tray design

The impression tray design depends on the type of impression coping selected by the clinician (see chapter 9). In the author's clinical experience, square impression copings (without ligation) produce the most accurate master casts. For square impression copings, an open custom impression tray is constructed with adequate clearance surrounding the copings (Fig 7-7). Proper seating of the tray during the impression procedure is reinforced by providing at least two stops with impression compound inside the tray. This step also ensures that adequate impression material surrounds each impression coping. Lubrication of the outside of the impression tray adjacent to the openings is recommended. (Various impression techniques are discussed in greater detail in chapter 9.)

Seating of square abutment copings

The provisional prosthesis is removed and the abutment screws are retightened to ensure complete seating (Fig 7-8). Before the square abutment copings are seated, it is important to visually confirm that no soft tissue is covering the abutment margins. Each abutment coping is then seated, and the guide pin is fully tightened (Fig 7-9). Periapical radiographs should be used to confirm the intimate fit of all the implant–abutment–impression coping interfaces. Without verification that all abutment screws have been completely tightened and visual as well as radiographic confirmation of the intimate fit of all interfaces, the success of the entire procedure is at risk.

Impression technique

Soft-bodied elastomeric impression material is injected around the soft tissue margins and impression copings. The impression tray is loaded with heavy-bodied elastomeric impression material and seated. It is helpful to locate each guide pin with a finger before the impression material sets. An angled periodontal scalpel is extremely useful in trimming the heavy-bodied elastomeric impression material from the guide pins; at least 2 mm of clearance is needed (Fig 7-10, *arrows*). The lubrication of the outside of the impression tray adjacent to the access holes facilitates complete access to the guide pins.

The guide pins are loosened but not removed from the impression. Freedom of vertical movement of each guide pin should be confirmed before the impression is removed. The guide pins and copings remain in the impression. After removal of the impression, the gingival surface of the impression copings should be fully exposed and the margins completely free of impression material (Fig 7-11, *arrows*). Abutment analogs (replicas) are then seated against the impression copings, and the guide pins are fully retightened with a screwdriver. (If the abutment is subgingival, placing the analog without impinging on the soft-bodied elastomeric impression material is critical.) The impression is then boxed and the cast poured in a high-quality stone (Fig 7-12).

Before the provisional prosthesis is replaced in the mouth, a preliminary centric relation record should be obtained over the abutments using wax or other suitable material. This record should be as close to the correct vertical dimension as possible. As described in chapter 3, a semi-adjustable articulator, which requires a facebow mounting of the maxillary cast (see Fig 3-42), should be used.

Second-Stage Provisional Prosthesis

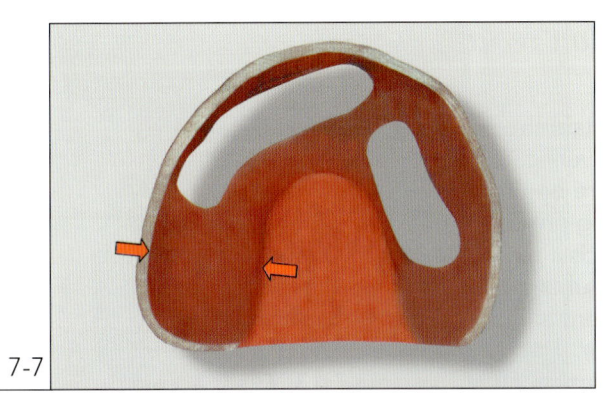

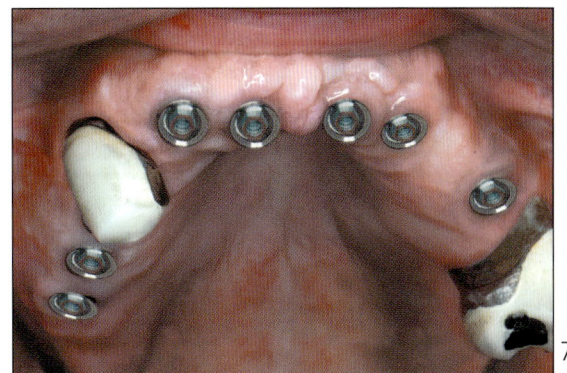

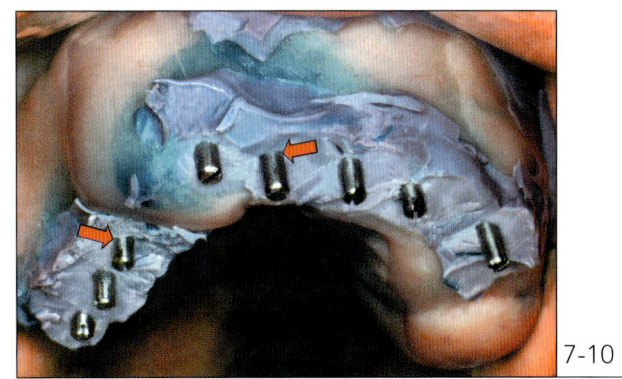

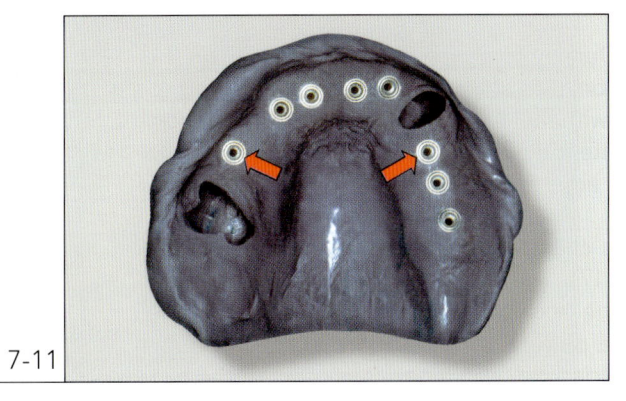

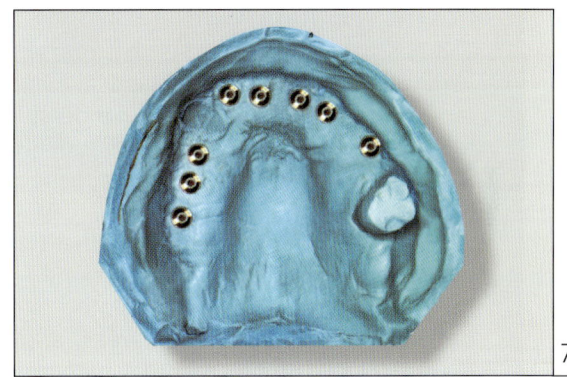

7-7

7-8

7-9

7-10

7-11

7-12

111

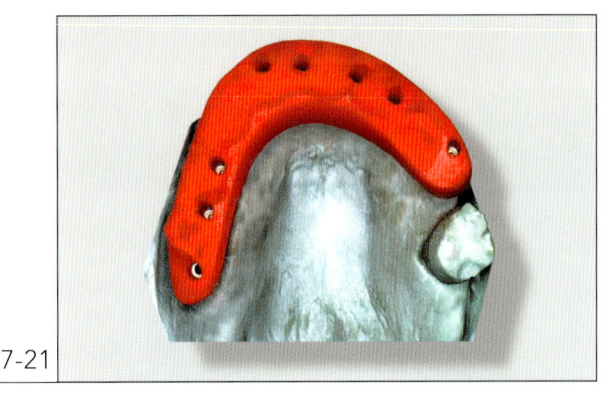

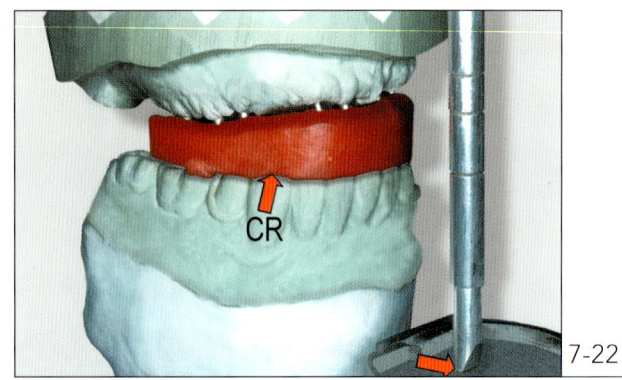

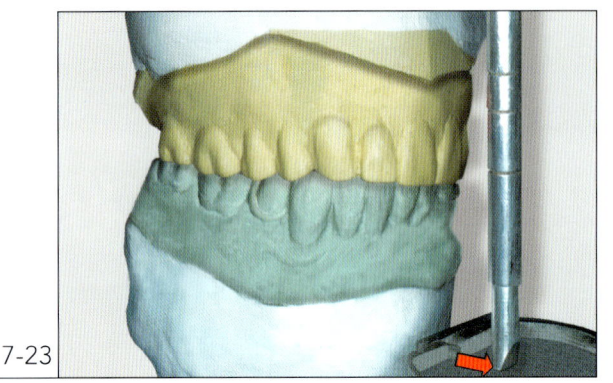

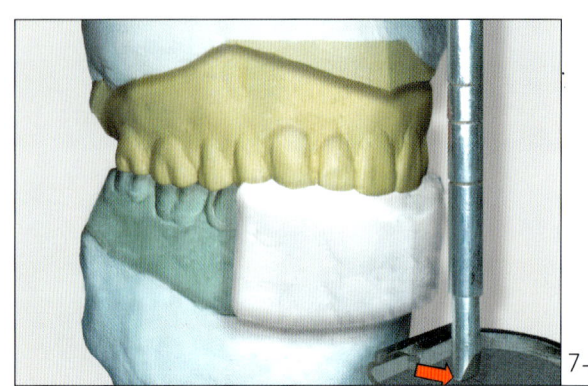

7 Clinical Procedures for Complete-Arch Osseointegrated Prostheses

7-21

7-22

7-23

7-24

Mounting and transfer procedures

Centric relation mounting
The verification jig and centric relation record are returned to the master cast and secured with the gold screws (Fig 7-21). The maxillary cast has been previously mounted to the articulator using a facebow and the split-cast technique. Any sharp edges should be removed from the acrylic centric relation record with a round diamond stone, and no debris should remain. Countercast inaccuracy is an avoidable cause of occlusal adjustment of the prosthesis upon completion. It is recommended that the countercast be obtained with an accurate elastomeric impression material rather than alginate. Any occlusal bubbles or artifacts will prevent complete seating of the centric relation record (CR), which will cause the countercast to rock. When precise fit is obtained, the mandibular cast is fixed to the articulator (Fig 7-22).

Esthetic incisal index transfer
Esthetic transfer to the master cast using an incisal index was discussed in detail in chapter 3. The maxillary master cast is removed from the articulator, and a cast of the planned provisional prosthesis is hand articulated with the mandibular cast and mounted to the upper member of the articulator (Fig 7-23). A plaster (or polysiloxane matrix putty) incisal index is obtained (Fig 7-24). The incisal index is trimmed occlusally until only slight indentations of the incisal surfaces remain to serve as an esthetic guide for the fixed-retrievable provisional (as well as the final) prosthesis (see Fig 7-24).

Second-Stage Provisional Prosthesis

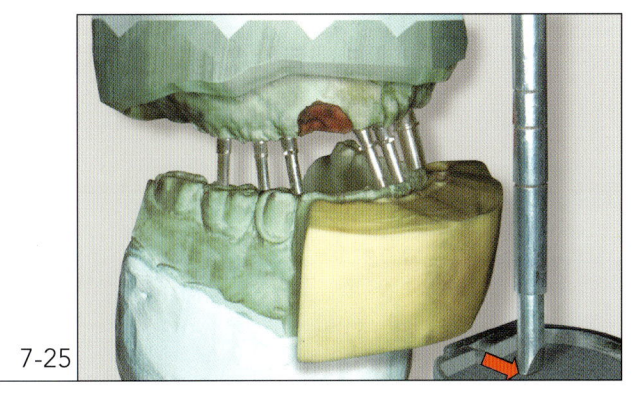

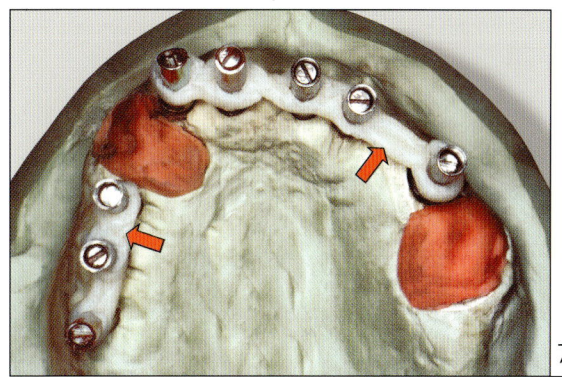

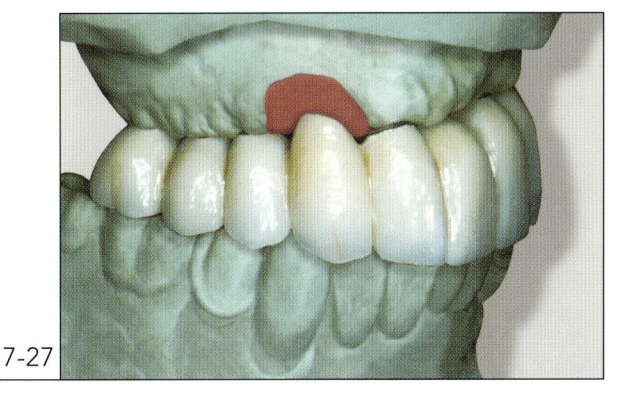

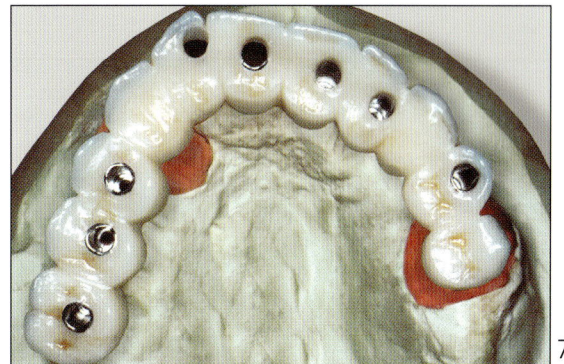

7-25

7-26

7-27

7-28

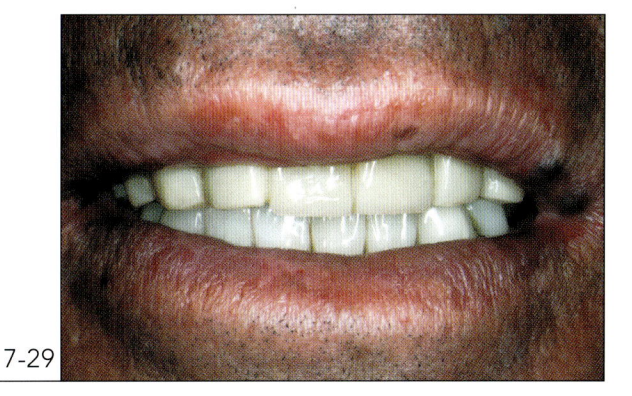

7-29

Provisional prosthesis construction

Temporary copings are seated on the abutment analogs with gold screws and adjusted to the vertical dimension of occlusion, which is maintained by the incisal pin of the articulator (Fig 7-25, *arrow*). Light-cured resin is placed around the temporary copings (*arrows*) to help maintain accuracy during the waxup and processing procedure (Fig 7-26). The acrylic provisional prosthesis is fabricated to the planned esthetics, exact centric relation, and vertical dimension (Fig 7-27). The temporary copings maintain access to the gold screws (Fig 7-28). The key to trouble-free insertion, minimal occlusal adjustment, and maximal esthetics (Fig 7-29) lies in the accuracy of the centric relation record at the planned vertical dimension (see Figs 7-15 to 7-22) and the incisal index transfer technique (see Figs 7-23 to 7-25). (In this case, the midline deviation was preserved from the pre-extraction location [see Fig 3-13] through the maxillary fixed prosthesis [see Fig 3-14], which was constructed 20 years before the implant-supported prosthesis.)

Final Implant-Supported Prosthesis

Framework fabrication

Framework fabrication should start with a complete full-arch waxup over the gold copings to ensure proper esthetics (Fig 7-30). The framework is carved to produce maximum occlusion and esthetics with the aid of the incisal index; note the controlled thickness of porcelain and orientation of the incisal plane when the waxup is related to the incisal index (Fig 7-31). The framework is cast to the gold cylinders and finished relative to the occlusion and incisal index (Fig 7-32). The type of metal used depends on the preference of the individual clinician; the author favors a precious metal content of at least 50%. The interface fit of the gold cylinders to the abutments is confirmed clinically and with the aid of periapical radiographs viewed through a magnifying loop, and the occlusion is adjusted (Fig 7-33, *arrows*).

Porcelain fusion

Porcelain is fused to the framework and the occlusion adjusted on the articulator; note the exact esthetic conformity to the incisal index (Fig 7-34). The biscuit-bake restoration is placed intraorally to confirm clinical and radiographic maintenance of all the interfaces, and the occlusion is adjusted once again. If the prosthesis is found to be satisfactory, it is glazed and stained (Fig 7-35). The gingival view of the final prosthesis is shown in Fig 7-36.

Final Implant-Supported Prosthesis

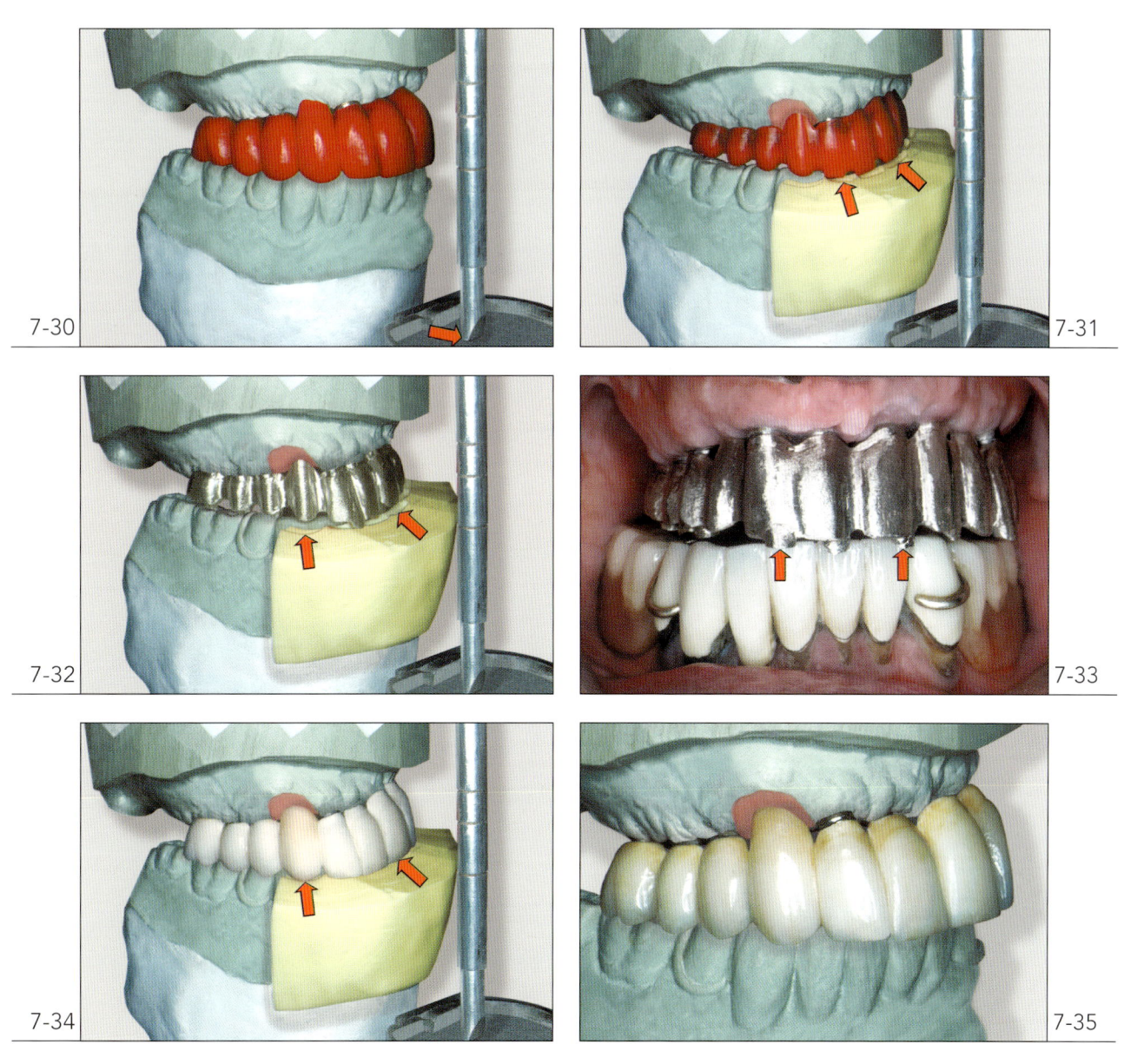

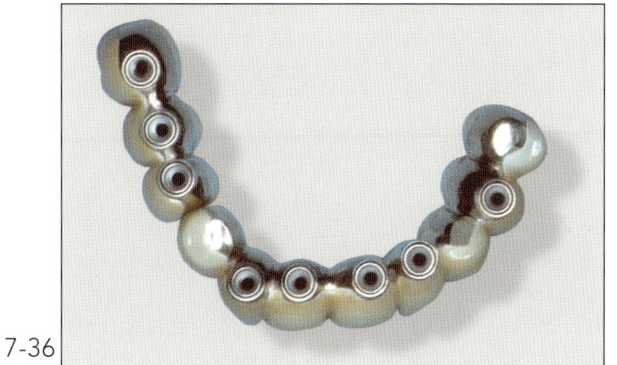

7-30
7-31
7-32
7-33
7-34
7-35
7-36

117

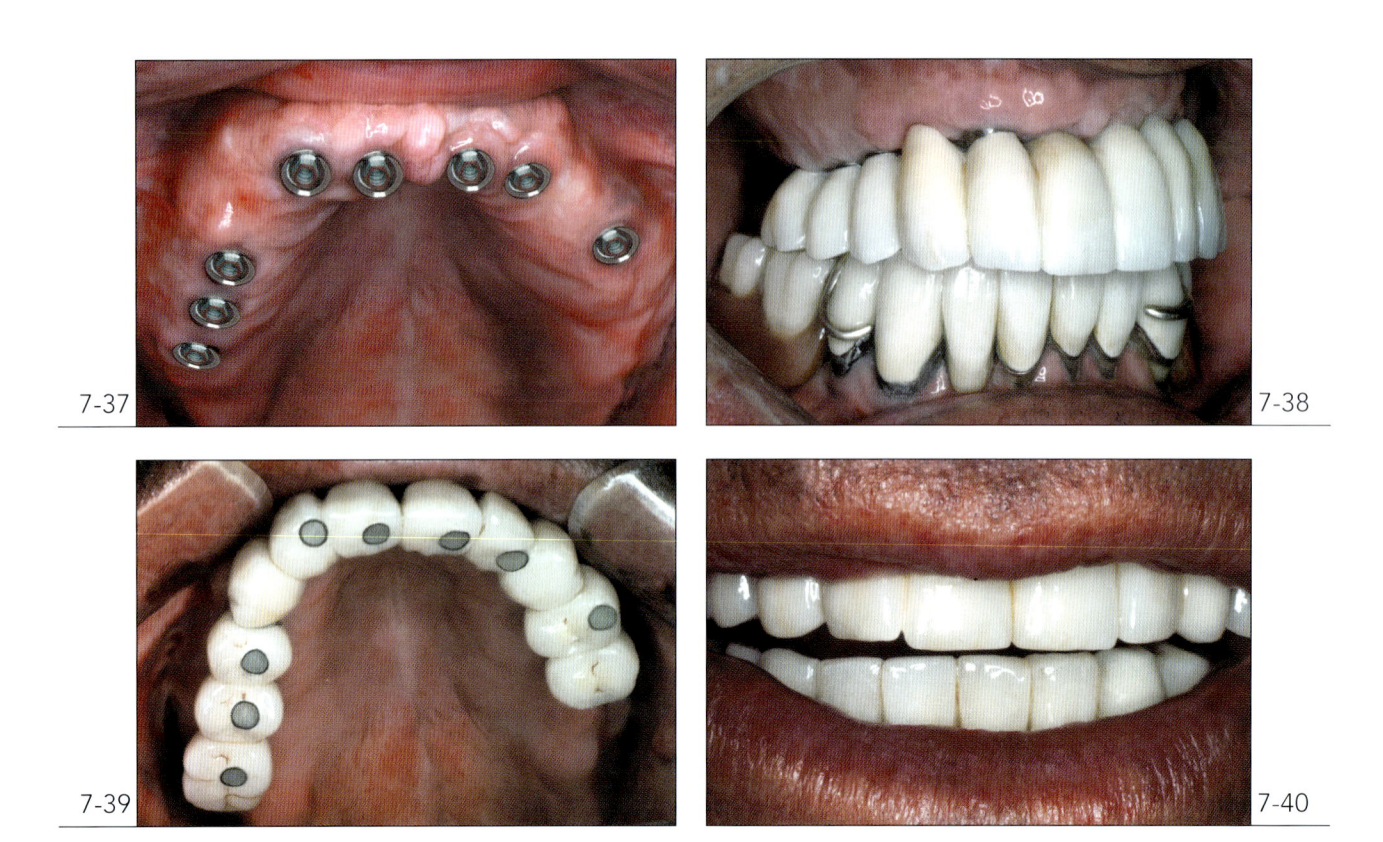

7 Clinical Procedures for Complete-Arch Osseointegrated Prostheses

7-37

7-38

7-39

7-40

Provisional placement

The provisional acrylic prosthesis is removed and all the abutment screws are checked for tightness (Fig 7-37). Seating of a large osseointegrated screw-retained prosthesis follows the special procedure previously described (see Fig 7-16). The clinical and radiographic integrity of all the interfaces, as well as the occlusion, must be confirmed again (Fig 7-38). The gold screws are protected with a small pellet of cotton and the access channels covered with temporary cement or other suitable elastic material.

Final placement

When the soft tissue response is healthy and the patient comfortable, the access channels can be covered with self- or light-cured resin (Fig 7-39). (The armamentarium, clinical procedures, and cementation regimen that eliminate the occlusal access channels are discussed in chapter 9.) The patient's original midline deviation through the fixed-retrievable provisional prosthesis (see Fig 7-29) has been reproduced in the final porcelain osseointegrated prosthesis (Fig 7-40).

Summary

The pitfalls of poor esthetics and occlusion can be avoided by strict adherence to sound clinical procedures that have been used successfully with full-arch tooth-supported prostheses (described in chapter 3). These clinical procedures maintain constant transferable references for the vertical dimension, centric relation, and esthetics from the original planning casts through all provisional prostheses (regardless of design or materials) and into the final prosthesis. Dedicating significant time and effort to planning, taking exact records, and transferring esthetics reduces the amount of time required chairside to produce the final prosthesis.

References

1. Brånemark PI. Osseointegration and its experimental background. J Prosthet Dent 1983;50:399–410.
2. Adell R, Lekholm U, Rockler B, Brånemark PI. A 15-year study of osseointegrated implants in the treatment of the edentulous jaw. Int J Oral Surg 1981;10:387–416.
3. Adell R, Eriksson B, Lekholm U, Brånemark PI, Jemt T. Long-term follow-up study of osseointegrated implants in the treatment of totally edentulous jaws. Int J Oral Maxillofac Implants 1990;5:347–359.
4. Lindquist LW, Carlsson GE, Jemt T. A prospective 15-year follow-up study of mandibular fixed prostheses supported by osseointegrated implants. Clinical results and marginal bone loss. Clin Oral Implants Res 1996;7:329–336.
5. Jemt T, Lekholm U, Adell R. Osseointegration in the treatment of partially edentulous patients: A preliminary study of 876 consecutively placed fixtures. Int J Oral Maxillofac Implants 1989;4:211–217.
6. Johns RB, Jemt T, Heath MR, et al. A multicenter study of overdentures supported by Brånemark implants. Int J Oral Maxillofac Implants 1992;7:513–522.
7. Jemt T, Pettersson P. A 3-year follow-up study on single implant treatment. J Prosthet Dent 1993;21:203–208.

8 Clinical Procedures for Tooth- and Implant-Supported Overdentures and Fixed-Retrievable Prostheses

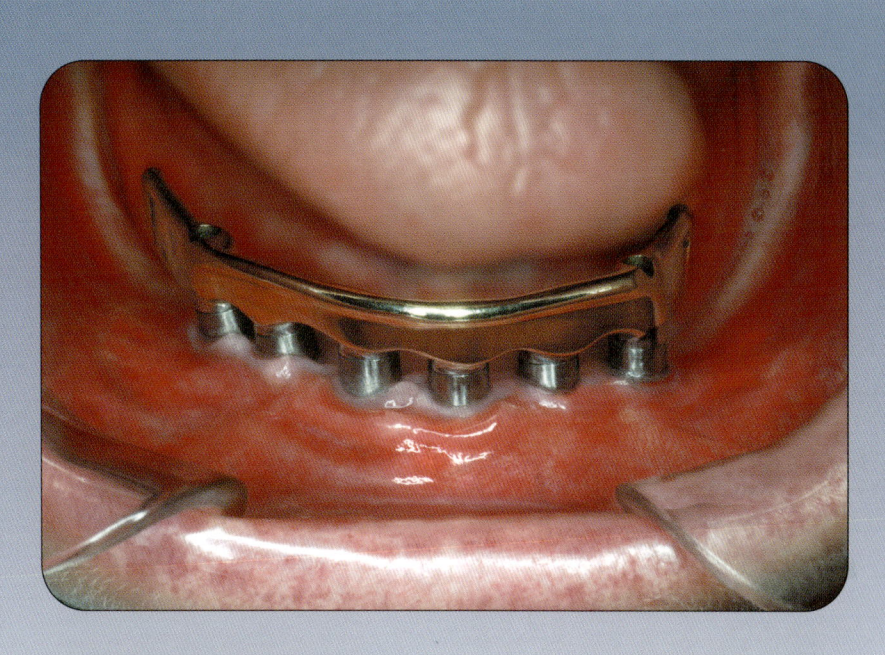

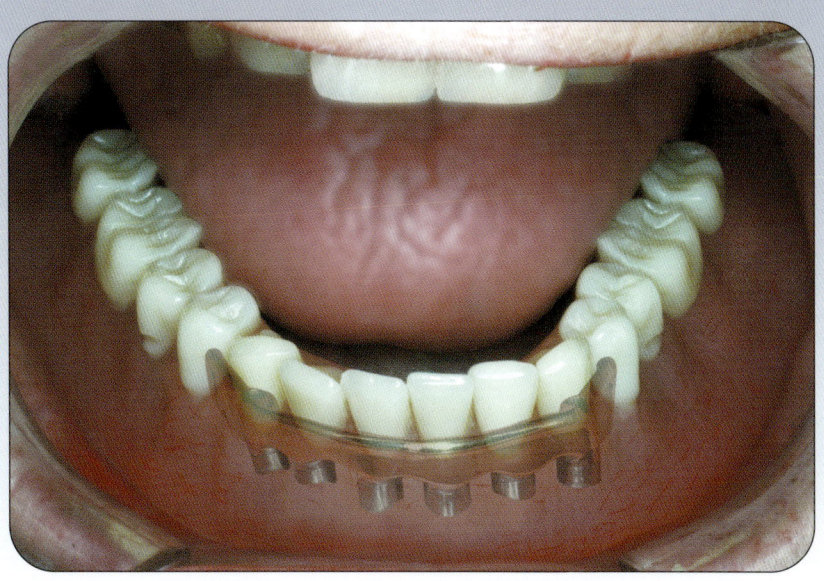

8 Clinical Procedures for Tooth- and Implant-Supported Overdentures and Fixed-Retrievable Prostheses

This chapter describes the step-by-step clinical procedures for tooth- and implant-supported overdentures and fixed-retrievable prostheses. In the interest of brevity, the fundamental prosthodontic procedures previously described have not been repeated; only the details critical to achieving a successful result are covered.

Tooth-Supported Clip Bar Overdenture

There are many different bar designs and retentive devices available; it is the responsibility of the individual clinician to determine which combination is most suitable for a specific clinical situation. The author prefers a simple bar design, with minimum vertical height of the retentive portion and simple replacement properties for long-term maintenance. In the case presented here, two anterior nonvital teeth were used with gold posts, which were positioned at the final cementation stage. The copings were cast separately to avoid the problem of parallelism of the posts and to improve retention and marginal adaptation.

Assemblage of the bar

A Dolder bar is cast and attached to the left coping while the right coping-bar interface remains open (Fig 8-1, *arrow*). The bar lightly touches the gingiva to prevent food impaction and ensure stability (Fig 8-2, *arrows*). Duralay (Reliance, Worth, IL) is painted in the interface (see Fig 8-1, *arrow*), and a direct plaster occlusal index is obtained for assemblage. Next, a complete elastic impression is obtained in the material of choice for fabrication of a custom impression tray, which must be adequately relieved anteriorly. Some clinicians prefer to combine these two steps, but the author prefers the accuracy of a plaster index because it facilitates assemblage and allows the clinician to return to the mouth to confirm fit (see Fig 8-2).

Final impression

To facilitate construction, the copings and bar are not yet cemented. Duralay acrylic is painted around the gingival areas buccolingually to ensure a good cast and provide undercut areas, which will enable removal of the clip bar with the impression. The borders of the impression tray are reduced to the beginning of the area where the mucosa will be reflected to provide space for border molding with compound. The posterior borders are determined by palpation of the pterygomaxillary notch laterally and by observation of the nature of the slope and movement of soft tissue of the palate, thus providing the outline of the postpalatal seal. This border-molding technique usually provides good results (Fig 8-3) when used with the swallowing technique.

Tooth-Supported Clip Bar Overdenture

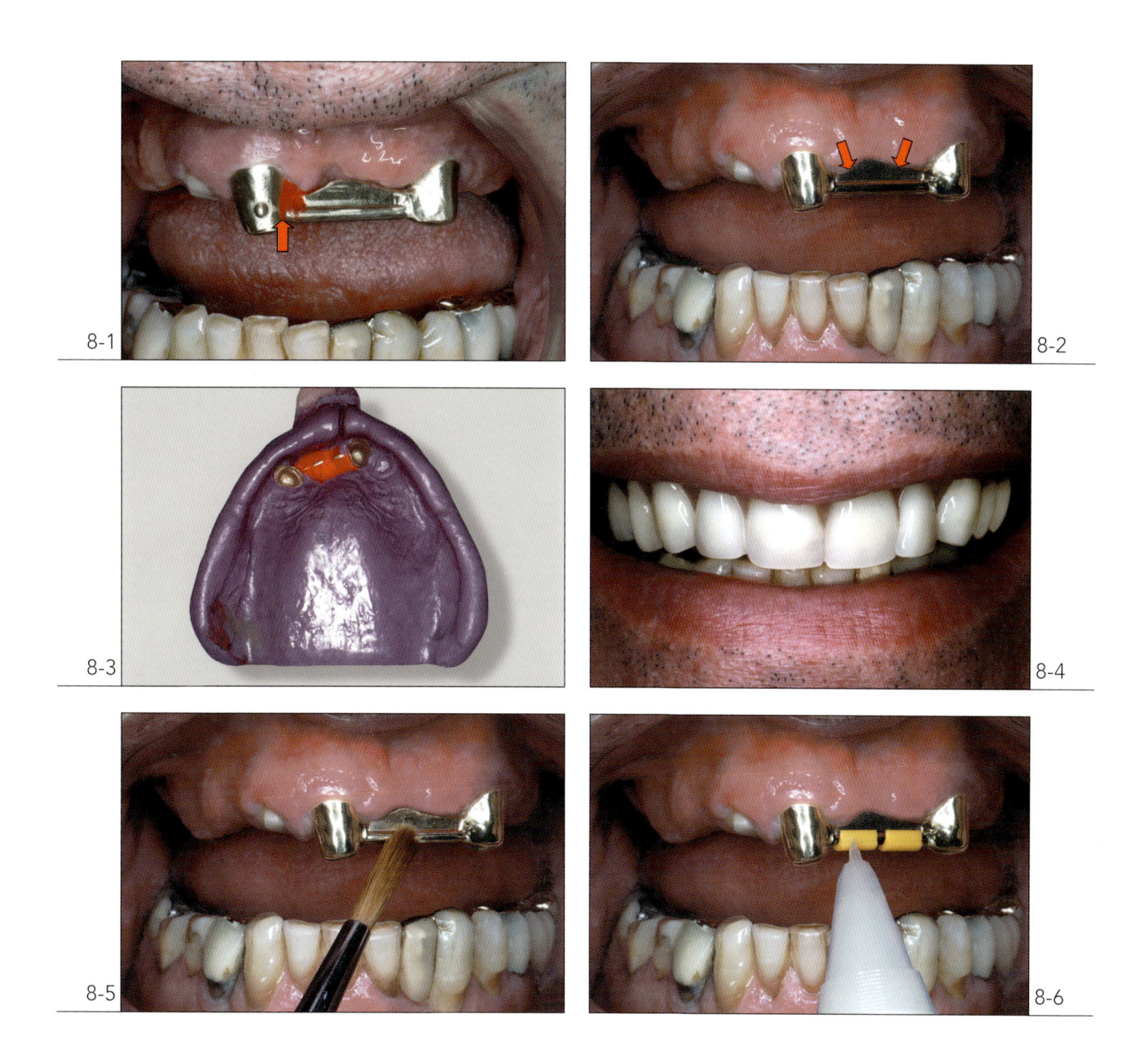

Attachment of retention clips to the denture base

Because of space limitations, it is usually necessary to use acrylic anterior teeth (Fig 8-4). The denture is processed with adequate relief over the bar and copings, using the hydrocolloid flasking technique to simplify removal. The copings and bar should be temporarily cemented and the denture allowed to settle without the retention clips attached. The occlusion may require adjustment; if so, this should be accomplished before the retention clips are attached. The copings and bar should not be permanently cemented until the clips have been attached to the denture base.

The copings and bar are thoroughly coated with oil as a safety precaution (Fig 8-5). The retention clips are seated on the bar, and one drop of cyanoacrylate is placed on the exposed occlusal surface of the clips (Fig 8-6).

Implant-Supported Clip Bar Overdenture

Even if a computerized tomography (CT) scan is available and the bone is adequate and compact, controlled placement of the implants using a surgical guide is advisable for a mandibular implant-supported clip bar overdenture for the following reasons: *(1)* The biomechanic forces produced by the location of the anterior teeth are affected by implant location (see chapters 4 and 5); *(2)* the bulk resulting from poor placement of the bar can cause serious esthetic problems; and *(3)* long-term prognosis is improved when a surgical guide is used. Treatment using an implant-supported clip bar overdenture is more complicated than the treatment modalities previously presented; therefore, step-by-step laboratory, surgical, and prosthetic clinical procedures are presented in the following sections.

Provisional complete dentures

The provisional dentures play an important role in the fabrication of the surgical guide and thus in the orientation of the implants, which will subsequently affect the success and esthetics of the final result. Therefore, a full denture setup is accomplished using denture bases on split-mounted final casts (Fig 8-17). The vertical dimension is preserved with the incisal pin on the table (see Fig 8-17, *arrow*). The waxed up dentures are tried in clinically and the esthetics and occlusion evaluated (Fig 8-18). A wrought-metal lingual bar (Fig 8-19) is waxed up in the mandibular denture to provide strength for subsequent procedures. The mandibular cast is invested in a flask (Fig 8-20), and a hydrocolloid pour is accomplished in the upper member (Fig 8-21). The same process is carried out for the maxillary denture (without the reinforcing bar), and the completed dentures are positioned intraorally and the occlusion adjusted (Fig 8-22).

Autostabilized denture bases

Three-dimensional surgical guides,[1-3] as described in chapter 6, require natural teeth or so-called immediate implants (not used in the prosthesis) to serve as fixed references from which radiographic and surgical guides can be related and firmly stabilized. When neither is available, special laboratory procedures can create *autostabilized* denture bases. In other words, the maxillary and mandibular denture bases stabilize themselves in vivo without clinical assistance. This can be accomplished if a removable physical connection (attached only to the maxillary denture base) is fabricated between the two denture bases when they are in a wide-open position. The only clinical problem is establishing sufficient space anteriorly between the maxillary and mandibular denture bases to facilitate surgical procedures.

Fabrication of the surgical guides

Duplicate clear acrylic dentures are processed on the same casts used to make the provisional dentures. The clear maxillary denture base is reduced anteriorly to 2 mm in thickness up to the second premolar bilaterally (Fig 8-23, *arrows*). The mandibular clear denture will serve as the surgical guide. A reinforcing lingual bar (*arrows*), similar to that processed in the provisional mandibular denture, was also processed into the clear duplicate denture (Fig 8-24). This permits the clear acrylic between the midlines of the second premolars to be removed, with the exception of a strut reduced to 3 mm in width that extends labially from the lingual bar to support an incisal tooth (see Fig 8-24).

Implant-Supported Clip Bar Overdenture

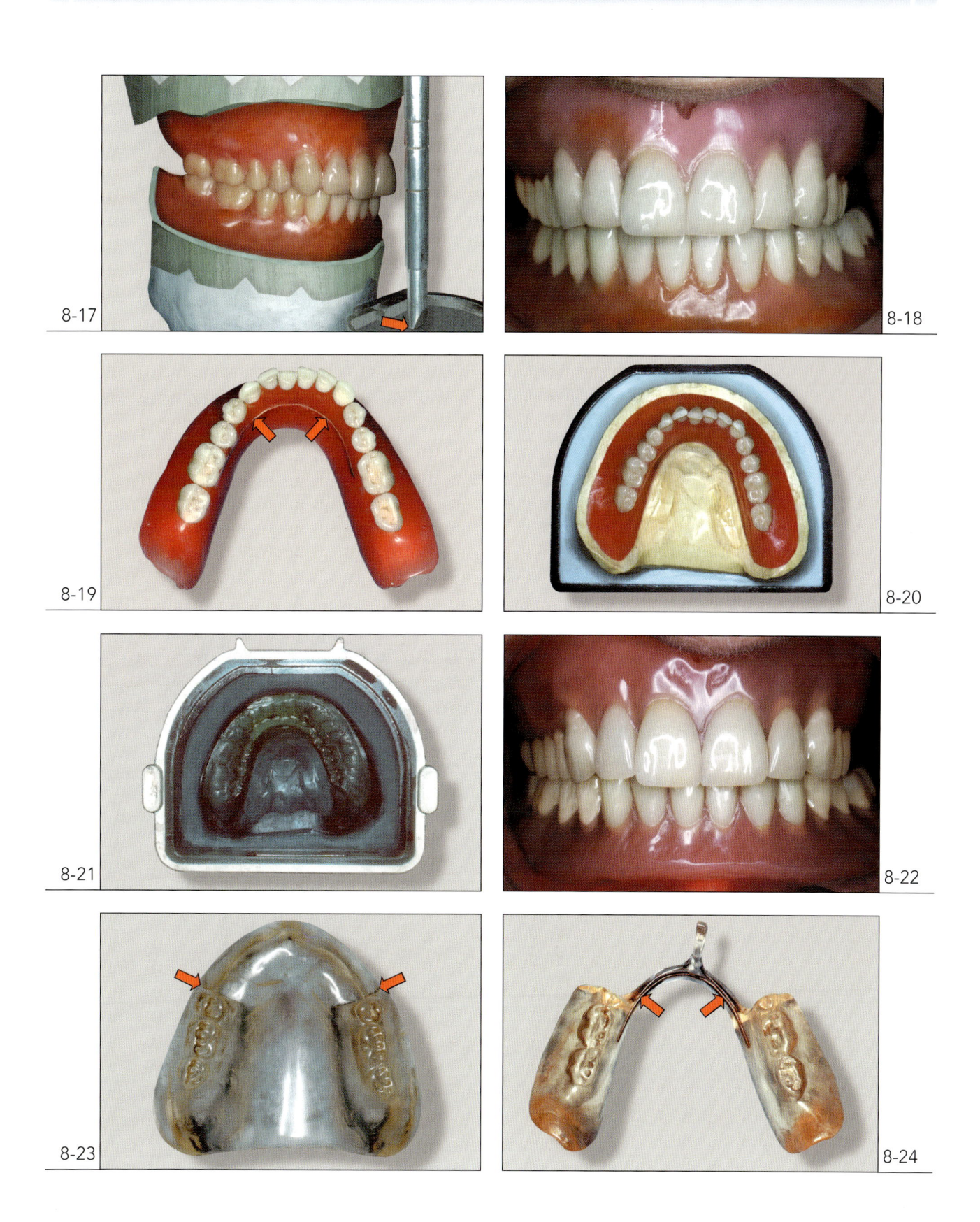

8-17

8-18

8-19

8-20

8-21

8-22

8-23

8-24

127

Intraoral records

The modified maxillary and mandibular dentures can be hand articulated. The lingual bar (*arrows*) connects the posterior segments of the mandibular surgical guide (Fig 8-25). The modified denture bases are placed intraorally, and stability is confirmed (Fig 8-26). Compound centric relation records are obtained at a comfortable wide-open vertical dimension (Fig 8-27). The modified dentures are hand articulated and luted together (*arrows*) with the compound centric relation records (Fig 8-28).

Mounting procedures and buccal strut fabrication

The assembled modified dentures with the compound centric relation records are mounted on a suitable instrument with an incisal pin (*arrow*) to maintain the increased vertical dimension (Fig 8-29). The compound centric relation records are removed, and buccal vertical struts (*arrows*) are fabricated in self-curing acrylic resin (Fig 8-30). These vertical struts are attached only to the maxillary denture and occlude with the reproduced occlusal anatomy of the posterior portions of the mandibular modified denture, providing excellent occlusal interlocking stability (Fig 8-31, *arrows*). This configuration creates more than adequate interocclusal space for surgical procedures on the anterior mandibular arch.

Diagnostic factors

Most often the bone in the anterior area of the mandible is compact, and the anatomic pitfalls that present themselves in other areas of the mouth (ie, nerves and sinuses) are not present. Moreover, the biomechanical requirements of an implant-supported overdenture are not as critical as those associated with an osseointegrated porcelain-fused-to-metal prosthesis[4,5] (see chapters 4 and 5). Therefore, the three-dimensional surgical guidance system described in chapter 6 usually is not required. However, as a precautionary measure, a full diagnostic workup, including a CT scan,[3] is required (Fig 8-32). In some rare overdenture cases or when a porcelain prosthesis is planned, three widely separated "immediate" implants can be inserted in nonstrategic areas to anchor the radiographic and surgical guides (as described in chapter 6). At the conclusion of the first-stage surgical procedure to place the implants for the prosthesis, these stabilizing implants are removed.

Implant-Supported Clip Bar Overdenture

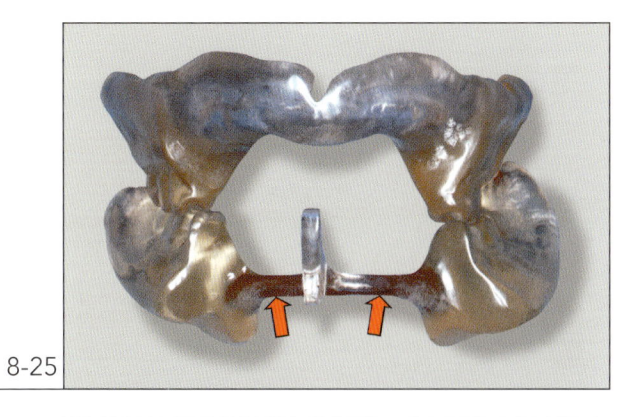

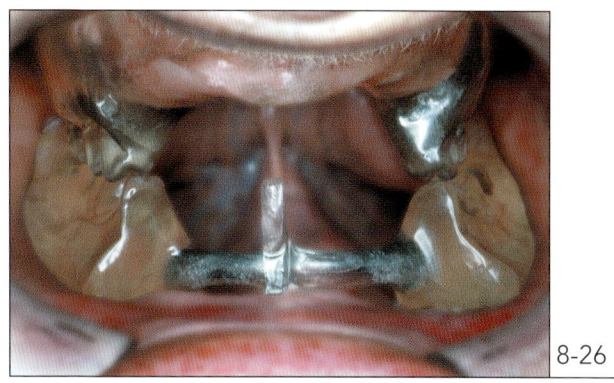

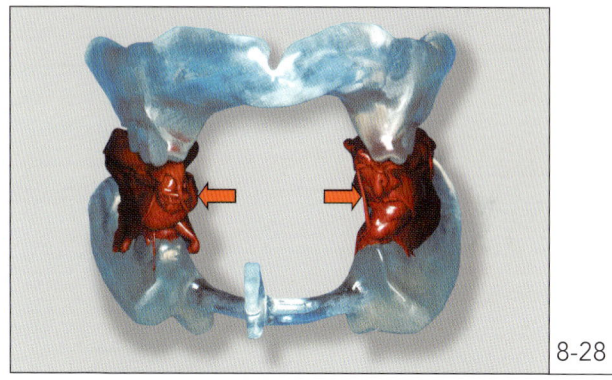

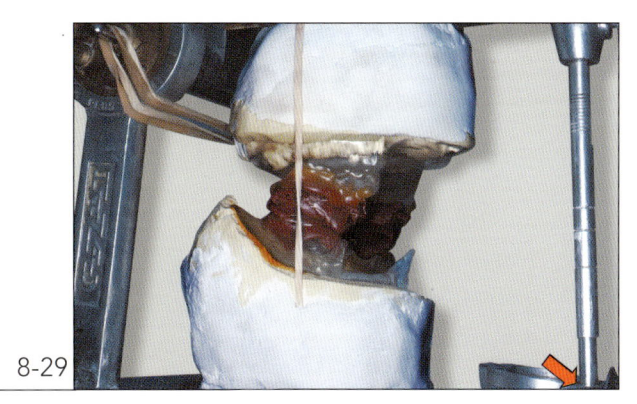

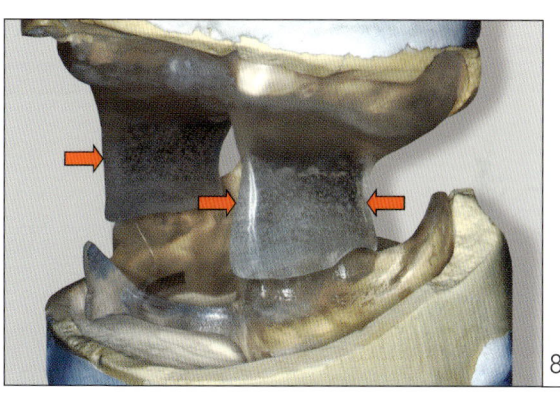

8-25

8-26

8-27

8-28

8-29

8-30

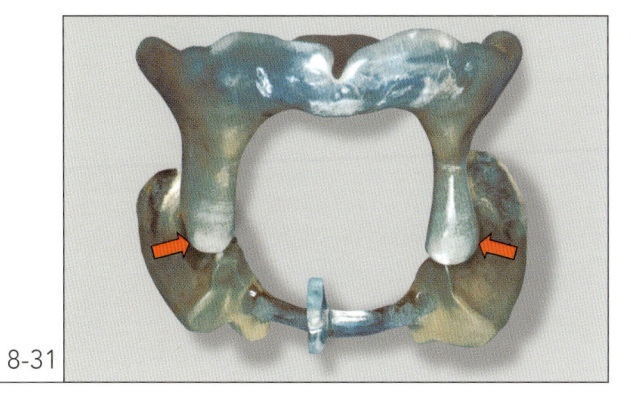

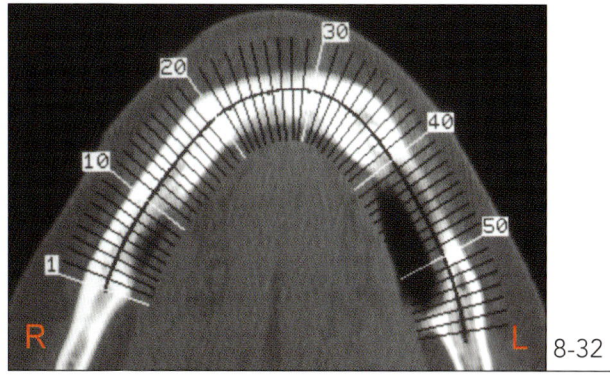

8-31

8-32

129

First-stage surgery

The modified dentures are inserted and tested for stability, first individually and then in occlusion in the wide-open position. Stability of the modified mandibular denture (surgical guide) is essential. To begin, both modified dentures are removed to facilitate reflection of the mandibular soft tissue. The maxillary modified denture is then re-inserted first, followed by the mandibular surgical guide (Fig 8-33). Often the lingual bar can be used to hold the reflected soft tissue out of the surgical field. Note how the vertical struts stabilize the mandibular surgical guide and provide excellent access to the surgical field (see Fig 8-33). The surgical guide is stabilized almost as effectively as if natural teeth were being used.

The first osteotomy is initiated adjacent to the long strut (*arrow*) connected to the lingual bar (Fig 8-34). The three-dimensional position of this strut on a stabilized base provides the surgeon with the anteriormost reference for the implants near the midline. The posteriormost landmark is the cross section of the second premolars bilaterally (see Figs 8-24 and 8-33). These landmarks form a curve (*red line*) representing the positions of the mandibular anterior teeth (Fig 8-35). The two central implants are placed first, followed by the posteriormost implants (see Fig 8-35). The remaining implants are then positioned using these central and posterior implants as guides (Fig 8-36).

Postsurgical soft tissue treatment

As discussed previously, a lingual bar was processed in the mandibular denture (see Fig 8-19) to provide strength for the extensive tissue surface relief that is required after first-stage surgery. The dentures are placed intraorally to confirm sufficient relief and stability (Fig 8-37). Soft tissue conditioning material is added to the mandibular denture, which is seated, placed in occlusion, and border molded. Any pressure areas that are revealed through the soft reline material should be generously relieved (Fig 8-38). It is advisable to remove all the soft tissue reline material and repeat the process. Figure 8-39 shows the 6-month postoperative view.

Second-stage surgery

A flap is created to expose the implants. Careful placement of the abutments is critical to prevent future problems with soft tissue impingement between the implant-abutment interfaces. An abutment holder should be used to seat the abutment, which is rotated to confirm the engagement of the hexes. Only then is the abutment screw inserted and tightened. Most often a panoramic radiograph is used to confirm seating; however, in the author's opinion, the level of detail provided by this technique is not adequate for this essential step. Therefore, use of standard periapical intraoral radiographs is preferred. The healing caps are positioned with a hex driver (Fig 8-40), and the denture is refitted to accommodate the vertical increase in height.

Implant-Supported Clip Bar Overdenture

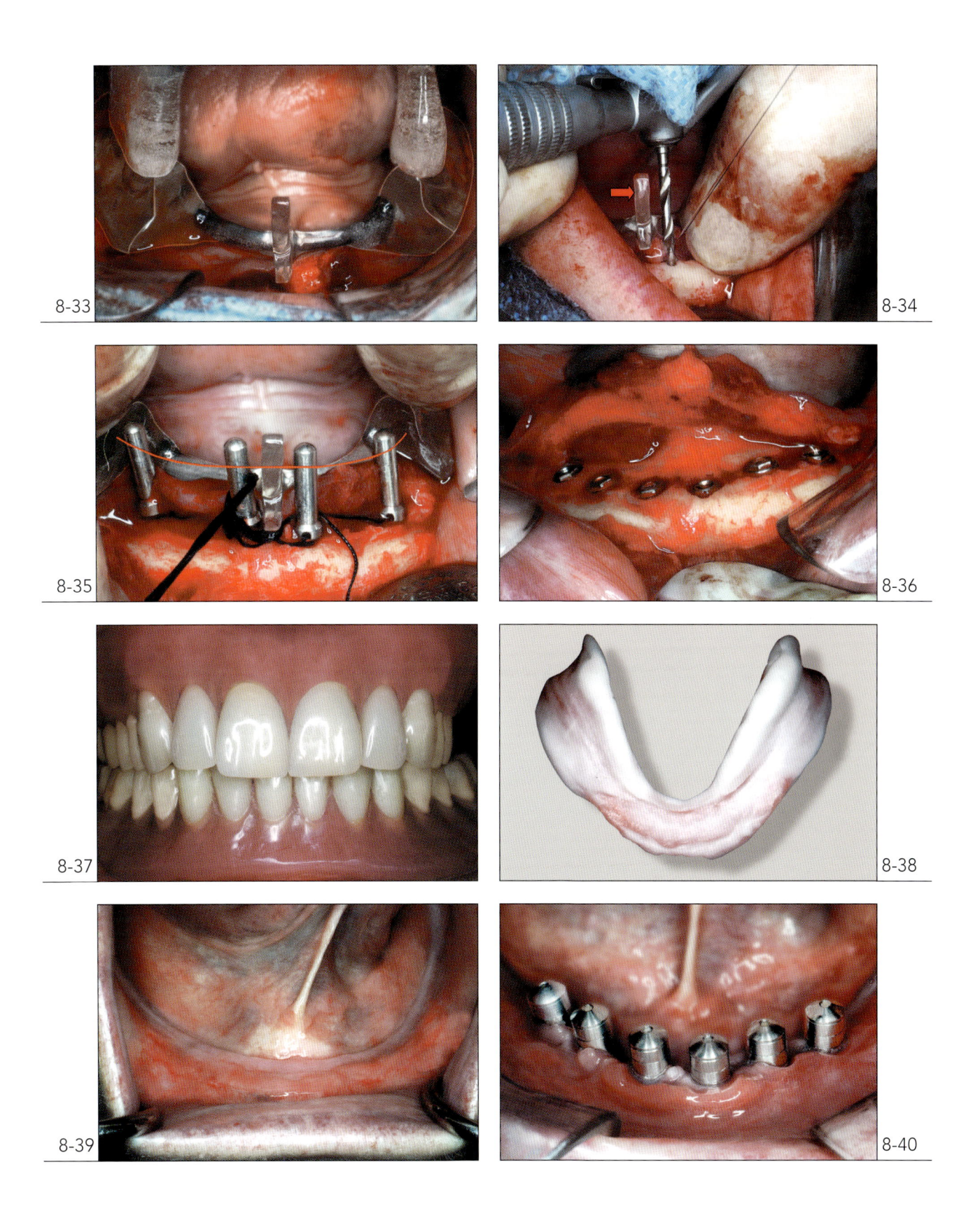

8-33

8-34

8-35

8-36

8-37

8-38

8-39

8-40

Soft tissue treatment

The need for the reinforcing lingual bar should be apparent at this stage of treatment. Extensive relief is now required to provide space for the abutments and healing caps. Disclosing wax helps to confirm sufficient relief as well as the relative stability of the mandibular denture and its occlusion with the maxillary denture. Soft tissue treatment material is used to reline the denture (Fig 8-41). As a general rule, this process should be repeated every other week for 6 to 8 weeks before the final impression is obtained, but the clinician should revise this regimen depending on the needs of the individual patient. All patients initially should be placed on a liquid diet; subsequently, soft foods can be gradually introduced.

Final impression

Impression copings, which transfer the orientation of the abutments to the cast, are placed over the abutments before the impression is taken and remain in place when the impression is removed (Fig 8-42). These copings are then repositioned in the impression to receive the abutment analogs before the cast is poured.

Tapered impression copings may have one of two different configurations, depending on the type of abutment used. If the abutment has a universal circular interface (ie, there are no interlocking interfaces between the abutment and the gold cylinder) (see Fig 8-42), the master impression will receive nonspecific (universal) impression copings (Fig 8-43) because the orientation of the copings in the impression is not important. On the other hand, if the abutment has a nonrotational female hex interface, then an impression coping with an interlocking male interface must be used.[6] This type of impression coping has a notched external surface that transfers its specific orientation to the impression. In this way, proper orientation of the coping in the impression, and thus proper orientation of the abutment analogs, is ensured.

Master cast and records

Once the impression copings are repositioned in the impression, brass abutment analogs are screwed into position and the cast is poured. Gold cylinders are positioned on the abutment analogs with gold screws (Fig 8-44). A denture base is fabricated on the cast and held in position by the gold cylinders, as shown through the superimposition of the denture base in Fig 8-45. Gold screws are used to position the denture base intraorally, and it is then tested for stability (Fig 8-46). The vertical dimension (Fig 8-47, VD) is obtained in black soft wax and subsequently reduced 2 mm to provide space for the wax centric relation record (CR). Wax occlusion rims are placed and reduced to this vertical dimension. Green occlusal recording wax is softened and flowed onto the occlusal surfaces of the posterior denture bases. The opposing occlusal surfaces are lubricated and the patient guided into centric relation closure to the predetermined vertical dimension (see Fig 8-47, VD). The centric relation record (CR) is chilled, and the denture base is removed, ready for mounting.

Laboratory procedures

Mounting
The mandibular cast is split-mounted on a semi-adjustable articulator with an incisal pin (Fig 8-48) to confirm and maintain the centric relation record transfer (CR) at the planned vertical dimension of occlusion (VD).

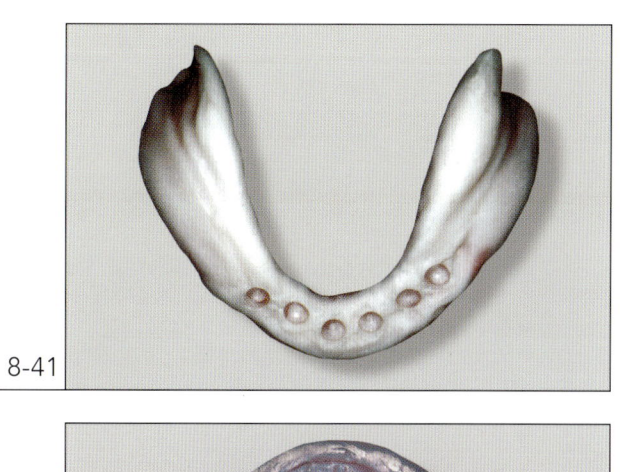

Implant-Supported Clip Bar Overdenture

8-41

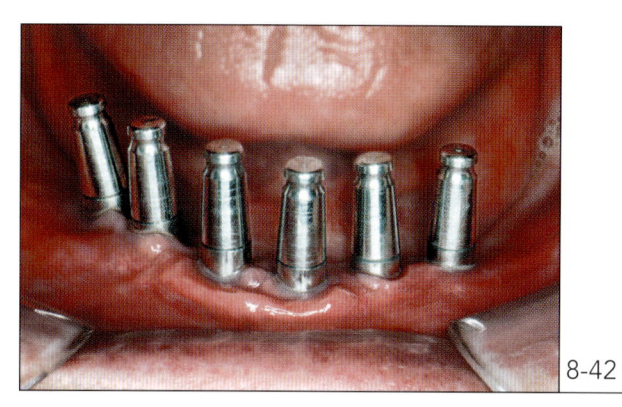

8-42

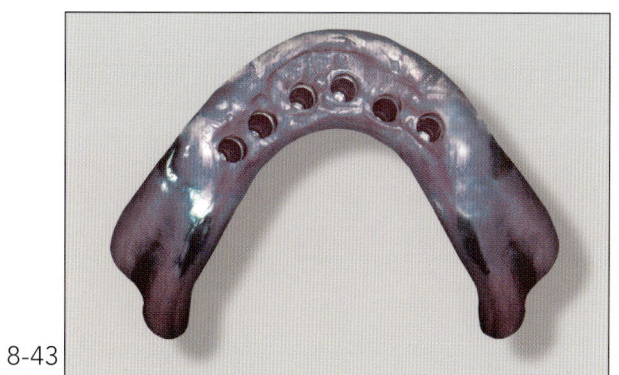

8-43

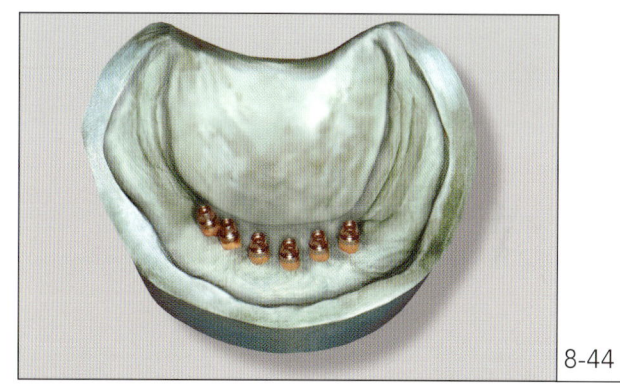

8-44

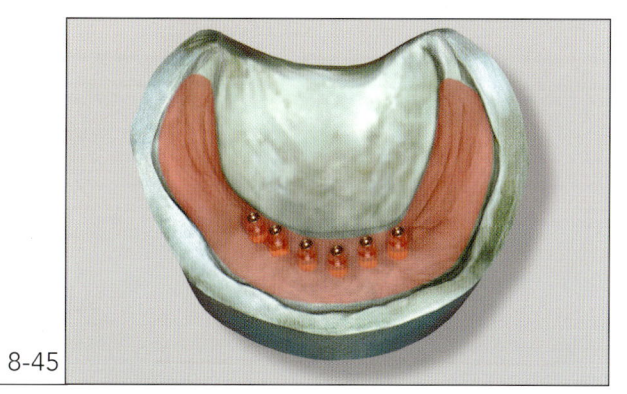

8-45

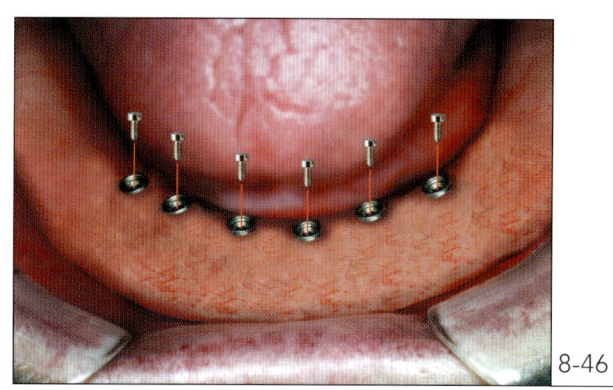

8-46

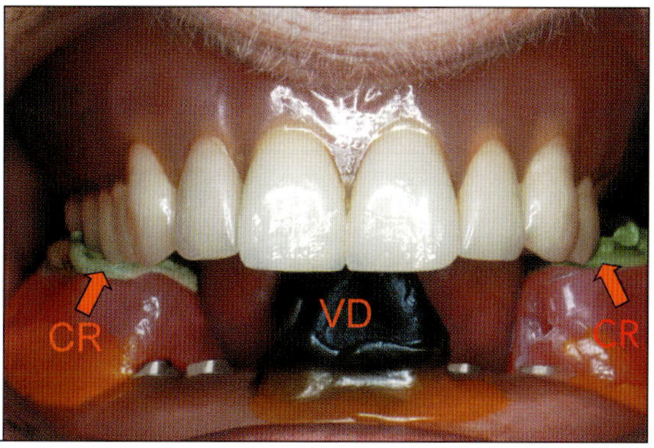

8-47

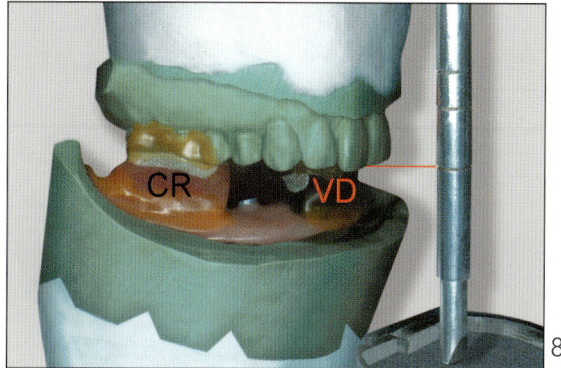

8-48

133

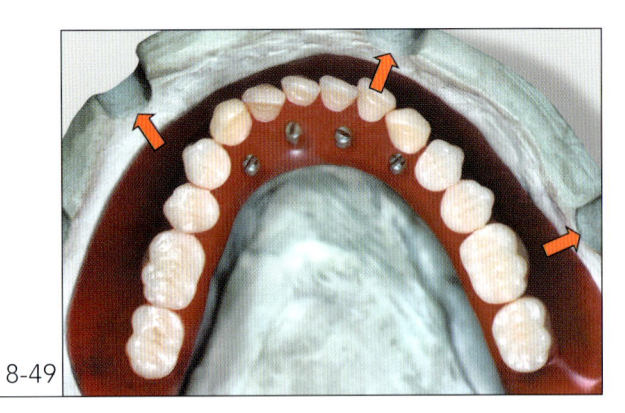

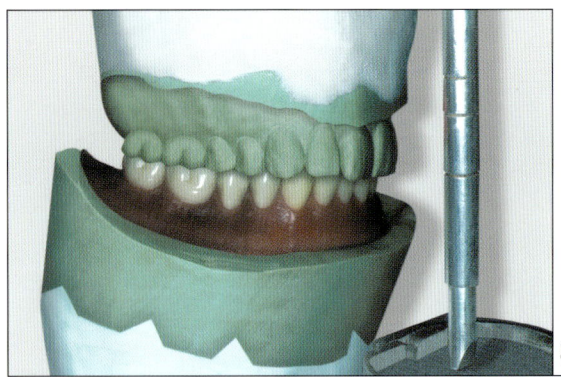

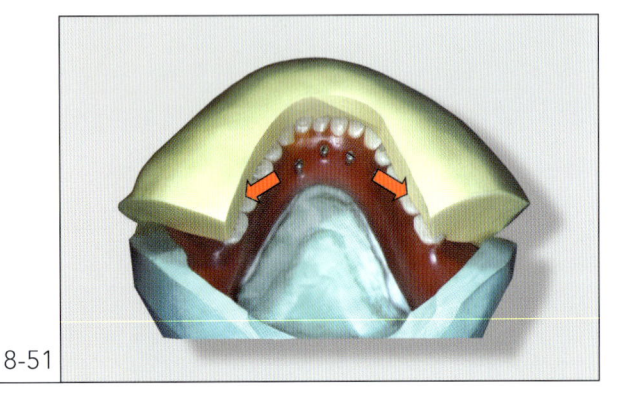

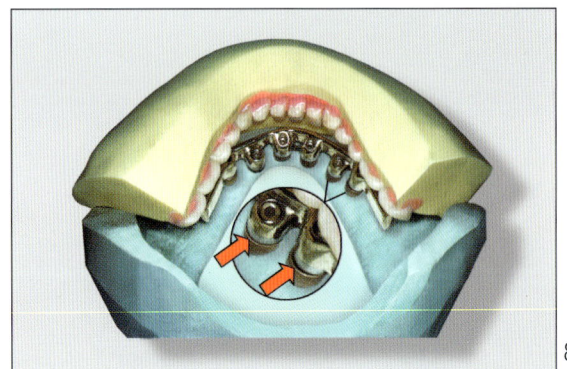

8 | Clinical Procedures for Tooth- and Implant-Supported Overdentures and Fixed-Retrievable Prostheses

8-49

8-50

8-51

8-52

Setup
The mandibular acrylic teeth are set up on the denture base. The denture base is stabilized on the cast using gold screws (Fig 8-49). (Note that lingual access channels are required to maintain access to the gold screws.) The mandibular cast is split-mounted on the articulator to facilitate all subsequent laboratory procedures (Fig 8-50). A cross occlusion is used[4,7] to reduce the posterior forces of occlusion on the implants and supporting bone (see Fig 8-50; for discussion, see Fig 8-69 and chapters 4 and 5).

Occlusal index
Notches (*arrows*) are placed on the stone border of the master cast (see Fig 8-49) to provide guidance for the occlusal index, which is obtained in polysiloxane modeling putty. The elastic occlusal index is trimmed to expose the lingual half of the acrylic teeth (Fig 8-51, *arrows*).

Fabrication of the clip bar
The clip bar is waxed up to the gold cylinders and cast in one piece. (Note that, as shown in the inset in Fig 8-52, discrepancies in the interface between the gold cylinders and the abutment analogs on the cast [*arrows*] often occur and require correction.) The clip bar is sectioned at strategic locations between each abutment to avoid interference with the bar configuration during repositioning and soldering procedures, which would affect the retention clips (Fig 8-53).

Assemblage procedures

As discussed earlier, when standard abutments are used there are no interlocking interfaces between the abutment and the gold cylinder (see chapter 9 for nonrotational designs). Therefore, when the sections of the clip bar are seated and the gold

Implant-Supported Clip Bar Overdenture

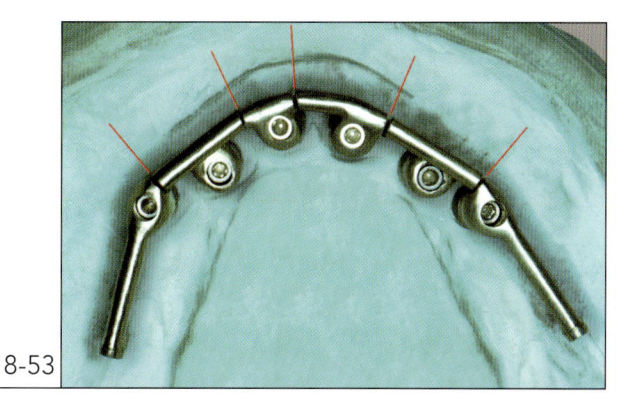

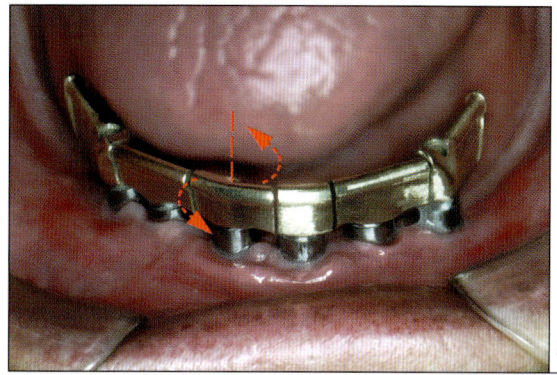

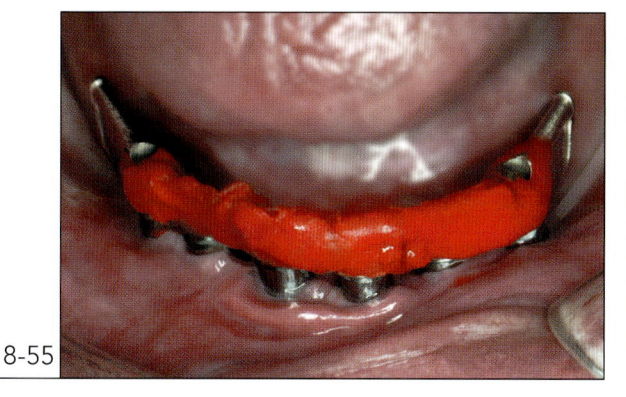

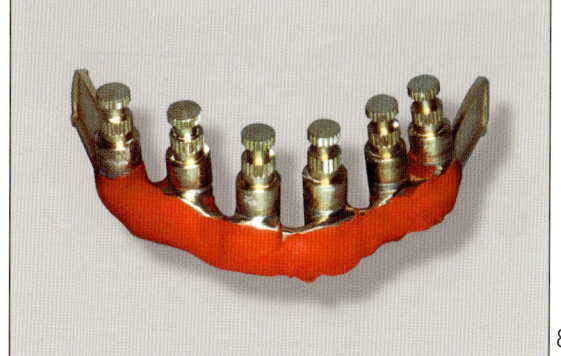

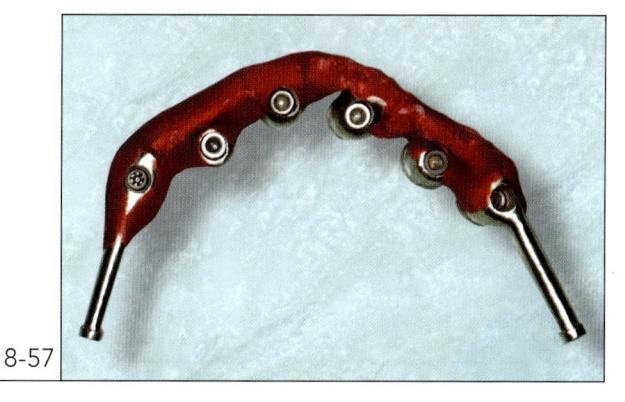

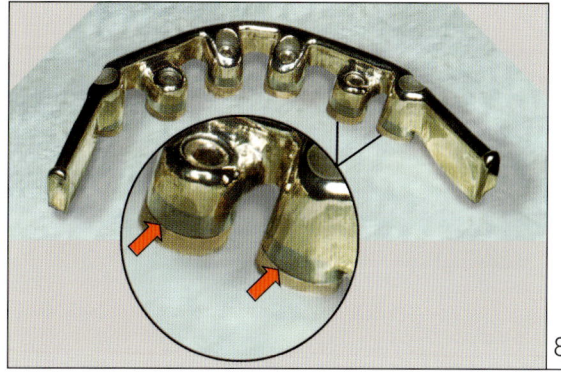

Figs 8-53 to 8-58

screws tightened, each individual section can rotate buccolingually (*arrows*) around the vertical axis of the gold screw (Fig 8-54). An acrylic index can be constructed to prevent this rotation (although the author prefers to use nonrotating abutments to eliminate this problem). Once all the interfaces have been confirmed clinically, the index is completed by painting Duralay acrylic around the entire bar while maintaining access to the gold screws (Fig 8-55).

Laboratory procedures

Abutment analogs are seated against the gold cylinders, and the gold screws are tightened (Fig 8-56). The assembled sections are invested in plaster (Fig 8-57). Before the soldering procedure, 1 mm of clearance should be provided between the abutment-cylinder interface and the plaster (Fig 8-58). The assemblage soldering technique follows standard procedures and is designed to correct the improper interface fit between the gold cylinders and the abutment analogs (see Fig 8-52, *inset*). The completed bar and the corrected abutment-cylinder interface (*inset*) are shown in Fig 8-58.

Intraoral placement

The assembled clip bar is seated intraorally to confirm passive fit (Fig 8-59), and the gold screws are tightened. All the observable interfaces are examined and periapical radiographs are taken to confirm the integrity of the implant-abutment interfaces (Fig 8-60, *arrows*).

Completion of the prosthesis

Framework construction

Even when corrections have been made (see Fig 8-58), most often the framework will fit acceptably on the master cast (Fig 8-61). When the discrepancies are too great, the technician must remove stone around the involved abutment analogs to free them from the cast, then reattach them in the appropriate position. A nonprecious metal framework is cast. This framework contains finger-like projections that fit over the clip bar (Fig 8-62) without interfering with placement of the clips (Fig 8-63).

Acrylic processing

With the assembled framework in place over the clip bar, the occlusal index containing the acrylic teeth is repositioned on the cast to confirm correct positioning of all components (Fig 8-64). The acrylic is processed at the laboratory bench without flask investment (Fig 8-65). The gingival view in Fig 8-66 shows the positioning of the nylon clips. (It is important to emphasize that clinical retention of the prosthesis requires only three widely separated clips. For stability, more clips were placed in the prosthesis shown in Fig 8-66. The technician will have to relieve the inside of many of the clips; otherwise, it will be difficult to remove the prosthesis from the cast and from the clip bar intraorally.)

Implant-Supported Clip Bar Overdenture

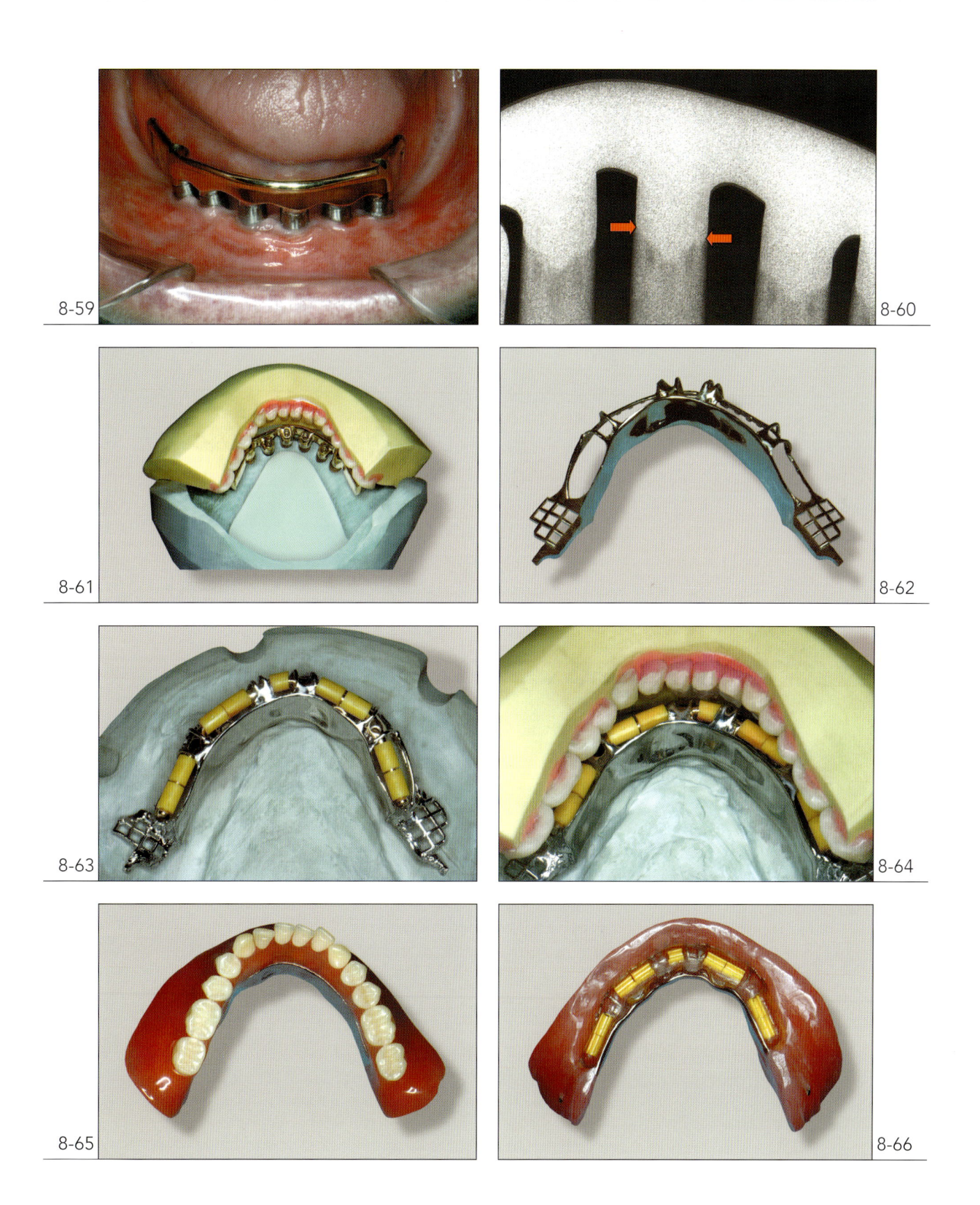

8-59

8-60

8-61

8-62

8-63

8-64

8-65

8-66

137

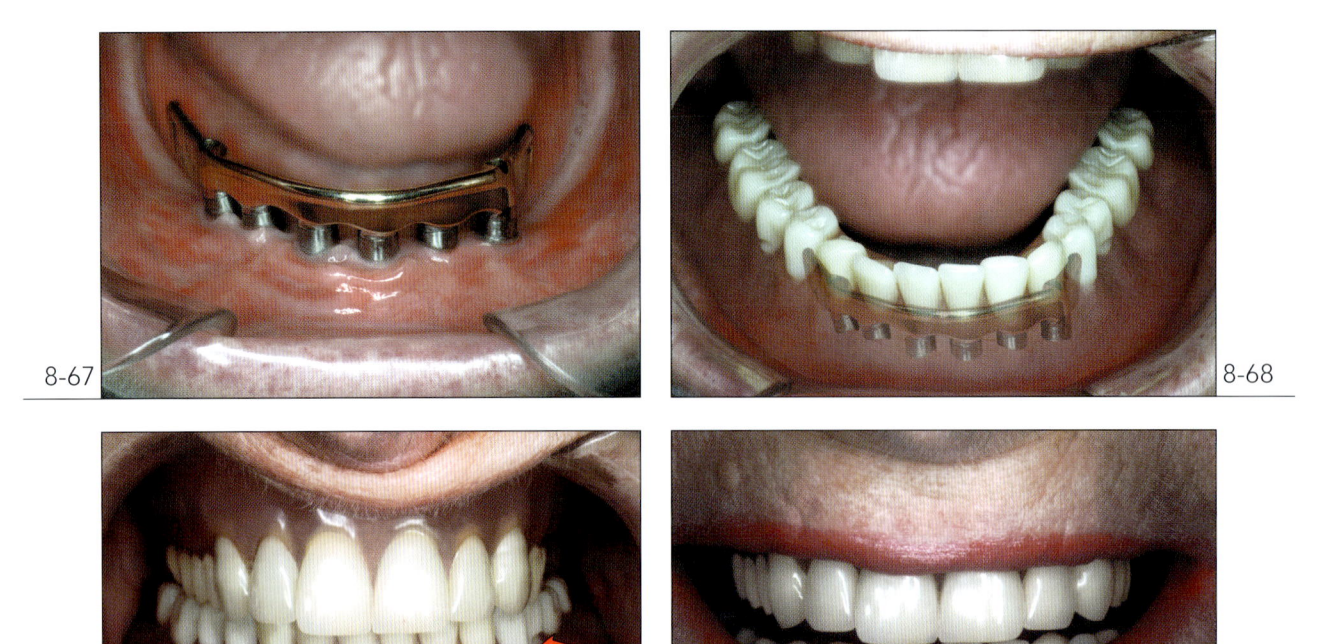

8 | Clinical Procedures for Tooth- and Implant-Supported Overdentures and Fixed-Retrievable Prostheses

Insertion of the final clip bar prosthesis

After the tightness of the abutment screws is confirmed, the clip bar is positioned on the abutments, and clinical and radiographic confirmation of proper interface fit is repeated (Fig 8-67). The finished prosthesis is firmly seated over the clip bar. The relationship between the clip bar and the seated prosthesis is illustrated by the superimposed image in Fig 8-68.

The occlusion is confirmed, and bilateral notches (*arrows*) are placed at the gingival aspect of the second premolars to make it easier for the patient to remove the prosthesis (Fig 8-69). Bilateral cross occlusion is usually recommended with advanced cases of alveolar atrophy[4,8–10] (see Fig 8-69 and discussion in chapter 5). The final esthetic result is illustrated in Fig 8-70.

Summary

Although there are some who feel that a surgical guide is not necessary for the placement of implants that support a mandibular clip bar prosthesis because of the quality of the bone, absence of critical hazards, and moderate occlusal forces, the author maintains that preplanning the optimum location of the implants will reduce implant loading and improve the esthetic result, the comfort of the final prosthesis, and the prognosis. In the author's experience, most patients are extremely pleased with the retention and stability that is achieved with a clip bar implant-supported overdenture that is constructed using the techniques presented in this chapter. This patient response is one of the most rewarding experiences in clinical practice, particularly because many of these patients have been struggling with a mandibular full denture and the associated negative impact on self-image for many years.

References

1. Weinberg LA, Kruger B. Three-dimensional guidance system for implant insertion: Part I. Implant Dent 1998;7:81–93.
2. Weinberg LA, Kruger B. Three-dimensional guidance system for implant insertion: Part II. Dual axes table—Problem solving. Implant Dent 1999;8:225–264.
3. Weinberg LA. CT scan as a radiologic data base for optimum implant orientation. J Prosthet Dent 1993;69:381–383.
4. Weinberg LA. Reduction of implant loading with therapeutic biomechanics. Implant Dent 1998;7:277–285.
5. Weinberg LA, Kruger B. Biomechanical considerations when combining tooth-supported and implant-supported prostheses. Oral Surg Oral Med Oral Pathol 1994;78:22–27.
6. Weinberg LA. Clinical utilization of non-rotational capability in osseointegrated prostheses. Int J Oral Maxillofac Implants 1994;9:326–332.
7. Weinberg LA. The biomechanics of force distribution in implant-supported prostheses. Int J Oral Maxillofac Implants 1993;8:19–31.
8. Weinberg LA. Reduction of implant loading using a modified centric occlusal anatomy. Int J Prosthodont 1998;11:55–69.
9. Gysi A, Clapp GW. Practical application of research results in denture construction (mandibular movements). J Am Dent Assoc 1929;16:199–223.
10. Weinberg LA, Kruger B. A comparison of implant/prosthesis loading with four clinical variables. Int J Prosthodont 1995;8:421–433.

9 Clinical Problems

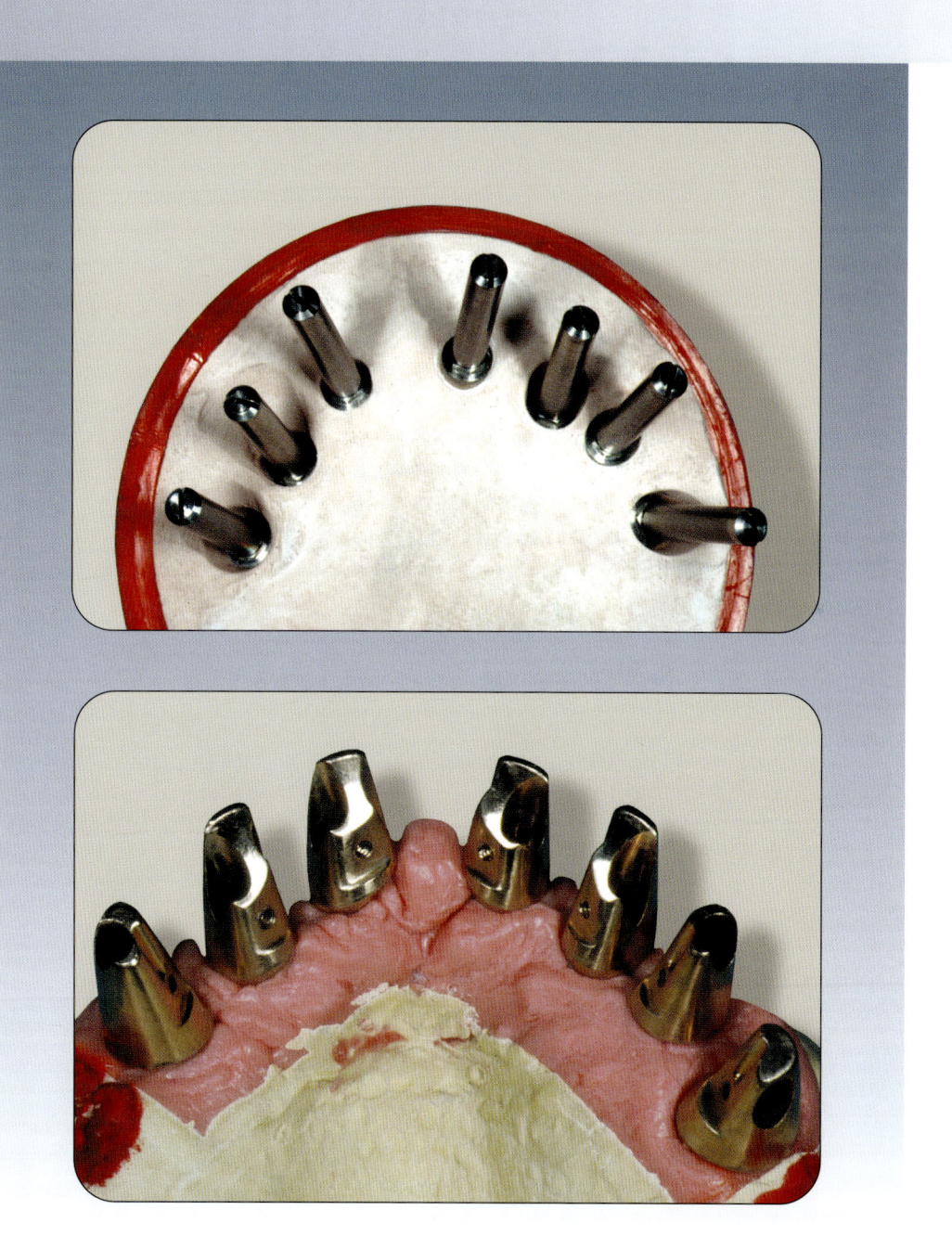

9 | Clinical Problems

It is appropriate to address clinical problems near the end of an atlas, where the myriad clinical variations and microtechnical details can be placed within a broader conceptual framework. To do otherwise would be to emphasize the trees and lose sight of the forest. An implant-supported prosthesis is the most technique sensitive of all restorative procedures in dentistry. Moreover, the increased demand for improved esthetics and the need for single-tooth restorations have led to a variety of original abutment designs, and some of these have been associated with specific clinical problems. Tooth-supported porcelain-fused-to-metal prostheses also have clinical problems associated with breakage and gingival impingement due to the location of the solder joint.

This chapter revisits some of the topics presented in previous chapters for the purpose of arming the reader with information (derived through trial and error) on how to avoid these types of clinical problems. The following topics will be addressed: *(1)* basic implant and abutment designs and alternative restorative concepts; *(2)* prosthesis construction; *(3)* rotational and nonrotational components; *(4)* compensating for implant divergence; *(5)* evolution of clinical procedures and armamentarium; *(6)* UCLA, CeraOne, and EsthetiCone abutments; *(7)* abutment-selection process; *(8)* maintenance and reproduction of gingival contours; *(9)* impression accuracy; *(10)* provisional and final osseointegrated prostheses; and *(11)* modified coping designs for porcelain-fused-to-metal (tooth-supported) restorations and anterior teeth.

Whereas previous chapters relied on generic terms as much as possible, in this chapter special abutment designs developed to solve esthetic problems require the use of brand name armamentaria. Nevertheless, it is important to remember that while implant designs undergo continual change, surface coatings evolve, and companies remain in flux, the generic market will always be a source for clinical alternatives.

Basic Implant and Abutment Designs and Alternative Restorative Concepts

Implants

There are two basic implant configurations (Fig 9-1): cylindrical (A, C) and screw-type (B). In addition, most implants are made with one of the three most common types of surfaces: plasma-sprayed titanium (A), which increases the surface area through its granular surface; machine-finished titanium (B), which is used mostly for screw-type implants; and hydroxyapatite (C), which is intended to increase osseointegration (see Fig 9-1).

Abutment screws

At second-stage surgery, the abutment (Fig 9-2, B) is placed on the implant (C) and held in position with the abutment screw (A). Abutment screws are generally made of titanium; however, there has been a recent increase in the use of special gold alloy screws, which offer greater control of torque application (usually electronically or mechanically driven) to reduce the incidence of loosening and thus increase the preloading force. (*Preloading force* is derived from the tightening of an abutment screw to bring two surfaces together.) When the preloading force of the abutment screw is sufficient, the resultant lateral occlusal forces are distributed directly to the abutment-implant interface rather than to the abutment screw.[1] Conversely, when the preloading force of the abutment screw is insufficient, the resultant inclined occlusal forces are distributed directly to the abutment screw itself, which can loosen or break as a result.

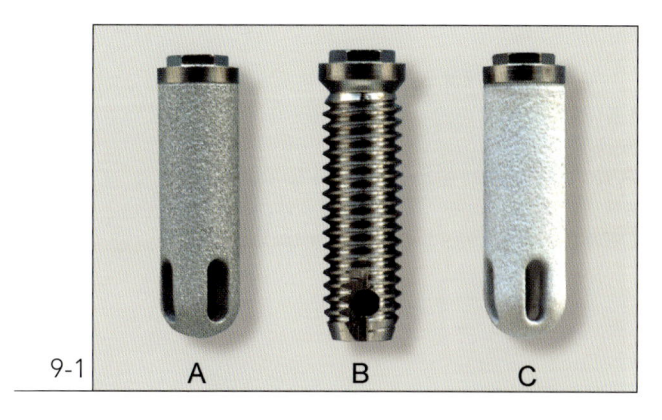

Basic Implant and Abutment Designs and Alternative Restorative Concepts

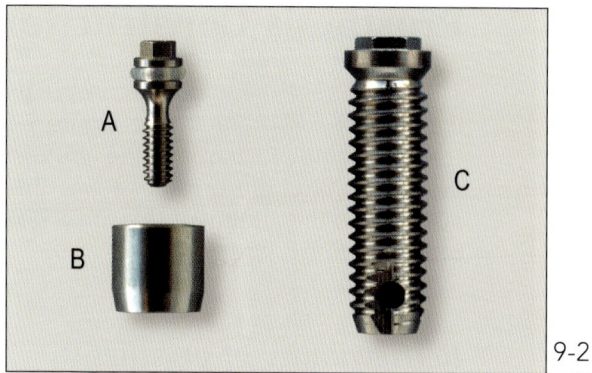

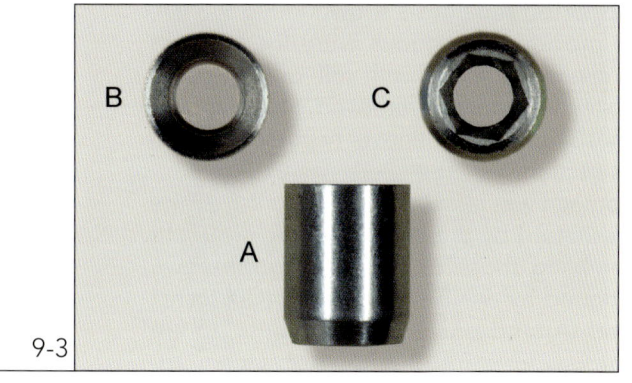

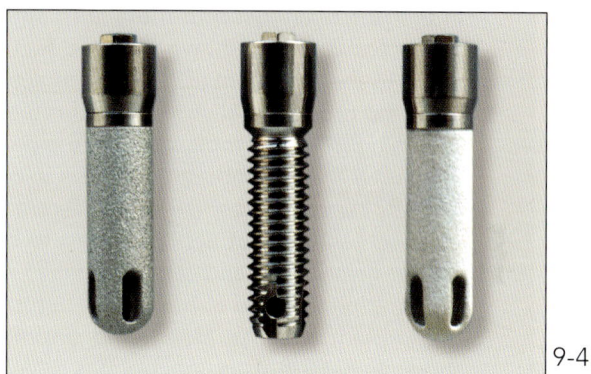

This concept applies to any interface held together by a retaining screw: Interlocking elements increase resistance to screw loosening or breakage, while poor interface fit increases damage to the retaining screw.

Abutments

As shown in Fig 9-2, the simplest abutment is cylindrical in shape (B) and is designed to fit over the male hex of the implant (C). The length of the abutment varies (Fig 9-3, A) depending on the thickness of the gingiva, esthetics, and available space. Figure 9-3 shows a common abutment configuration, which has a circular (rotational) surface (B) that connects with the prosthesis and a female hex (nonrotational) surface (C) that interlocks with the male hex of the implant (see Fig 9-2, C). A variety of abutments are manufactured to interface with any implant design and surface coating (Fig 9-4).

143

9 Clinical Problems

Nonrotating square impresssion copings

In Fig 9-10, the nonrotating square impression coping (A) has a male hex on the abutment interface (*arrow*), whereas the standard square impression coping (B) does not. A tapered impression coping that remains on the abutment after impression removal can also be designed to be nonrotating providing it has *(1)* a female hex on the abutment interface, *(2)* a short retaining screw, and *(3)* an external notched surface that will transfer the orientation of the implant hex to the impression.

When there is inadequate vertical space or when esthetic problems require that no abutment be used, square or tapered impression copings for the implant head are available. Each must have a female hex at the implant interface. Special esthetic clinical problems and their solutions are discussed in considerable detail later in the chapter.

Impression procedures

Because square copings remain embedded in the impression material, the impression tray must have an access hole opposite each implant site (Fig 9-11, *arrow*). It is advisable to provide more than adequate clearance, as well as tissue stops in three separate areas, to ensure proper seating of the tray. The custom impression tray should be tried in the mouth to confirm stability and proper relief around the impression copings (Fig 9-12).

Heavy-bodied elastomeric impression material is used in the tray, and thin-bodied elastomeric impression material is injected around the gingival margins and copings. Once the tray is loaded and seated, the guide pins should be located with the finger before the material has time to set (Fig 9-13). The hardened impression material is cut away from the guide pins, and the guide pins are loosened, as described in chapter 7 (see Fig 7-10), and the impression is removed from the mouth.

The brass analog for each nonrotating abutment is seated against the nonrotating impression coping, and the abutment screw is firmly tightened (Fig 9-14). Most often, a removable soft tissue material (ie, vinyl polysiloxane) is used around the implant analogs to provide flexibility and/or a controlled emergence profile. It is critical to note that the nonrotating interfaces of components made by various manufacturers are *not* interchangeable. If components from two different manufacturers were used in one patient, careful examination of the internal pattern of the hexes would reveal two completely different configurations (Fig 9-15).

Nonrotating gold cylinders

Standard gold cylinders have a circular (universal) abutment interface (Fig 9-16, A), whereas nonrotating gold cylinders feature a male hex abutment interface (B and C). Note the difference in the interface configuration in the two nonrotating gold cylinders, which were produced by different manufacturers. This demonstrates the principle described above, ie, that all implants (A), abutments (B), and gold cylinders (C) must be produced by the same manufacturer to be compatible (Fig 9-17). Similarly, rotational components cannot be mixed with nonrotational components, regardless of whether they are made by the same manufacturer.

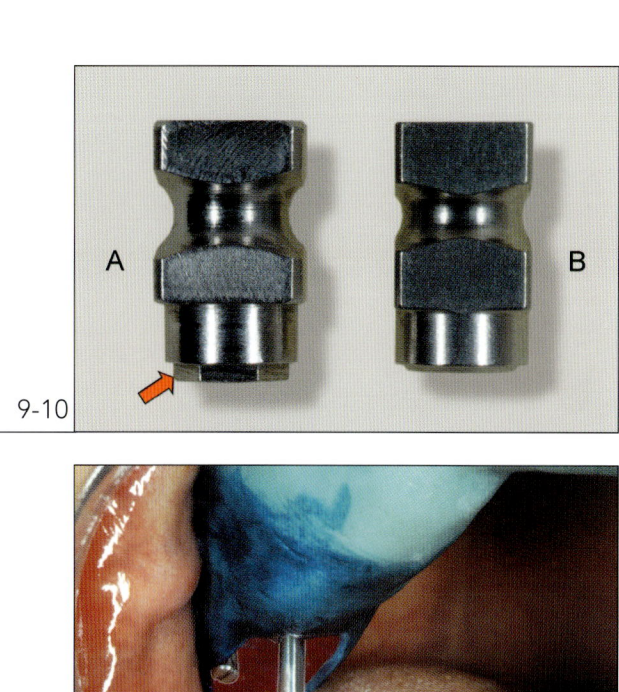

Rotational and Nonrotational Components

9-10

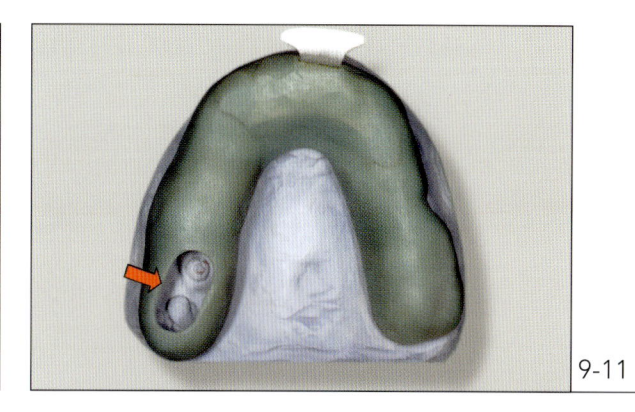

9-11

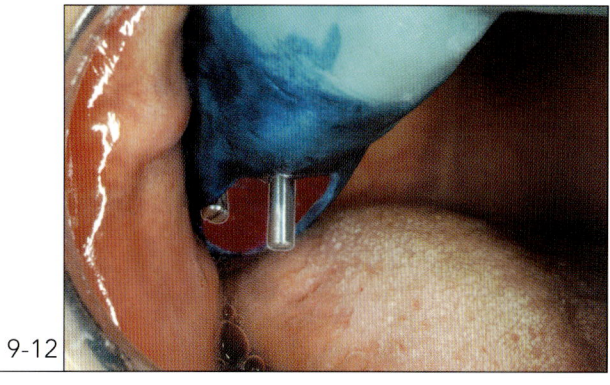

9-12

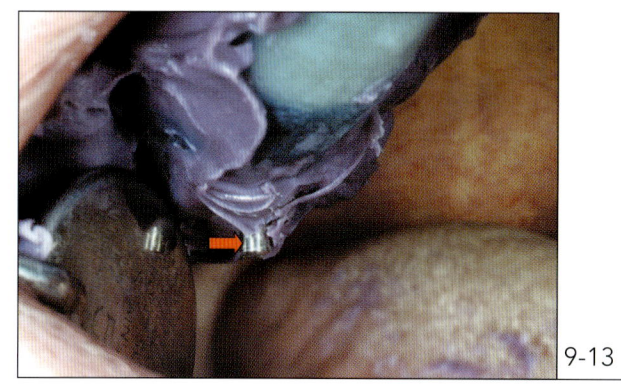

9-13

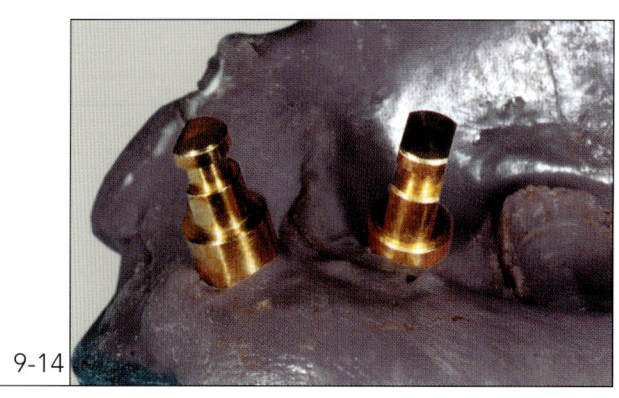

9-14

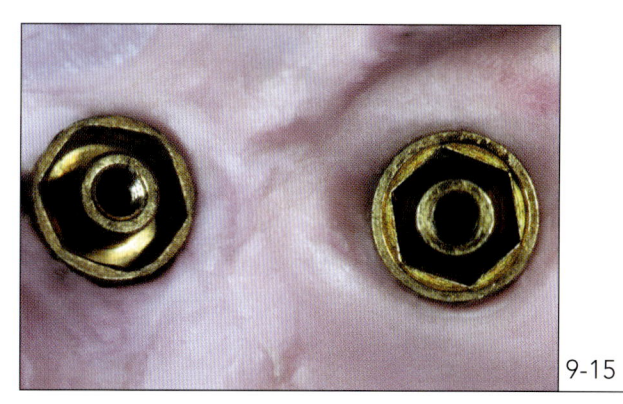

9-15

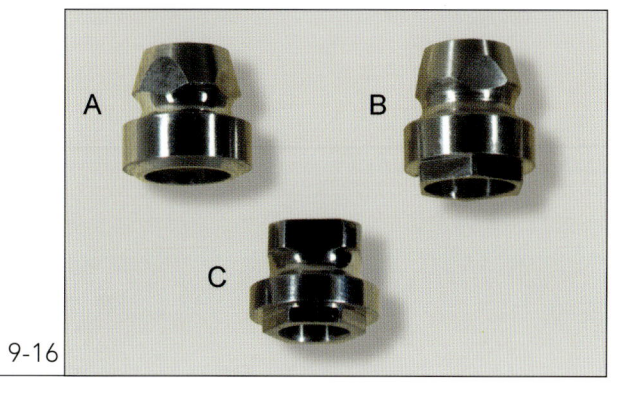

9-16

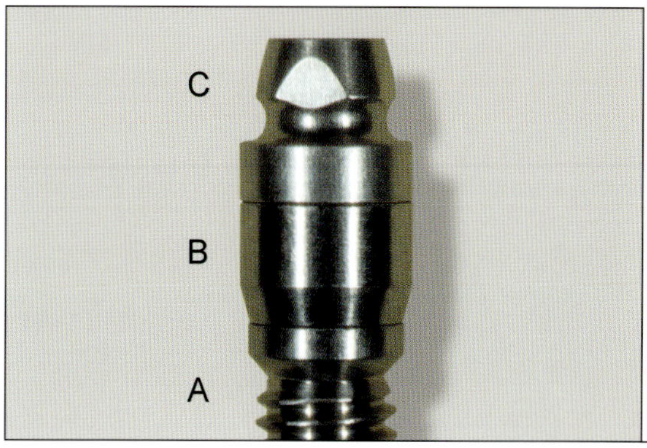

9-17

147

Compensating for Implant Divergence

Standard procedure

Implants need not be completely parallel when interlocking (nonrotating) interfaces are used. In Fig 9-18, the guide pins of two posterior abutments clearly indicate a divergence rather than a parallelism. The impression copings were held together with Duralay (Reliance, Worth, IL) acrylic prior to the impression procedure and subsequently transferred to the master cast (Fig 9-19).

Once the guide pins were unscrewed, the encased impression copings were easily removed in one piece (Fig 9-20). The reason for this apparent contradiction is that the length of the male hex of the gold cylinders (among various manufacturers) ranges from 0.7 to 1.0 mm (Figs 9-20 and 9-21, *arrows*), which is not sufficient to establish a precise path of insertion for each gold cylinder. The necessary tolerances built into all manufactured implant armamentaria also contribute to this phenomena. Thus, the seemingly divergent paths of insertion do not impede construction and seating of the prosthesis in one piece. (It should be noted that use of nonrotational abutments would simplify assemblage procedures for clip bar overdentures, as discussed in chapter 8. Note also that Figs 9-20 and 9-21 clearly illustrate the different male hex configurations from various manufacturers.)

The finished prosthesis is placed in position using the fixed-retrievable procedure (Fig 9-22). In this case, the surgeon used an exaggerated posterior inclination for the most distal implant in order to avoid the sinus and make use of the pterygomaxillary bone. The postoperative radiograph confirms complete seating and interface integrity (Fig 9-23).

Compensating for Implant Divergence

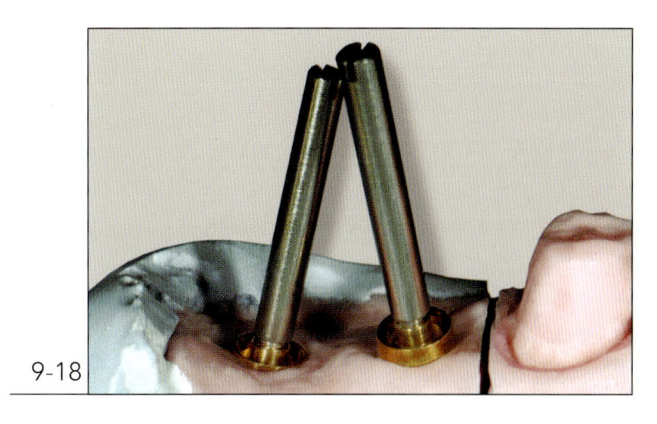

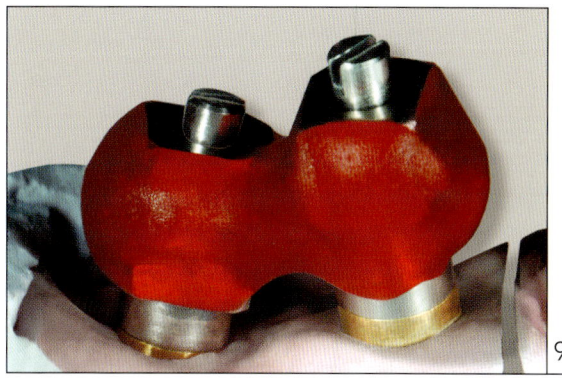

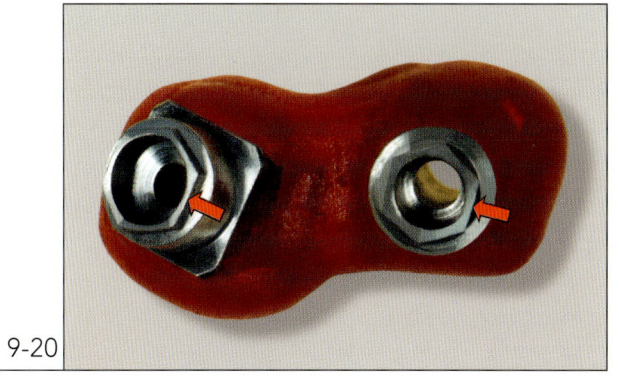

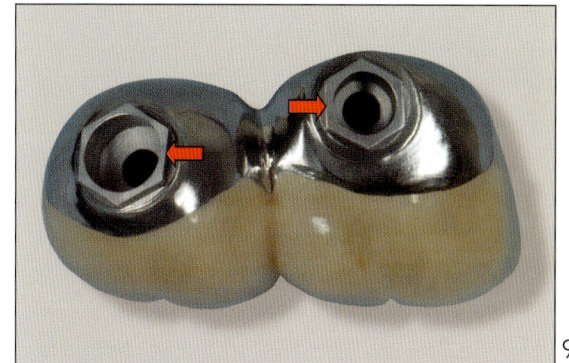

9-18

9-19

9-20

9-21

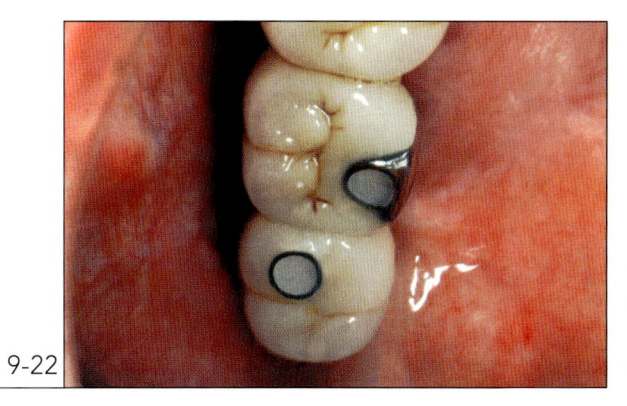

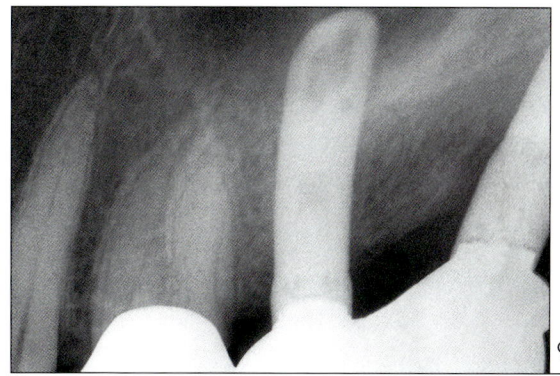

9-22

9-23

Reangulation

There are two types of reangulation procedures. The first is to use prefabricated angulated abutments that are designed to reangulate the path of insertion of the implant. The second, which is to construct a custom-reangulated abutment in the laboratory with a gold casting, is discussed in detail later in the chapter.

Prefabricated angulated abutments

In the 1990s many implant manufacturers began supplying prefabricated titanium angulated abutments, usually in two inclinations and in various designs for prosthesis construction (Fig 9-24). In general, the inclinations ranged from 15 to 35 degrees and were secured with special gold alloy abutment screws (see Fig 9-24, 3 to 6). Other implant systems used a "split" abutment design that featured offset hexes to provide more flexibility (see Fig 9-24, 1 and 2). However, this system declined in popularity because the laboratory technician was required to glue the components together once the most favorable position was obtained (Fig 9-25, 1 and 2). All angulated abutments provided the required nonrotating interface with the implant (see Fig 9-25, *arrows*). Most systems provided abutments with female hex interfaces for the male hex implant head (see Fig 9-24; 3,4, and 6), while others provided abutments with a male nonrotating configuration to interface with the female nonrotating design of the implant (see Fig 9-24, 5). Still others made either configuration available, depending on the implant configuration (see Fig 9-24, 1 and 2).

Most prefabricated angulated abutments are designed to be prepared by the technician after placement to meet the specific needs of the patient (Fig 9-26). One implant system (6) supplies a prefabricated tapered cylinder to which the prosthesis is waxed up and cast, precluding the need for abutment preparation (see Fig 9-26).

The two-part angulated abutment shown in Fig 9-27 was used to reangulate an implant that had an exaggerated labial and mesial inclination (Fig 9-28, *arrow*). The appropriate angulated abutment was positioned on the implant analog and reshaped for the restoration (Fig 9-29). (Note the finish line [*arrow*].) All three crowns were completed as single-tooth restorations (Fig 9-30). A lingual gold screw (*arrow*) was used to stabilize the restoration and to allow fixed-retrievability (see Fig 9-30).

Evolution of Clinical Procedures and Armamentarium

Single-stage surgery

There has been a recent increase in the popularity of single-stage surgery with immediate loading. Although an in-depth discussion of this procedure, including osseointegration factors, is beyond the scope of this text, some of the related prosthodontic aspects, particularly in relation to abutment angulation, are addressed below.

During surgery, the surgeon must address any reangulation problems by selecting the appropriate implant-abutment combination since components of the various systems are not interchangeable. In the author's opinion, this approach is unlikely to result in optimum esthetics or biomechanics since it is based on the clinician's judgment rather than being planned before surgery. Preplanning enables the clinician to coordinate the occlusion with the optimum implant location, thereby reducing implant loading (as described in chapter 6). With single-stage surgery, the clinician has less control over the gingival relationship and resulting esthetics, as discussed later in this chapter.

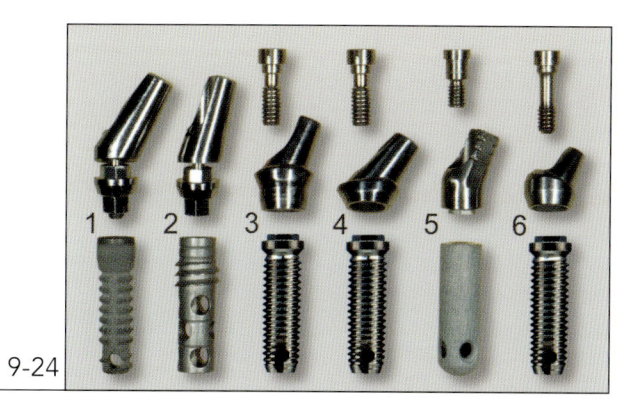

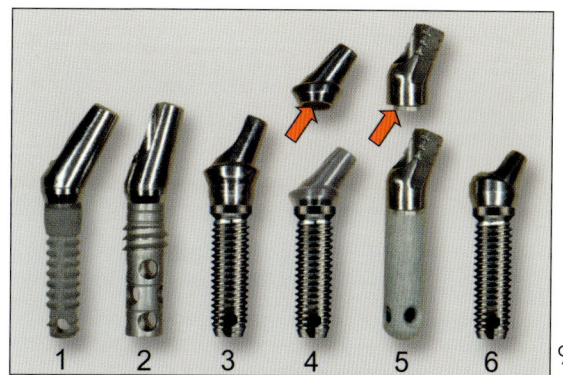

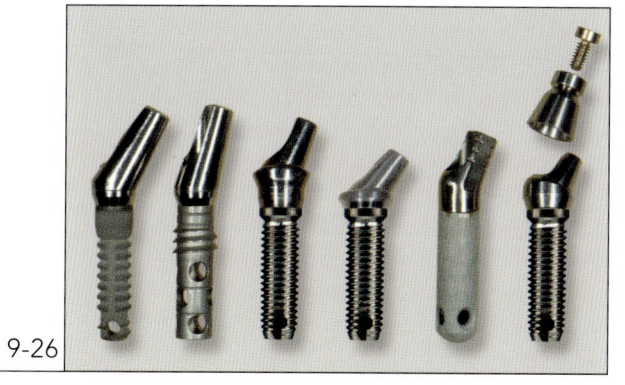

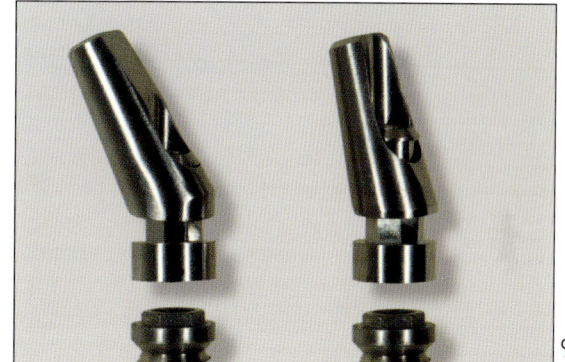

Evolution of Clinical Procedures and Armamentarium

9-24

9-25

9-26

9-27

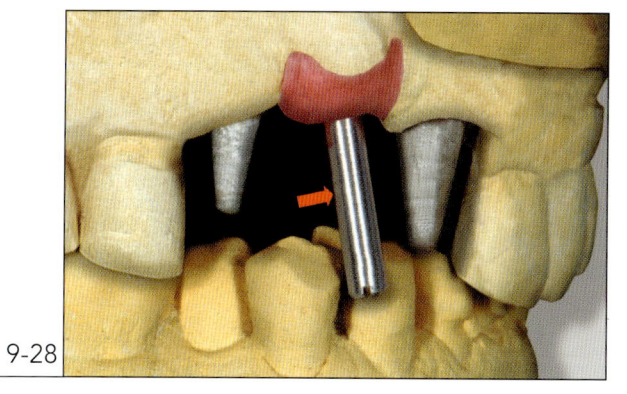

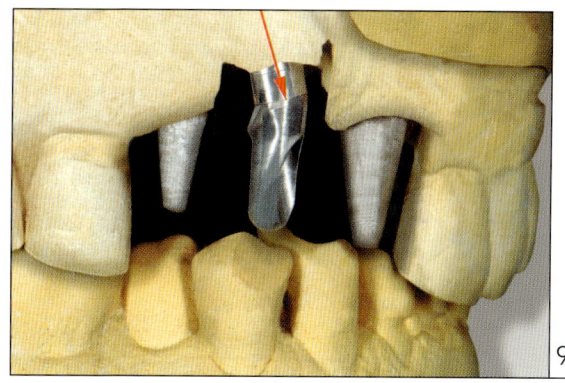

9-28

9-29

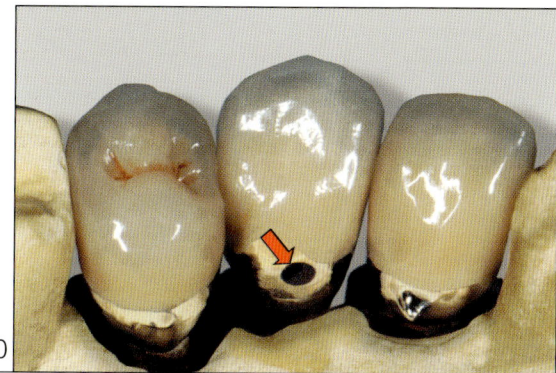

9-30

151

Implant design

Over the years, the diameter of implants has been increased to provide a wider platform for the prosthesis. This increases the resistance both to torque-induced breakage and to loosening of the implant and abutment screws. Moreover, increased diameter provides a larger surface area for osseointegration with the supporting bone, which increases resistance to implant overload.

Another recent innovation in implant design is providing expansion capabilities, while new surgical approaches to implant site preparation have been developed in an attempt to reduce heat-induced bone damage.

Abutment design

As shown in Figs 9-24 to 9-27, the early emphasis of implant-supported prosthesis armamentaria was on more, rather than fewer, pieces and parts. Subsequent evolution of abutment design emphasized simplicity, a trend that was motivated by the development of the UCLA configuration.[2] This design, a complete departure from the original protocol,[3] eliminates the use of a prefabricated abutment, instead providing a one-piece cast gold abutment (resembling a natural tooth preparation) that interfaces directly with the implant. Specific innovations in abutment design, namely the UCLA abutment, CeraOne abutment, and EsthetiCone abutment, are discussed in greater detail in the following sections.

UCLA Abutment

Although the UCLA abutment[2] originally was designed to improve esthetics for anterior teeth, it soon became the technique of choice for many clinicians when a custom-reangulated abutment was required in any location. The custom-reangulated (UCLA) abutment has many advantages: *(1)* it eliminates the need for a prefabricated angled abutment, *(2)* it simplifies construction, and *(3)* it results in better esthetics. The UCLA abutment also has advantages related to interface fit and resistance to lateral force, which are discussed later in the chapter. For the sake of clarity, it is appropriate to first describe posterior and anterior UCLA abutments (with or without reangulation), then introduce their use in anterior multiple implant–supported fixed prostheses.

Posterior UCLA custom-reangulated abutments

When implants are not parallel (Fig 9-31), the custom-reangulated abutments must provide parallelism for the final prosthesis. The technique used to achieve this has a direct effect on the resistance to lateral force and screw loosening. For example, the UCLA custom-reangulated abutment is fabricated to interface directly with the implant (Fig 9-31, *left, arrow*) using a premachined gold palladium cylinder (Fig 9-32, A), to which the custom-reangulated abutment is cast. It originally was secured with a titanium abutment screw (Fig 9-32, C), but this has since been replaced with a gold alloy abutment screw that can be tightened electronically or mechanically to 32 Ncm. The premachined internal hex (Fig 9-32, D) interfaces with the implant male hex (B), which provides maximum resistance to lateral force and screw loosening. The lingual surface of the custom-reangulated abutment is tapped to receive a gold screw, which provides fixed-retrievability (Fig 9-33, *left*).

UCLA Abutment

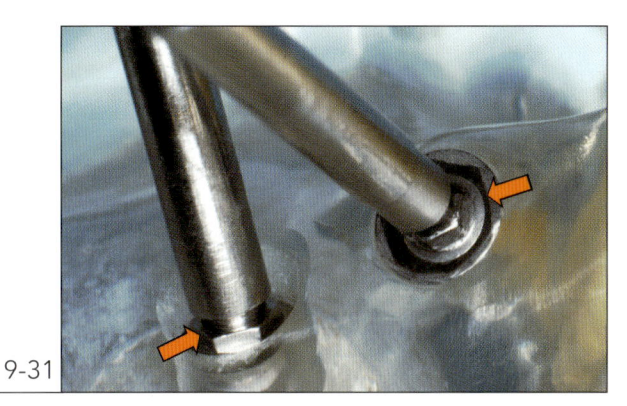

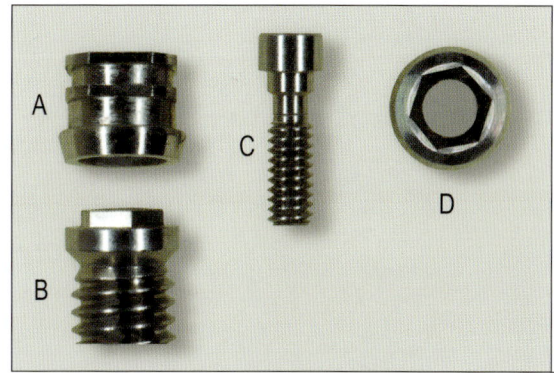

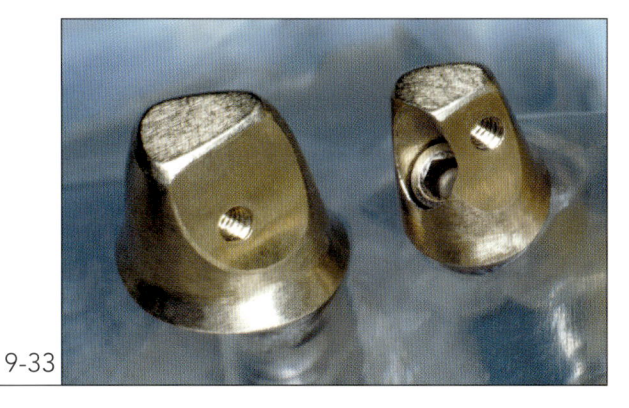

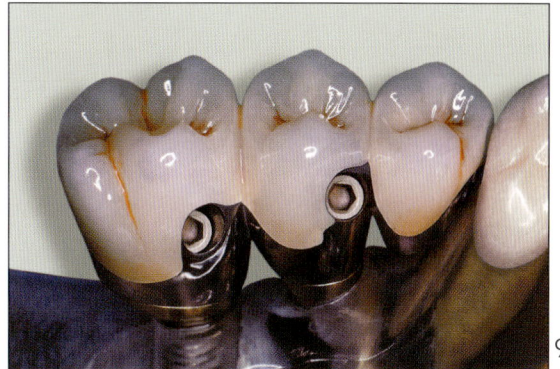

9-31

9-32

9-33

9-34

It is important to note that when a prefabricated nonrotating abutment is positioned over an implant (Fig 9-31, *right, arrow*), a nonrotating gold cylinder is required, to which the custom-reangulated abutment is waxed up and cast (Fig 9-33, *right*). With this configuration a gold retaining screw with a maximum of 10 Ncm must be used to position the custom-reangulated abutment. Therefore, the resistance to lateral force and/or screw loosening is far less than that achieved with the UCLA procedure, which uses an abutment that interfaces directly with the implant (see Figs 9-31 and 9-33, *left*) and a much larger gold alloy abutment screw that can be tightened to 32 Ncm for even greater retention.

The superstructure copings are waxed up to include an anterior pontic. The framework provides lingual gold retaining screws. The porcelain is baked to the framework, the occlusion is adjusted, and the porcelain is glazed. The finished restoration is shown on a clear acrylic cast in Fig 9-34.

9 Clinical Problems

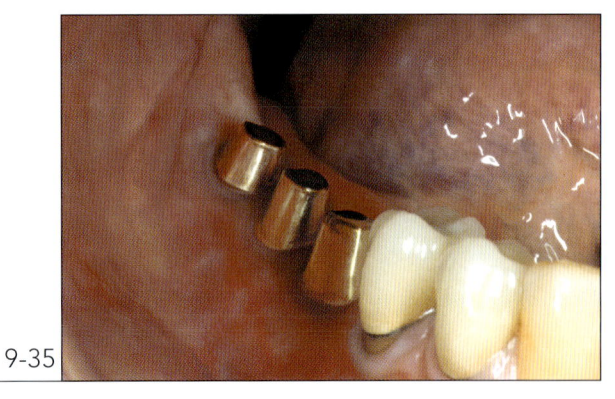

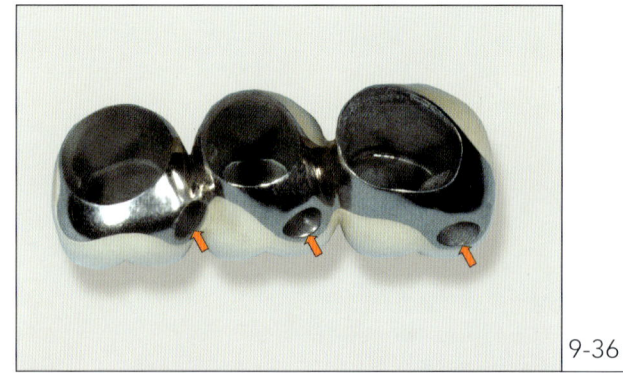

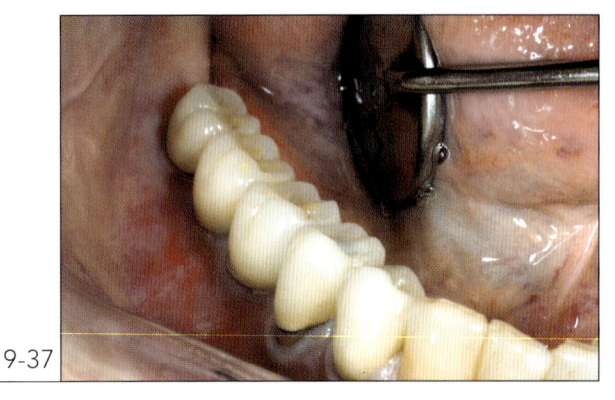

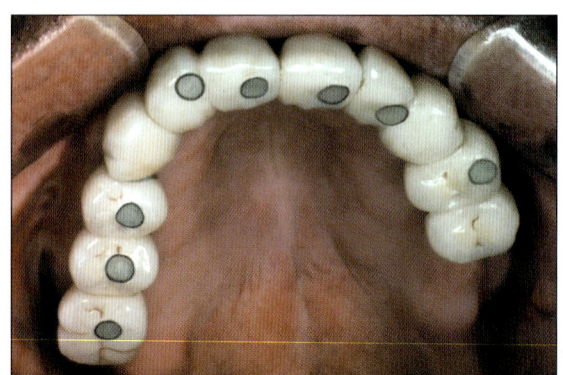

9-35

9-36

9-37

9-38

Posterior UCLA abutments (without reangulation)

The UCLA abutment also can be used when reangulation is not required. The same UCLA gold cylinder (see Fig 9-32, A) interfaces directly with the implant (B) and is positioned with a titanium or gold abutment screw (C). The nonrotating implant interface (D) provides excellent torque resistance. In this case the abutment screw is vertical with occlusal access. The resultant abutments resemble prepared natural teeth (Fig 9-35).

There are two main options for assemblage of the ceramometal copings. The indirect procedure calls for assemblage from the master cast. The author prefers the direct method, in which the crowns are seated intraorally and a plaster occlusal index is obtained to assemble the castings. The finished restoration, illustrated from the gingival view in Fig 9-36, resembles a tooth-supported prosthesis, with the exception of the lingual screw preparations (*arrows*). When seated intraorally, the prosthesis resembles natural tooth esthetics (Fig 9-37) since the need for occlusal access channels, which are required with standard abutments (Fig 9-38), is eliminated.

9-39

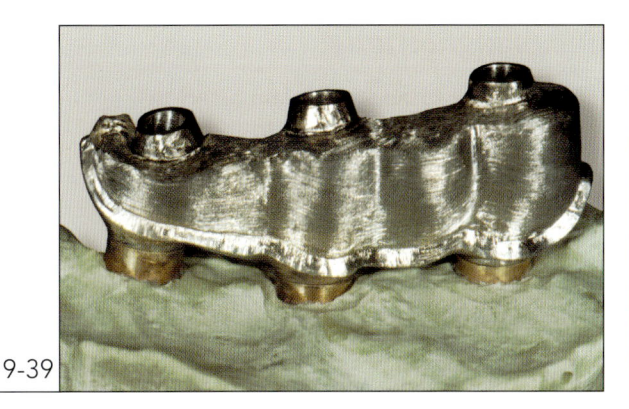

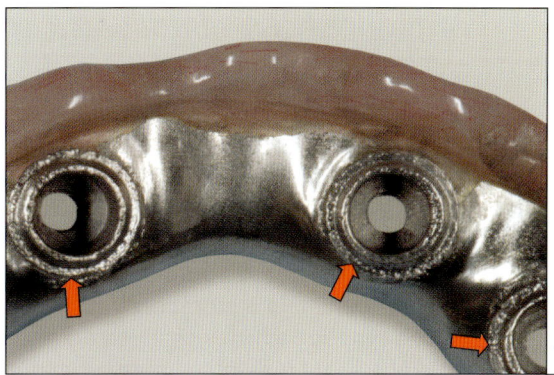

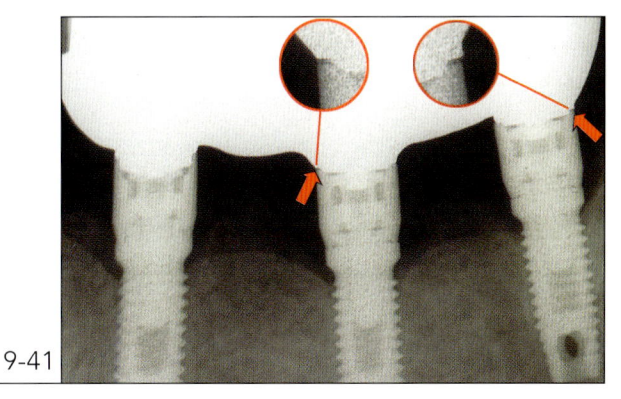

9-40

9-41

Disadvantages of multiple standard (titanium) abutments

The standard abutment configuration presents difficult laboratory problems that are not often acknowledged. For example, because the gold cylinders are waxed up together and cast in one piece (Fig 9-39), a great volume of molten metal, which shrinks on cooling, is required. Regardless of the investment material, this shrinkage is difficult to control. Single-crown units, which have a small volume of metal and a large hollow core, avoid this disadvantage. Moreover, the distortion factor requires laboratory technicians to section and resolder the prosthesis many times before it has acceptable fit on the master cast. As a result, the gold cylinders become pitted (Fig 9-40, *arrows*). Another problem is inaccurate fit (*arrows*), which can be best observed with periapical radiographs under magnification (Fig 9-41).

Anterior UCLA abutments (without reangulation)

Figure 9-42 shows an anterior UCLA gold cylinder (UCLA) and porcelain-fused-to-metal crown in cross section. An access channel (AC) maintains entrance to the abutment screw. Based on the relationship of the bone (B) and gingiva (G), the porcelain extends to within approximately 1.5 mm of the head of the implant (*arrow*), which maximizes esthetics (Fig 9-43).

Originally the UCLA cylinder was made of plastic, as shown in cross section on the implant with the abutment screw seated (*left, arrow*) and superimposed on the finished porcelain restoration (*right*) in Fig 9-44. The waxup was completed on the plastic cylinder, which was invested and cast in gold. When the resulting UCLA cast gold abutment was introduced, there was some concern about the effect of the difference in electric potential between the gold and titanium; however, this factor has not proven to have any measurable negative effect.

Anterior UCLA custom-reangulated abutments

The same armamentarium required for posterior restorations is used for anterior restorations (see Fig 9-32). Figure 9-45 shows an implant with a vertical orientation. For esthetic purposes and because the hex head is positioned very close to the free margin of the gingiva, a reangulated UCLA abutment is required. The reshaped abutment and the abutment screw (*arrow*) can be seen from the labial view in Fig 9-46. A ceramometal superstructure coping is then cast with lingual gold screw retention (*arrow*), and the porcelain is fused to it (Fig 9-47). The UCLA abutment is shown superimposed over the finished restoration from the labial in Fig 9-48. In the author's opinion, the UCLA reangulated abutment, which also helps prevent abutment screw loosening, is the preferred esthetic solution in these topographical circumstances.

UCLA Abutment

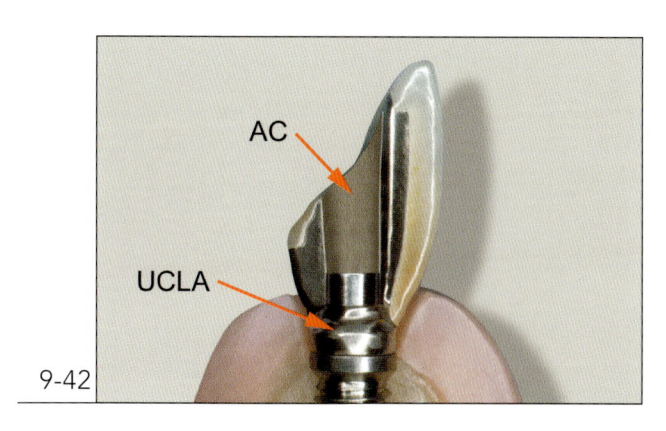

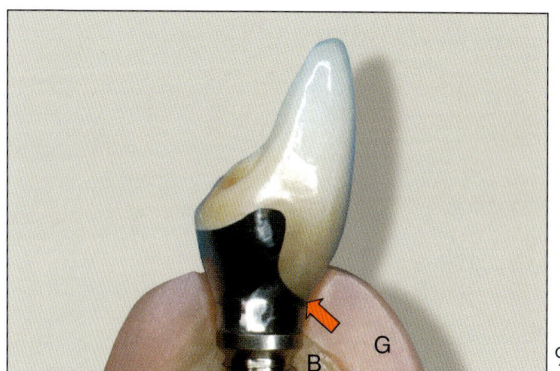

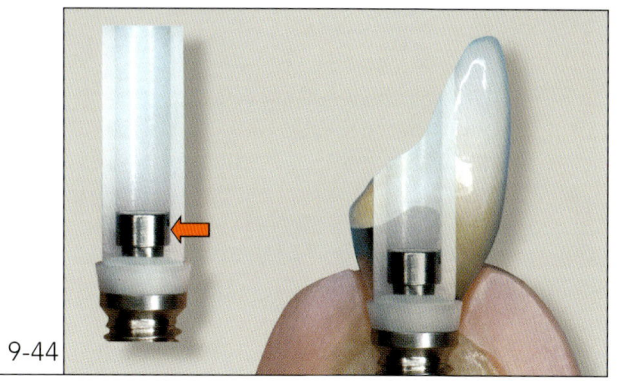

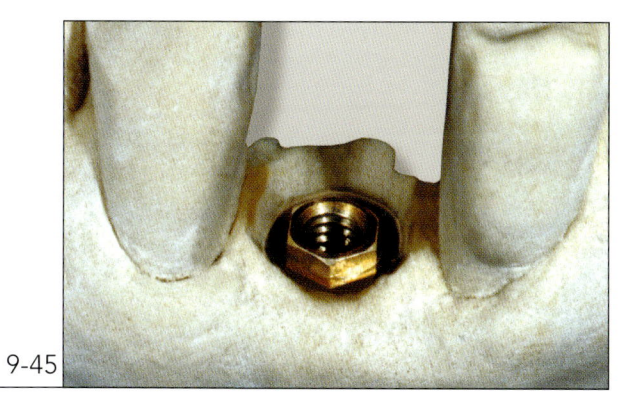

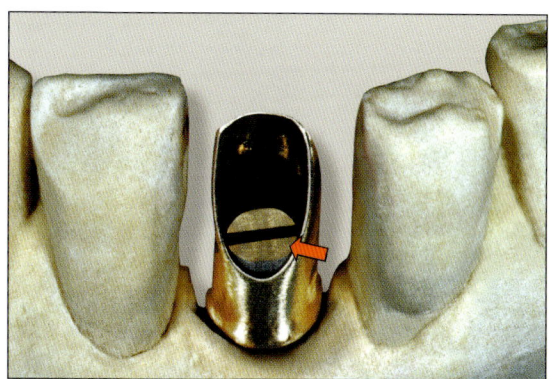

9-42 AC UCLA

9-43 B G

9-44

9-45

9-46

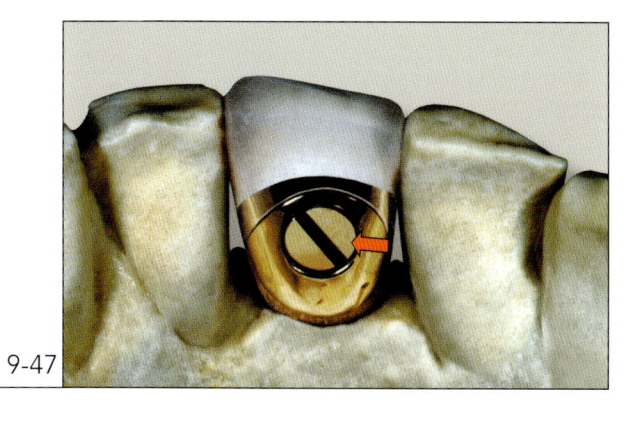

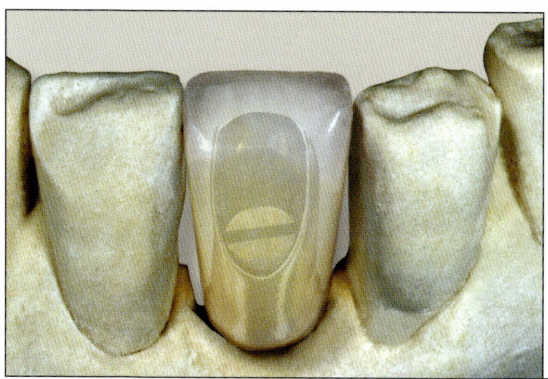

9-47

9-48

157

UCLA abutments in multiple implant–supported fixed prostheses

The need for reangulation is illustrated in Fig 9-49. Custom-reangulated UCLA abutments were fabricated with lingual gold retaining screws to provide fixed-retrievability (Fig 9-50). The finished restoration, shown from the gingival view in Fig 9-51, is seated intraorally and positioned with the lingual gold screws (Fig 9-52, *arrow*).

Summary of UCLA abutment design

The UCLA abutment for custom reangulation (using a UCLA gold cylinder) has more flexibility and is more esthetic than a prefabricated angulated abutment. Furthermore, the resultant abutment casting (either angled or straight) has the same configuration as a natural prepared tooth (see Fig 9-35). As a result, the prosthetic units look like individual crowns (see Fig 9-36) and can be assembled directly from the mouth, providing more accurate fit. The tapered restorative crown interface of a UCLA abutment provides much better adaptation than the butt joint of the gold cylinder to the prefabricated abutment (see Fig 9-41, *arrows*). In addition, the UCLA abutment-crown configuration (see Figs 9-35 and 9-36) provides multiple approaches to cementation.

When the UCLA abutment is used, the fixed-retrievable technique is simplified because the occlusal access channel is replaced with a lingual gold screw. Therefore, no provisional restoration is required to cover the lingual access channel. The clinician may choose to eliminate the lingual gold screw and use final cementation. However, the author prefers to use a thin marginal provisional sealer on the restoration margins in combination with a lingual gold screw. This enables periodic inspection of the abutment screw, troubleshooting, and repair, while also offering improved esthetics and avoidance of the time-consuming clinical procedures associated with occlusal fixed-retrievable techniques (see Fig 9-38).

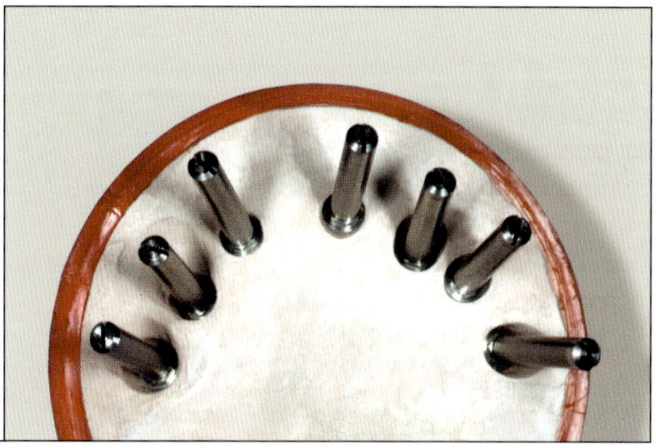

UCLA Abutment

9-49

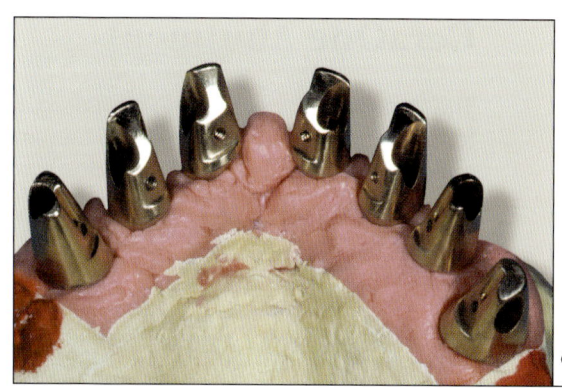

9-50

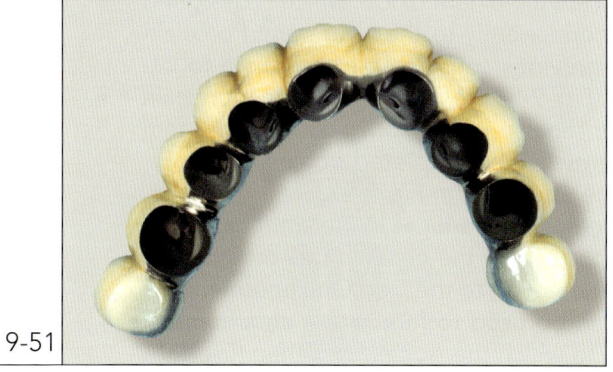

9-51

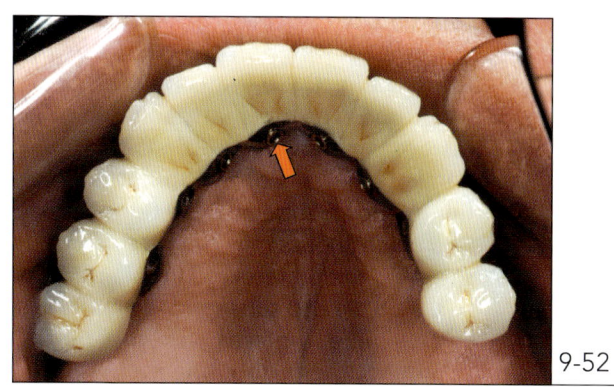

9-52

159

9 | Clinical Problems

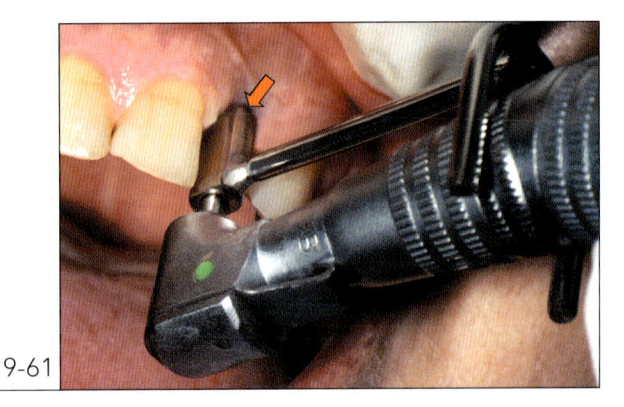

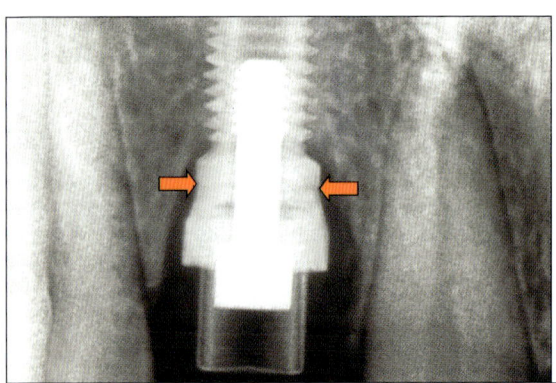

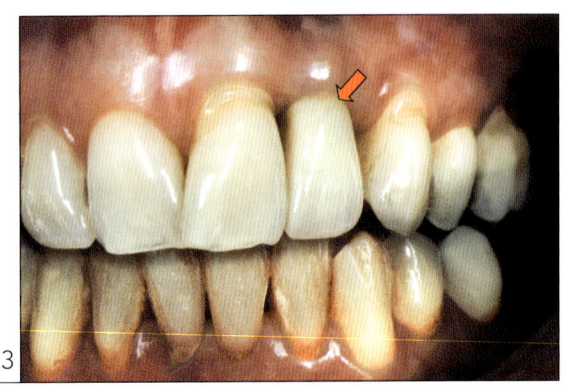

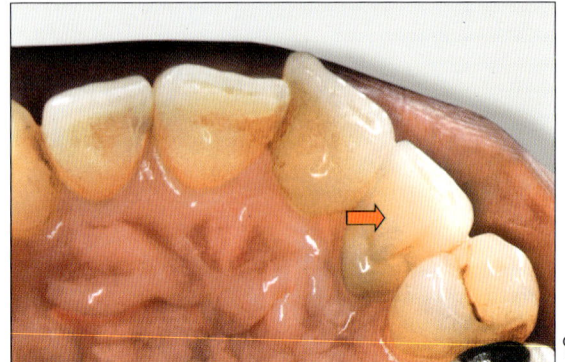

|9-61|9-62|
|9-63|9-64|

Nontorque bone-implant interface procedure

The CeraOne abutment's 3.61-mm hex configuration allows for placement of a gold abutment screw with 32 Ncm of torque without distributing torque to the bone-implant interface. Using a contra-angle handpiece, an internal hex holder is placed over the abutment (*arrow*) to engage the male hex (Fig 9-61). This prevents torque distribution to the bone-implant interface while the gold abutment screw is seated under 32 Ncm of torque by an electronic controller. A periapical radiograph reveals complete seating of the abutment to the implant (Fig 9-62). The porcelain restoration (*arrow*) is shown from the labial in Fig 9-63 and from the lingual in Fig 9-64.

Posterior CeraOne abutment with ceramometal coping

The CeraOne abutment (*arrow*) is seated with the gold abutment screw as previously described (Fig 9-65). A plastic impression coping (Fig 9-66, A) is designed to fit over the CeraOne abutment (B). To ensure that no section of the plastic impression coping bends during the impression procedure, Duralay acrylic (*arrows*) should be used for reinforcement (Fig 9-67).

The reinforced plastic impression coping is seated on the abutment, and complete marginal adaptation (*arrow*) is confirmed (Fig 9-68). No portion of the impression coping should contact the adjacent teeth. A custom impression tray is then seated and adequate relief confirmed (Fig 9-69, *arrows*). Light-bodied elastomeric impression material is syringed around the gingival areas, and the tray containing heavy-bodied impression material is seated. The gingival view of the impression should reveal that no impression material covers the internal portion of the impression coping (Fig 9-70). A plastic abutment analog (*arrow*) is seated into the impression, the gingival contours are duplicated in vinyl polysiloxane, and the cast is poured in stone (Fig 9-71).

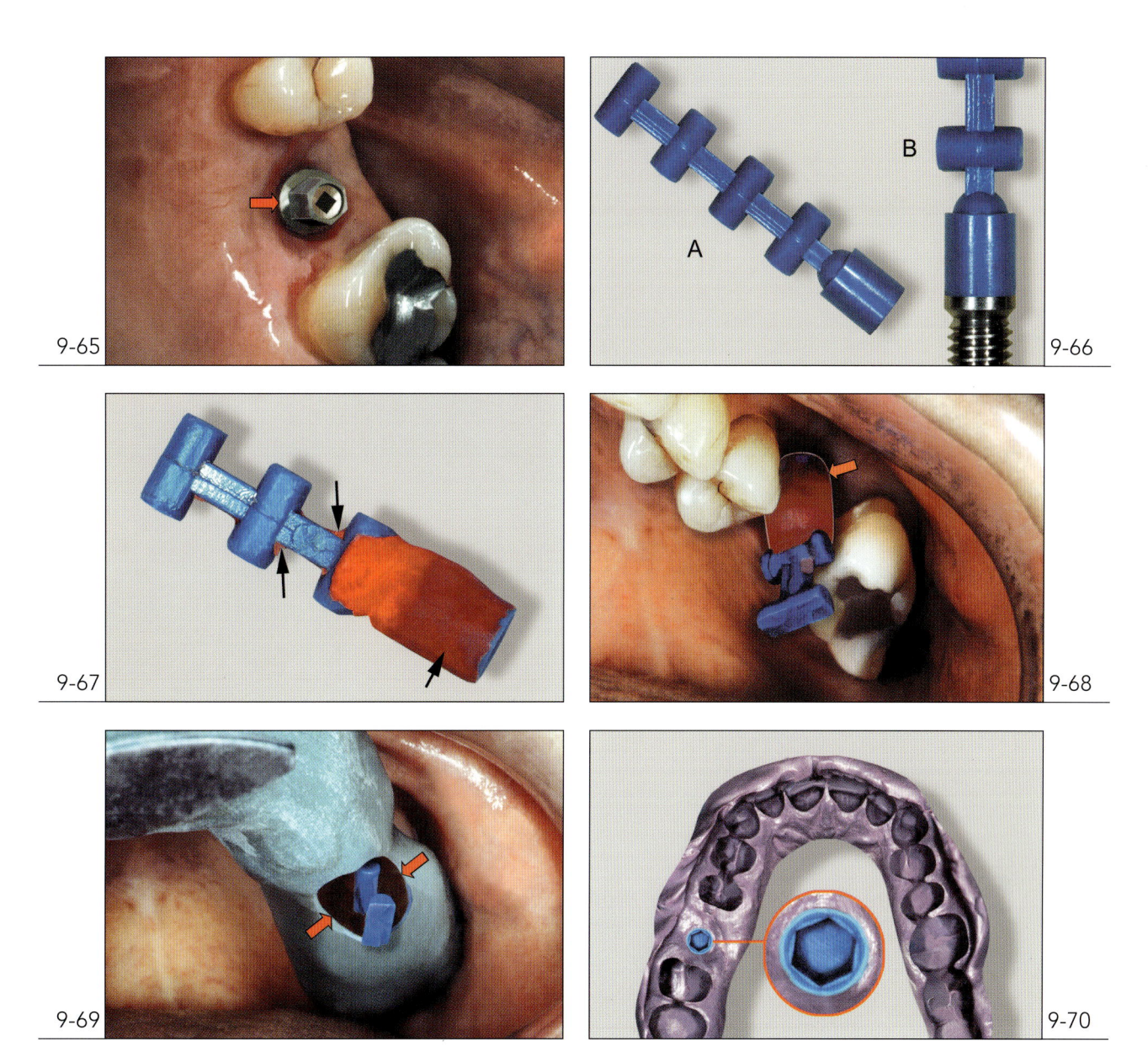

CeraOne Abutment

9-65

9-66

9-67

9-68

9-69

9-70

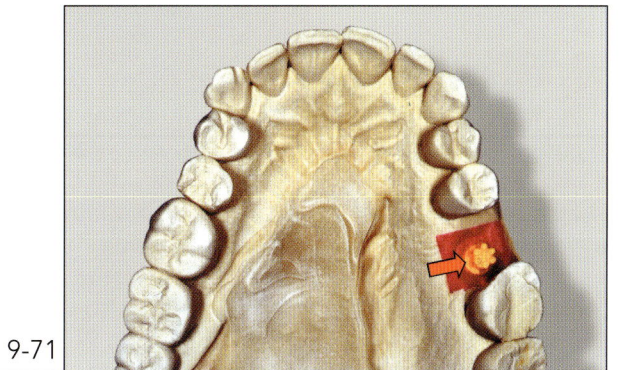

9-71

9 Clinical Problems

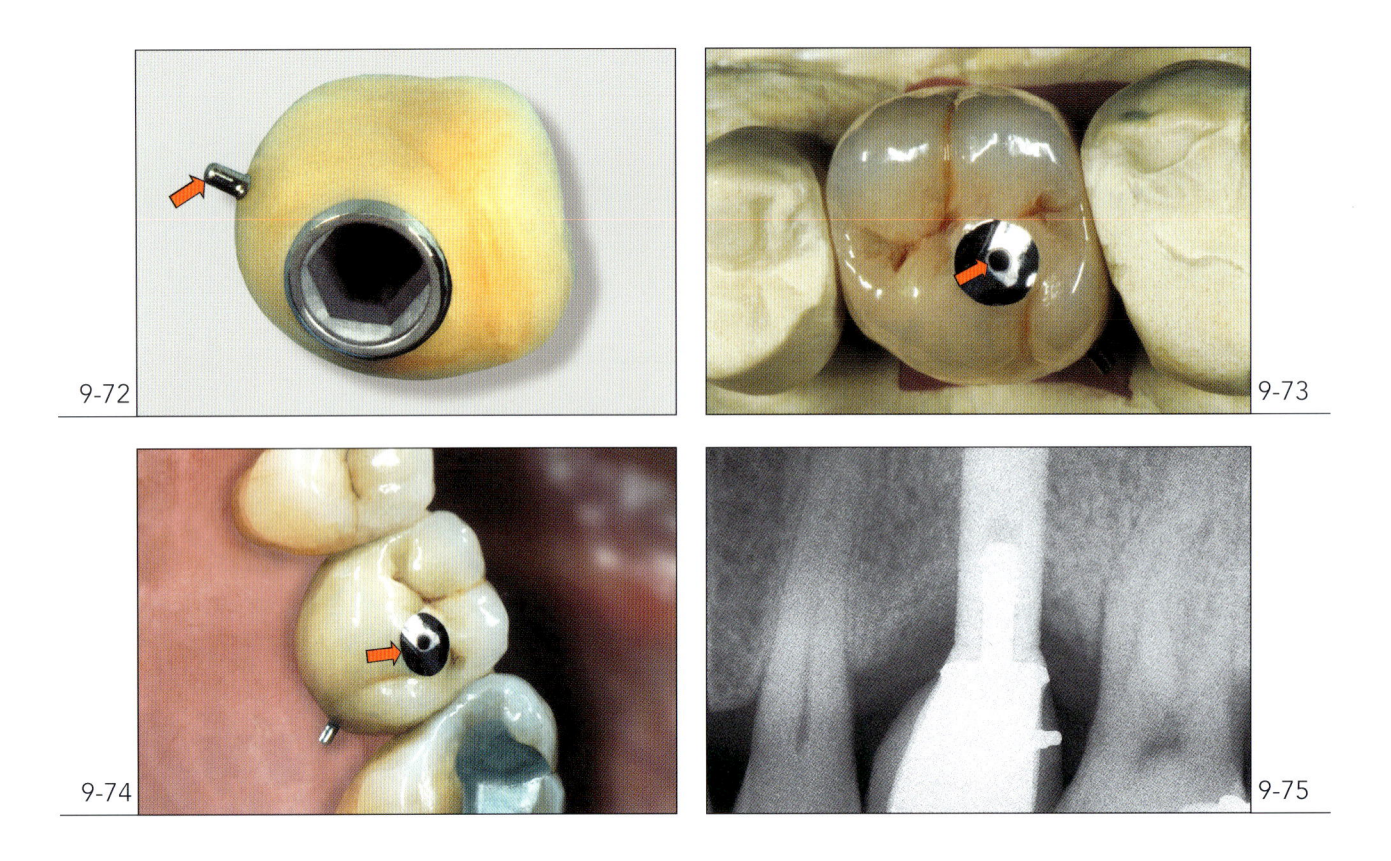

9-72

9-73

9-74

9-75

CeraOne restoration with modified access channel

The cast ceramometal coping shown in Fig 9-60 (B) is the preferred material for the posterior areas, as previously described. However, to facilitate troubleshooting, the author adds a lingual removal button (*arrow*), as shown in the gingival view of the finished restoration in Fig 9-72. As an additional precautionary measure, a narrow occlusal access channel (*arrow*) is fabricated in gold to facilitate re-entry if subsequently required (Fig 9-73).

The restoration is seated intraorally, and the contact areas and occlusion are adjusted as necessary. After final glazing is accomplished, the restoration is seated with final cement. The space immediately over the abutment screw is obturated with a cotton pellet and gutta percha to allow widening of the access channel without damage to the abutment or abutment screw. Self- or light-curing resin is used to seal the occlusal opening (*arrow*) to allow access to the abutment screw if there are any postoperative problems (Fig 9-74). If such measures are not taken, the crown has to be destroyed to gain access to the abutment screw. This is traumatic to the patient, time consuming, and likely to result in damage to the abutment. The radiograph reveals proper abutment-implant interface fit (Fig 9-75).

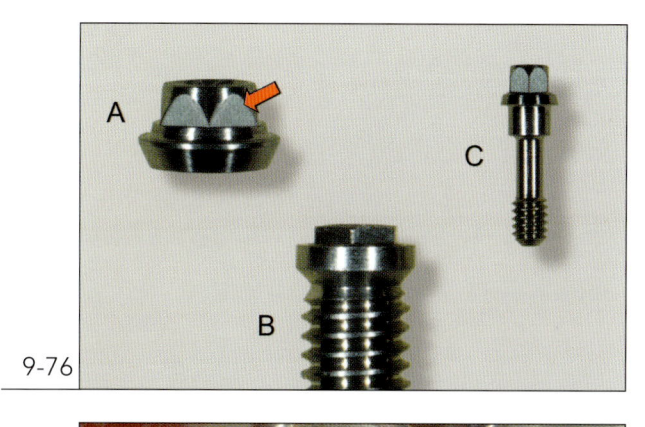

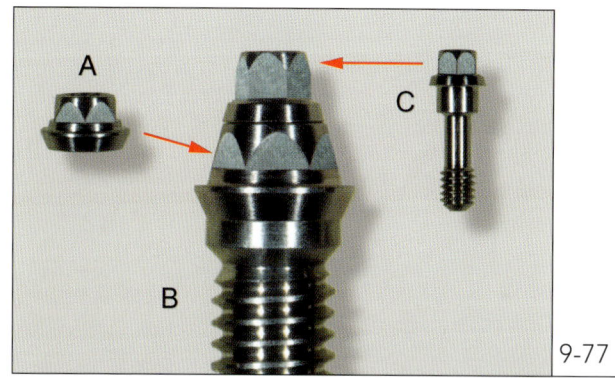

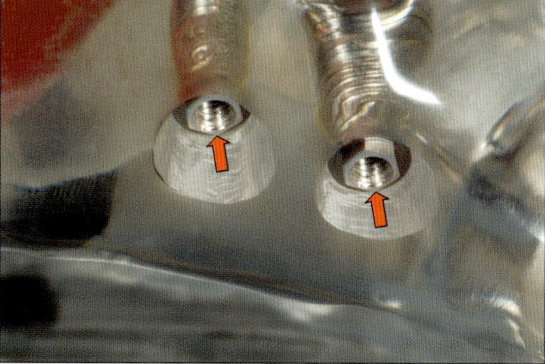

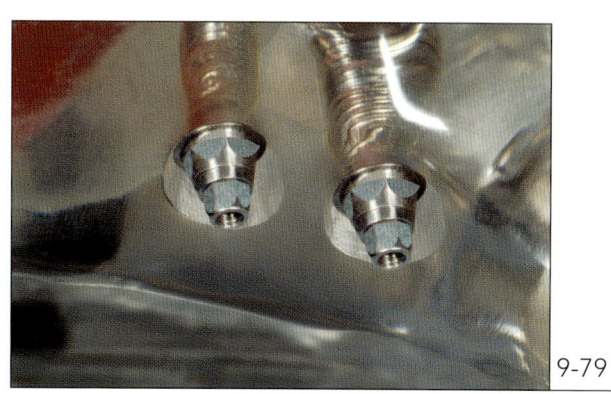

EsthetiCone Abutment

The EsthetiCone (Nobel Biocare) abutment has hex-shaped, tapered sides (Fig 9-76, A, *arrow*); features a female hex interface with the implant male hex head (B); and is secured by a titanium abutment screw (C).[4,5] The assembled abutment is shown in Fig 9-77, and two implants (*arrows*) in a transparent cast are shown in Fig 9-78. In Fig 9-79, two EsthetiCone abutments have been positioned on the cast by the abutment screws. Note the relationship of the "gingiva" to the topography of the abutments.

9 Clinical Problems

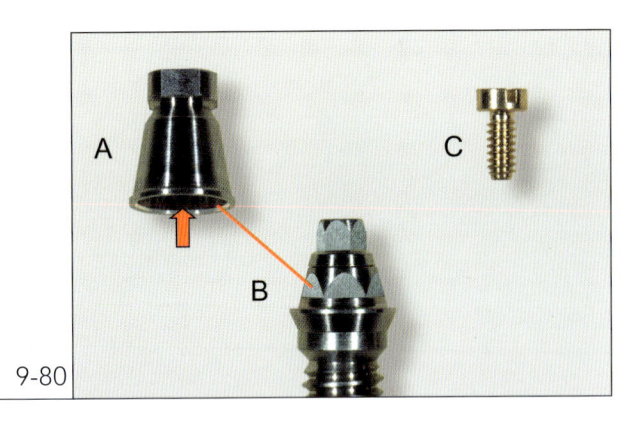

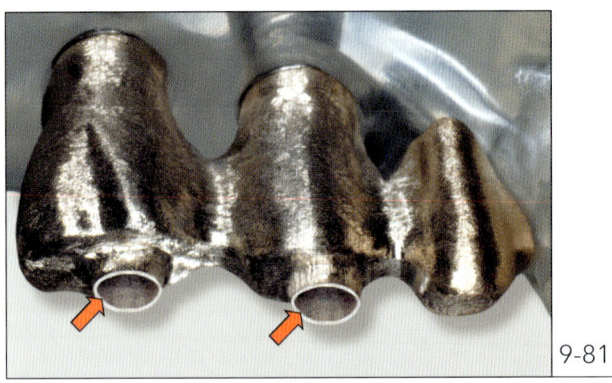

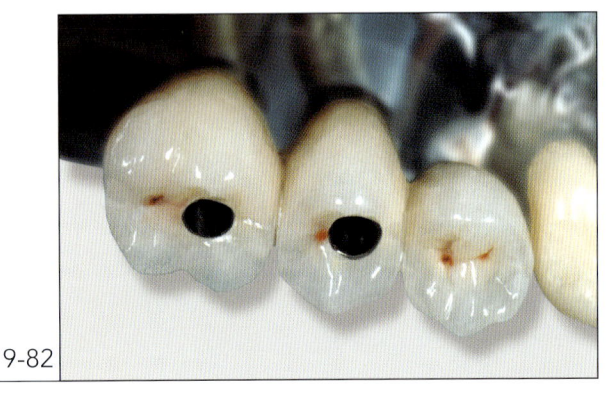

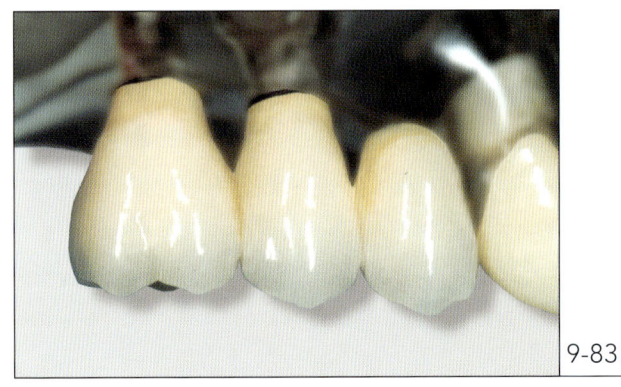

|9-80|9-81|
|9-82|9-83|

Prosthesis construction procedures

The prosthesis is waxed and cast to a tapered gold cylinder (Fig 9-80, A), which is positioned and seated over the assembled abutment (B) with a gold retaining screw (C). It is important to note that the tapered gold cylinder's interface with the abutment is circular (see Fig 9-80, *arrow*), ie, it lacks a nonrotating configuration, and therefore is intended to be used with prostheses supported by multiple implants (Fig 9-81). Access channels (see Fig 9-81, *arrows*) are required to seat the prosthesis on the abutments. Although the tapered gold cylinder also is available with a nonrotating abutment interface (internal hex), the EstheticCone should not be used as a single-tooth abutment because of the weakness of the gold screw. The finished prosthesis is shown from the occlusolingual and buccal views in Figs 9-82 and 9-83, respectively.

Abutment-Selection Process

Comparative configuration versus function

The functional and esthetic requirements of the restoration relative to implant location, gingival contours, available space, number of implants, and biomechanics all affect the choice of abutment. For instance, if the restoration is supported by multiple implants and esthetics is not the primary concern, then the standard rotational cylinder (Fig 9-84, A) can be used with the standard abutment screw (B). On the other hand, a clinical situation calling for a single-tooth restoration in the anterior maxilla would indicate use of the CeraOne abutment (C) secured by the gold screw (D) with 32 Ncm of torque.

Abutment-Selection Process

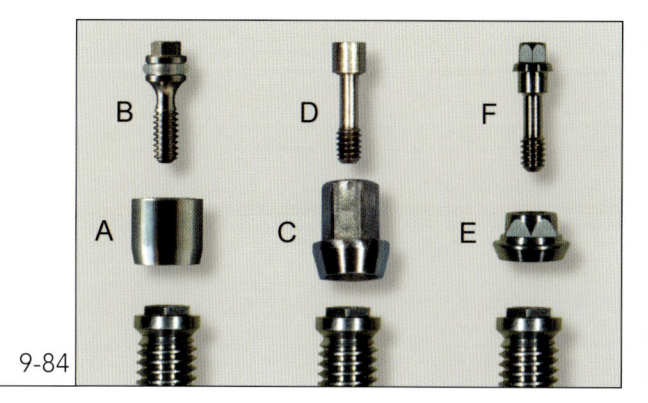

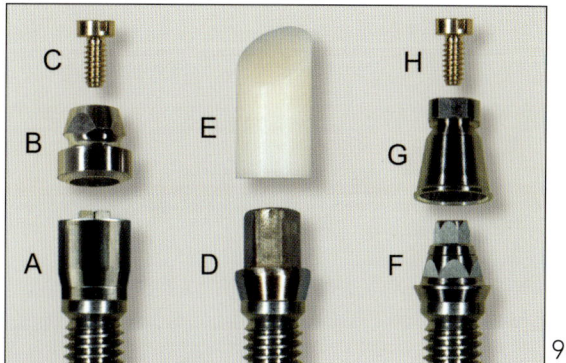

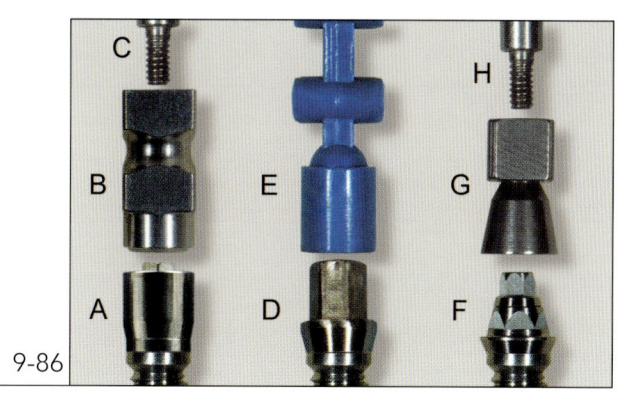

9-84

9-85

9-86

Prostheses supported by multiple implants with critical esthetic gingival areas can best be treated with a tapered abutment such as the EsthetiCone (see Fig 9-84, E and F). As discussed earlier, when reangulation is required, a UCLA custom-reangulated abutment (see Figs 9-50 to 9-52) is indicated. UCLA abutments without angulation (see Figs 9-35 to 9-37), or prefabricated reshapeable titanium abutments (see Figs 9-7 and 9-8), should be used if posterior esthetics are extremely important, contraindicating occlusal access channels (see Fig 9-38).

Prosthesis comparison

Each abutment configuration requires a different prosthesis construction. Figure 9-85 shows the abutments seated on the implants (A, D, and F). When the standard cylindrical and tapered abutments (A and F) are used, the restoration is waxed and cast to the gold cylinders (B and G), which are retained with gold screws (C and H). The CeraOne has a porcelain cap (E) to which the porcelain restoration is fused.

Impression copings

Each abutment has its own impression coping. The standard cylindrical abutment (Fig 9-86, A) requires a square impression coping (B) that uses a guide pin (C) or a tapered impression coping as previously described (see Fig 8-42). The CeraOne abutment (see Fig 9-86, D) uses a plastic impression coping (E) as illustrated previously (see Figs 9-66 to 9-71). The EsthetiCone abutment (see Fig 9-86, F) is used with a square impression coping (G), which is stabilized with a guide pin (H).

167

9 | Clinical Problems

9-87

9-88

9-89

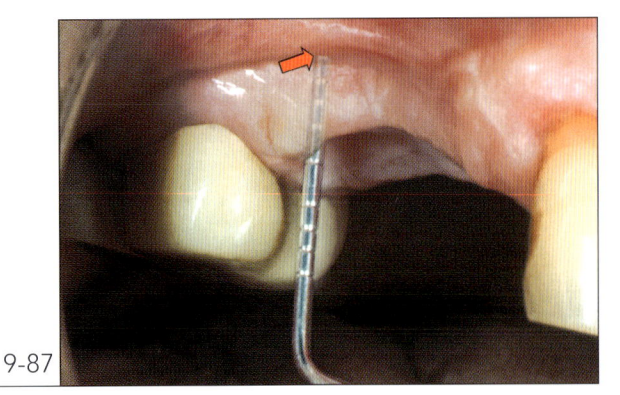

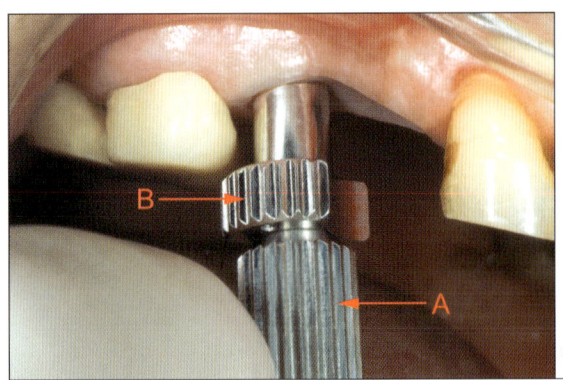

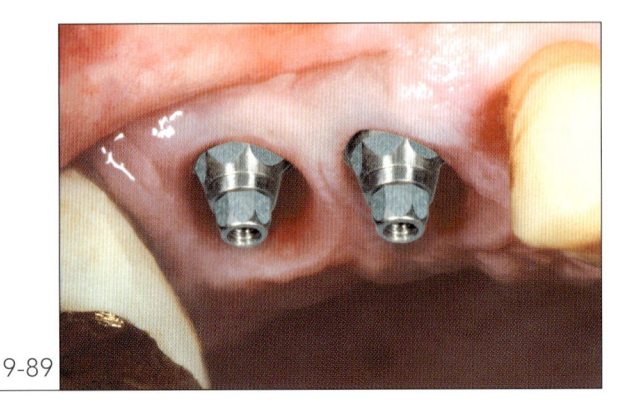

Gingival depth

The gingival depth is measured from the free gingival margin to the head of the implant using a periodontal probe, as shown through the superimposed gingiva in Fig 9-87. Favorable gingival depth provides flexibility in abutment selection.

The abutment should be seated using an abutment holder (B), which is rotated until the hex of the implant is engaged (Fig 9-88). The position of the abutment is maintained by the abutment holder while the driver (A) tightens the abutment screw. The bucco-occlusal view in Fig 9-89 illustrates the gingival space relative to the seated abutments. An electronic or mechanical torque driver (see Fig 9-54) can be used once the abutment seating is confirmed clinically and radiographically.

Maintenance and Reproduction of Gingival Contours

Gingival healing

There are several ways to create controlled gingival healing prior to impression procedures. At second-stage surgery, the abutment (Fig 9-90, A) can be placed on the implant and covered with a healing cap (B). If abutment selection is delayed because the implant location is more critical (C), a healing abutment (D) can be used instead. Healing abutments are available in varying shapes and sizes (A to C) to improve the emergence profile of the gingiva (Fig 9-91).

Maintenance and Reproduction of Gingival Contours

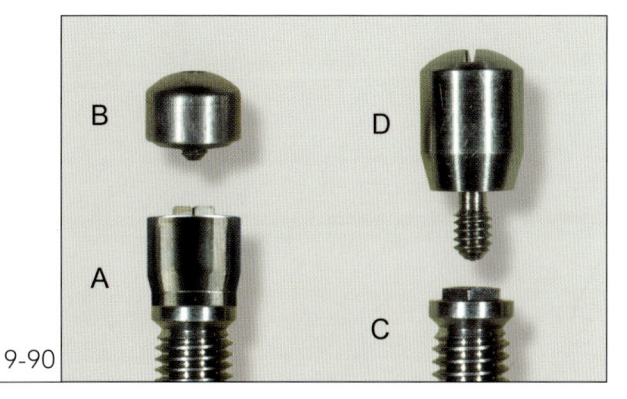

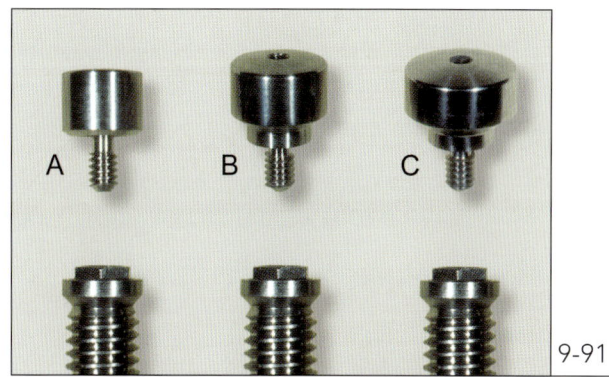

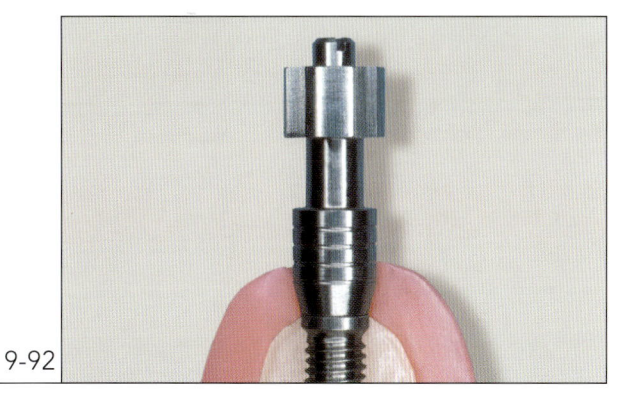

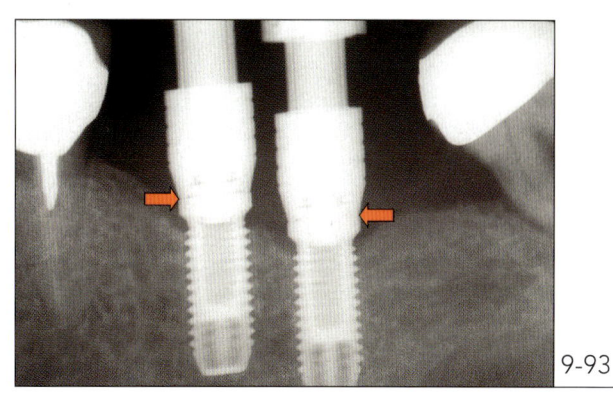

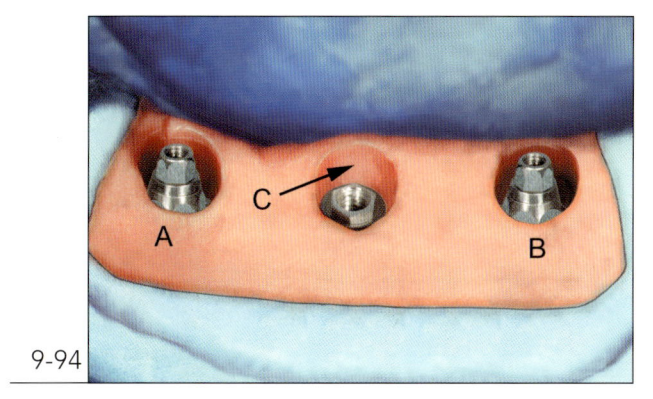

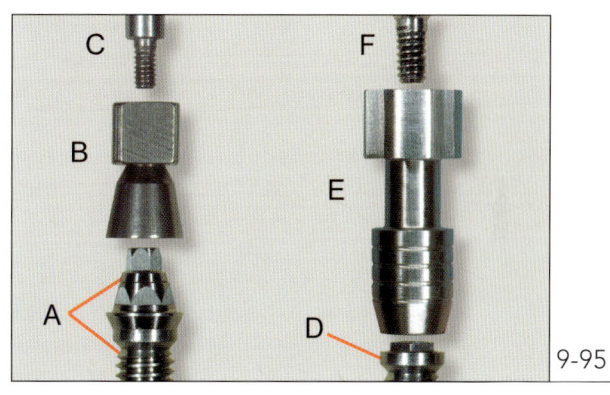

Gingival reproduction

Gingival healing is not always predictable; however, the final gingival height and contour are extremely important to abutment selection and ultimate esthetics. Therefore, many clinicians use the following technique to ensure a favorable result.

Healing abutments are positioned at second-stage surgery to provide an improved emergence profile. Impression copings are used to reproduce the implant head and the relationship of the healed gingival sulcus (Fig 9-92). As always, the abutment–impression coping interface (*arrows*) must be confirmed radiographically (Fig 9-93).

The three-dimensional gingival relationship relative to the implants is reproduced on the master cast with vinyl polysiloxane (Fig 9-94). Using this approach, EsthetiCone abutments were selected and seated in the lab at (A) and (B), but the buccogingival depth at (C) suggested a UCLA abutment. The clinician may choose to position the abutment on the implant (A, Fig 9-95) and make the impression with the appropriate (tapered) impression coping (B) positioned on the abutment with a guide pin (C).

169

However, if the gingiva does not heal as predicted, the entire impression procedure may have to be repeated. Therefore, some clinicians feel the clinical situation is better controlled when impression procedures are delayed and healing abutments, rather than final abutments, are placed until complete healing has been achieved. After complete healing, an impression coping (E) is positioned on the implant (D) using a guide pin (F), and an impression is made to reproduce the implant position relative to the surrounding gingival contours (see Fig 9-95).

Laboratory reproduction

Laboratory analogs (replicas) are available for each impression configuration. Figure 9-96 shows the replicas to be used with a tapered impression coping with (A) or without (B) a nonrotating internal hex configuration. In those cases where the implant itself is impressioned, a brass replica is used (C). An example of the abutment replica in Fig 9-96 (A) is shown in situ in Fig 9-97, illustrating an accurate duplication of the gingival relationship to the abutments.

Impression Accuracy

Square and tapered impression copings

Both square and tapered copings and the associated clinical procedures are described in detail in chapters 7 and 8, respectively. The one-piece tapered impression coping (A) that screws into the abutment has a circular interface (Fig 9-98). If the abutment has a nonrotating interface, a positioning screw is required to position the male hex of the impression coping with the female hex of the abutment replica (B). The nonrotating abutment replica maintains this relationship providing that the outside surface of the tapered impression coping is notched to transfer its specific orientation to the impression, which ensures that it will be reinserted into the impression in the proper position.

Research[6] and clinical experience have shown that square impression copings, which remain within the elastomeric impression material when the impression is removed, produce the most accurate master casts. The square impression coping with a circular interface (C) and the nonrotating square impression coping (D), which is shown seated on the abutment replica in Fig 9-98, produce equally accurate casts.

Unpublished research by the author, reinforced by long-term clinical experience, indicates that ligation between impression copings does not increase the accuracy of the impression and in fact may decrease the accuracy very slightly.

Impression technique

Tapered impression copings can be used provided there is reasonable alignment of the implants (Fig 9-99). Exaggerated divergence might distort the impression material enough to warrant the use of square impression copings. One of the most serious errors in accuracy is to forget to check the tightness of the abutment screws every time

Impression Accuracy

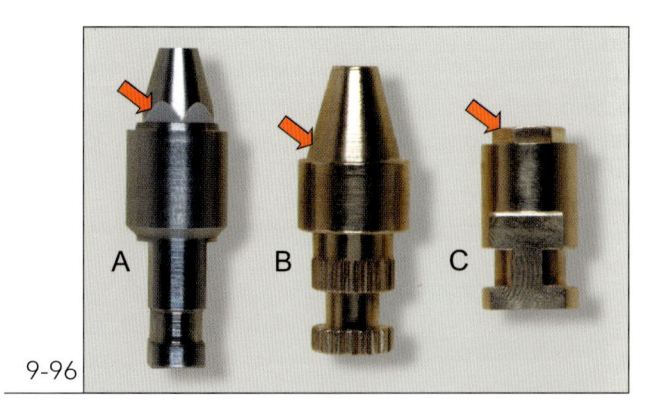

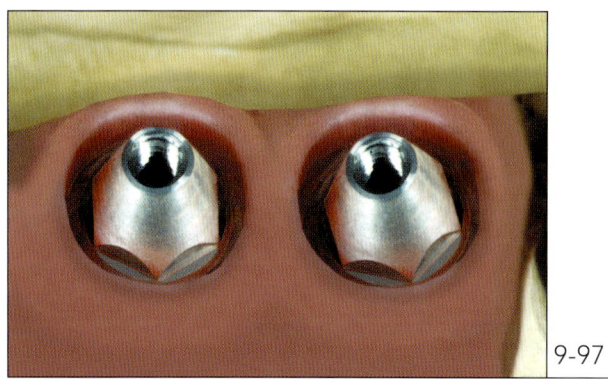

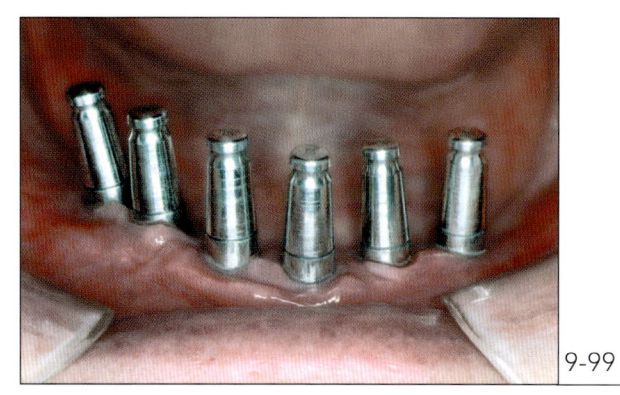

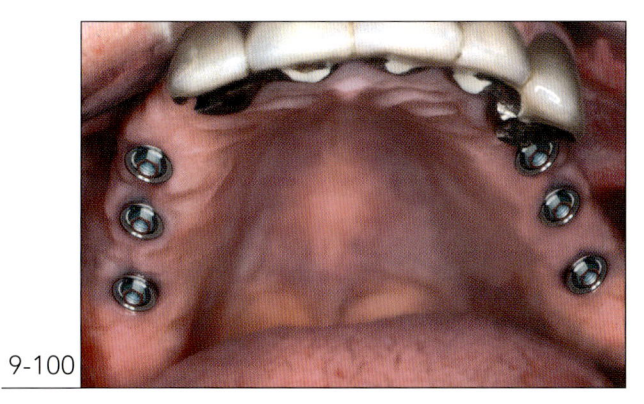

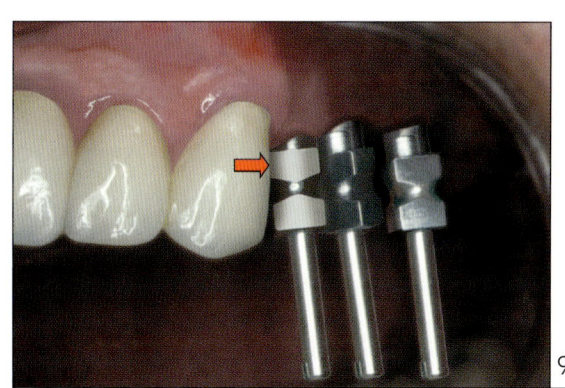

9-96

9-97

9-98

9-99

9-100

9-101

a clinical procedure involves their exposure (Fig 9-100). During the positioning of a square impression coping, it is essential to confirm clearance with an adjacent natural tooth (Fig 9-101). Without sufficient clearance, the patient will feel pressure on the natural tooth as the impression coping guide pin is tightened because of the stiffness of the osseointegrated interface compared with the flexion of the periodontal ligament.

Final Osseointegrated Prosthesis

Temporary cementation

The temporary cementation of a multiple implant–supported prosthesis (Fig 9-108) follows clinical procedures similar to those previously described for an acrylic provisional prosthesis (see Figs 9-106 and 9-107).

Fixed-retrievable cementation

A cotton pellet protects access to the abutment screw as before. Selection of the material to be placed under the final occlusal sealant is a matter of clinician preference. The author prefers warm gutta percha, which can be applied and removed easily and cleanly. A self- or light-cured resin is used to seal the access channels (see Fig 9-38). As always, the final step is to radiograph all interfaces (*arrows*) to confirm complete seating (Figs 9-109 to 9-112).

Alternative methods

There is an increasing trend to use final cementation rather than the fixed-retrievable procedures that have been described. Again, this is a matter of personal preference. The author is more conservative because of the tremendous amount of time and financial cost invested in extensive osseointegrated prostheses. However, there are disadvantages to the fixed-retrievable configuration, ie, compromised esthetics and time- and effort-consuming procedures, that could be solved by a completely different approach to construction that would offer the advantage of sectional repair as an alternative to complete remake.

UCLA abutments for prostheses

As previously described (see Figs 9-32 to 9-38 and 9-42 to 9-52), the UCLA construction with a prefabricated gold cylinder has many advantages, including fixed-retrievability. The laboratory procedure requires slightly more initial expense, but a great deal less chair time for assemblage and cementation problems. The advantages are:

1. Esthetics are improved (no occlusal access channels are required).
2. Gold alloy abutment screw retention increases the preloading force.
3. Abutments can be custom reangulated.
4. Abutments have improved esthetics.
5. All abutments have a nonrotating configuration.
6. Abutments have improved emergence profiles.
7. Abutments have natural tooth preparation configurations.
8. Each restoration has a tapered interface similar to that of a standard fixed partial denture restoration.
9. There are no large, one-piece castings to cause distortion or require resoldering.
10. Assemblage impressions can be made directly in the mouth (similar to a standard fixed partial denture).
11. Soldering procedures cause very little distortion and require few remakes.
12. Multiple butt joint prosthesis-abutment interfaces are avoided.
13. Lingual screw retention for fixed-retrievable capability is practical and esthetic.
14. Provisional marginal seal is a practical alternative to permanent cementation.
15. User-friendly procedures are similar to those associated with a standard fixed partial denture.

Final Osseointegrated Prosthesis

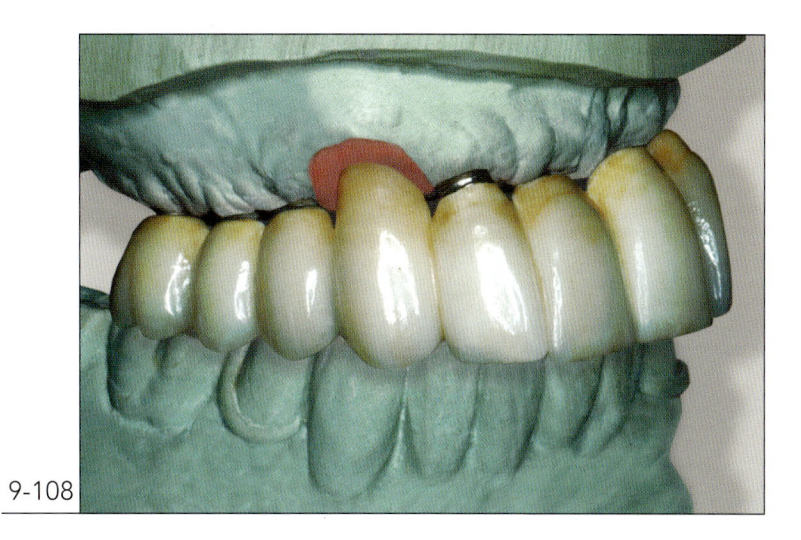

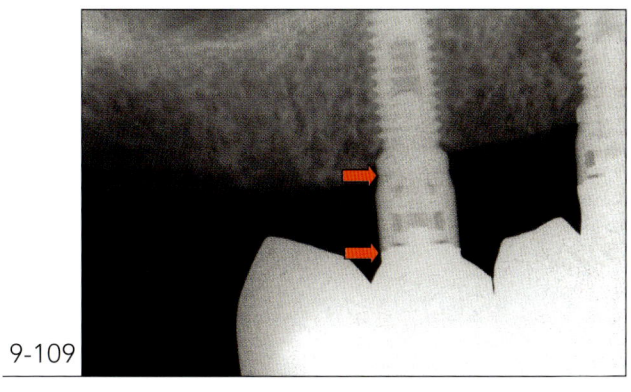

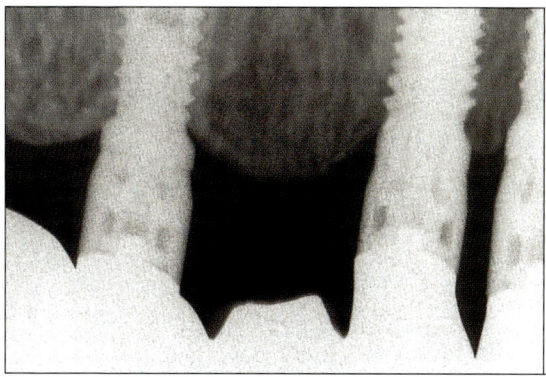

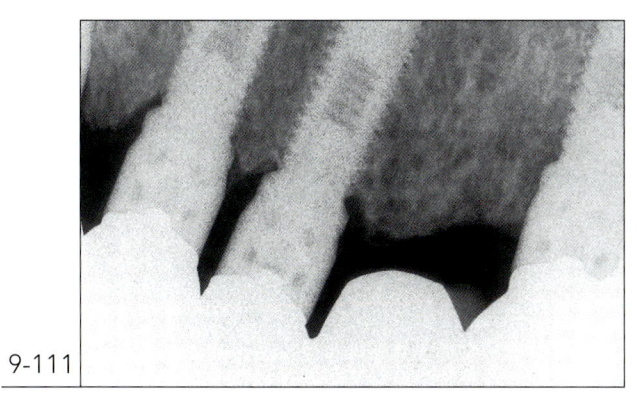

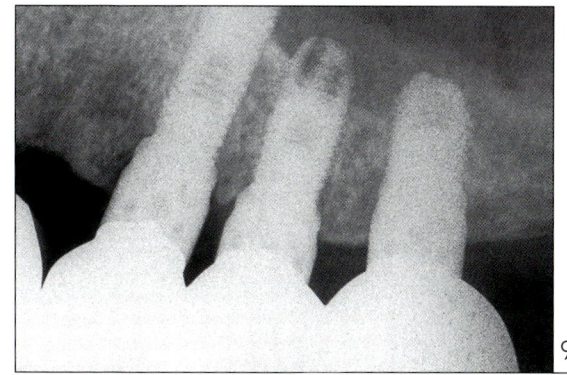

9-108

9-109

9-110

9-111

9-112

175

9 Clinical Problems

Modified Coping Design for Porcelain-Fused-to-Metal (Tooth-Supported) Restorations

There are two basic disadvantages associated with porcelain-fused-to-metal prostheses: gingival impingement and porcelain fracture. A modified coping design[7] that effectively minimizes these hazards is described below. Extensive clinical research has explored the nature of the bonding phenomenon and coping design.[8-16] However, first it is necessary to establish the parameters of a standard coping design.

Standard coping design

The standard coping is approximately 0.5 mm thick on the occlusal, buccal, and lingual surfaces. The buccogingival area is of minimum thickness and provides a porcelain butt joint for esthetics, whereas the linguogingival portion provides slightly more thickness (Fig 9-113). The proximal solder joint area (connecting strut) extends approximately 1 mm buccal and 2 mm lingual to the center line. This ensures that the solder joint is covered with porcelain.

Owing to the standard coping design, the assembled framework is subject to three-dimensional substructure flexion because the bulk of metal provided is insufficient to ensure the required stiffness (Fig 9-114). As a consequence, porcelain is subject to fracture and solder joints can fail, particularly when the interocclusal height is limited. Another unavoidable problem is gingival impingement caused by limited gingival space coronal to the solder joint (Fig 9-115). The finished prosthesis is shown in Fig 9-116 from the linguo-occlusal view, revealing minimal gingivolingual metal.

Modified coping design

The modified coping design provides the best protection against gingival impingement and substructure flexion. These objectives are obtained by placing the solder joint at the occlusal surface without covering it with porcelain (Fig 9-117, *buccal view*). Furthermore, the 3- to 4-mm lingual metal shoulder provides sufficient stiffness for the casting (*lingual view*). (Note that the lingual height of contour of the porcelain is sufficient to hide the metal.)

The proximal connecting strut extends occlusally, beyond the level of the occlusal surface of the coping, to the opposing occlusion (see Fig 9-117, *proximal view*). No porcelain will cover this portion of the metal substructure. The connecting strut extends 1 mm buccal and 2 mm lingual to the center line of the coping. The solder joint is located occlusally, in contact with the opposing occlusion (Fig 9-118). The only area that resembles the standard abutment design is that of the buccal shoulder (see Figs 9-113 and 9-117, *proximal view*). The coping should provide a porcelain square butt joint of sufficient bulk to ensure good porcelain esthetics.

Principle of corrugation

Increased stiffness of the substructure framework is obtained by means of the engineering principle of corrugation, in addition to added bulk. This principle states that the strength of a given material can be increased merely by changing its shape. An ordinary corrugated cardboard box is a simple example. Corrugation and meshwork are also used in all supersonic aircraft to increase strength without increased weight. In the modified coping design, the substructure consists of a continuous rigid bar of metal in a corrugated shape (Fig 9-119, *red line*).

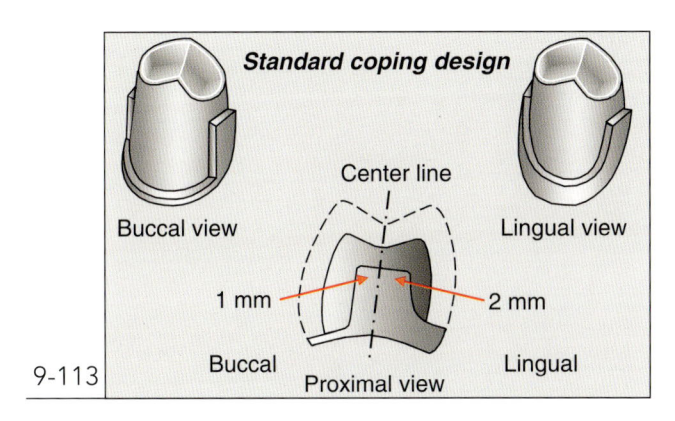

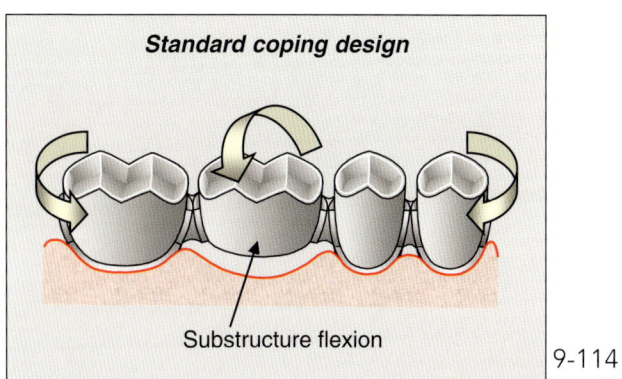

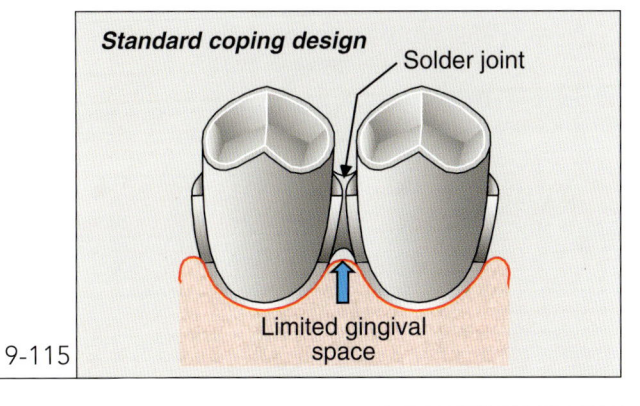

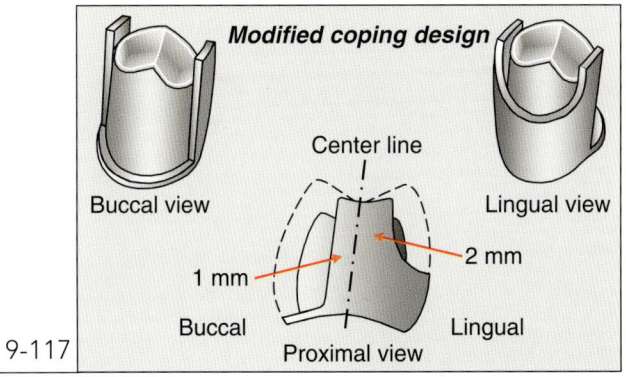

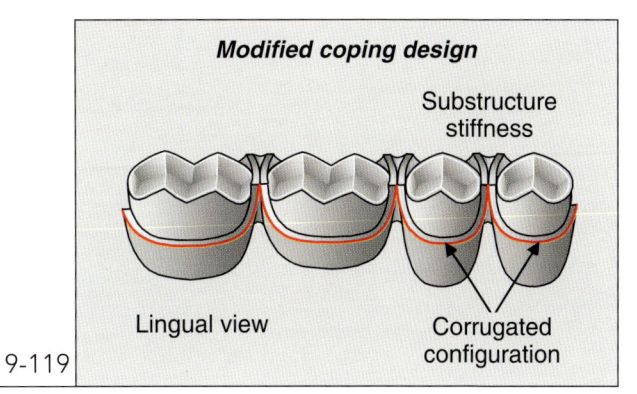

Modified Coping Design for Porcelain-Fused-to-Metal (Tooth-Supported) Restorations

9-113 Standard coping design — Buccal view, Lingual view, Proximal view (Center line, 1 mm Buccal, 2 mm Lingual)

9-114 Standard coping design — Substructure flexion

9-115 Standard coping design — Solder joint, Limited gingival space

9-116 Standard design for porcelain-fused-to-metal restorations — Lingual view of metal framework

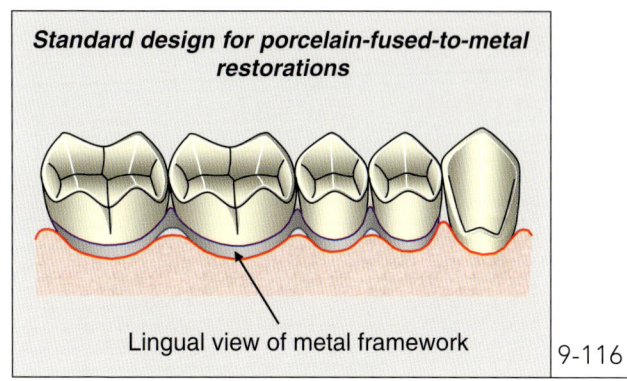

9-117 Modified coping design — Buccal view, Lingual view, Proximal view (Center line, 1 mm Buccal, 2 mm Lingual)

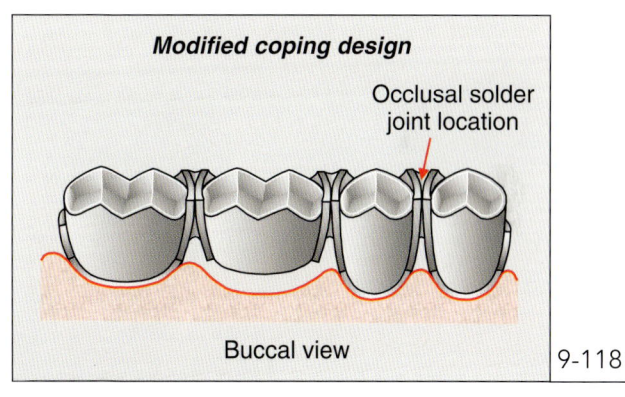

9-118 Modified coping design — Occlusal solder joint location, Buccal view

9-119 Modified coping design — Substructure stiffness, Corrugated configuration, Lingual view

177

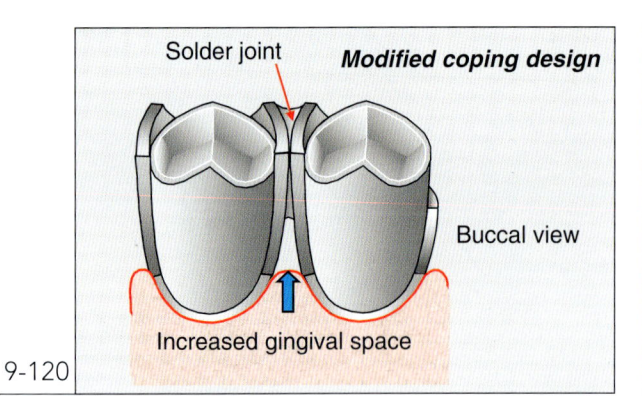

9 Clinical Problems

9-120 Solder joint — Modified coping design — Buccal view — Increased gingival space

9-121 Solder joint reshaped — Modified coping design — Buccal view — Maximum gingival space

9-122 Solder joint reshaped — Modified coping design — Lingual view — Maximum gingival space

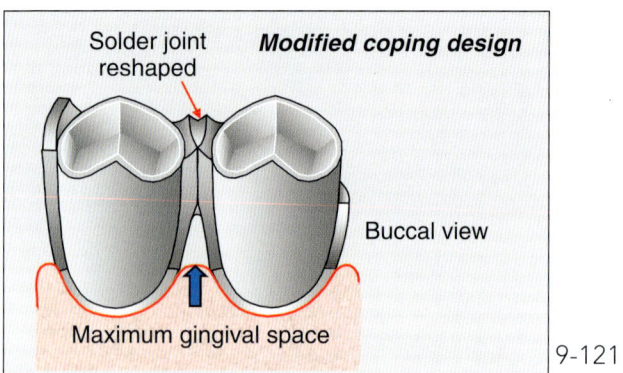

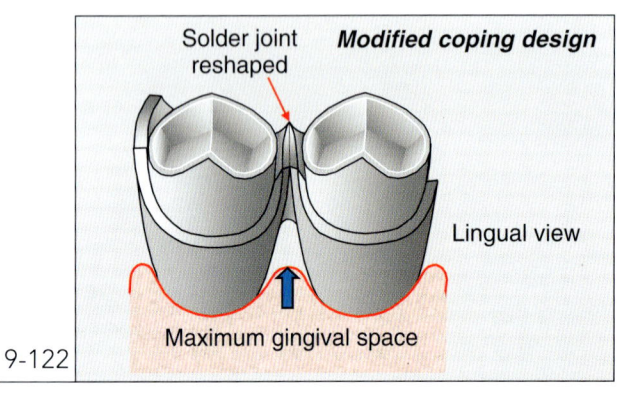

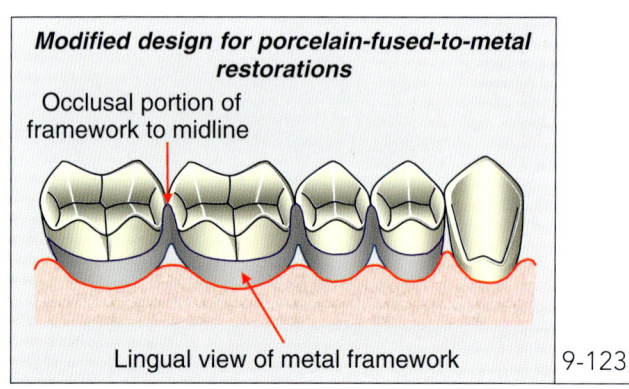

9-123 Modified design for porcelain-fused-to-metal restorations — Occlusal portion of framework to midline — Lingual view of metal framework

9-124 Pontic design: Gingival contact — Buccal — Standard design — Porcelain butt joint — Complete porcelain contact

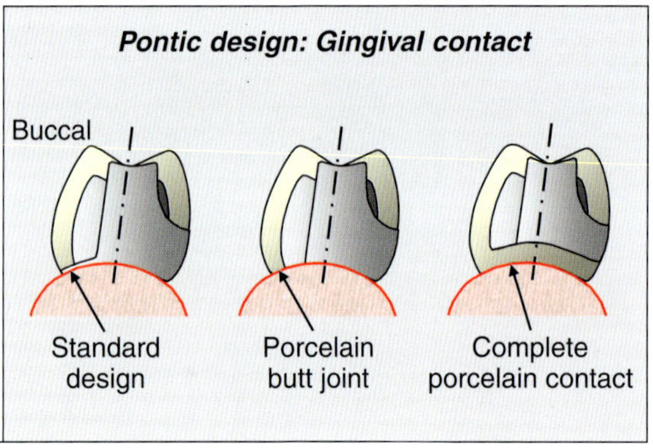

Solder joint reshaping

The occlusal location of the solder joint allows for increased gingival space (Fig 9-120). The solder joint is reshaped and tapered mesiodistally toward the occlusal without weakening its structure (Fig 9-121). The solder joint begins at the midline occlusally and extends lingually, not exceeding 1.5 to 2 mm in mesiodistal width (Fig 9-122). The lingual view shown in Fig 9-122 demonstrates the added bulk of lingual metal for strength, as well as the maximum gingival space interproximally, due to the occlusal location of the solder joint.

Pontic design

When porcelain is fused to the metal substructure, only the lingual view reveals the metal framework (Fig 9-123). Depending on the available vertical space, three pontic configurations are possible (Fig 9-124). If space is limited, the metal can be extended buccally to be in direct contact with the gingiva (*left*), or a porcelain butt joint can be used for maximum esthetics (*middle*). When space permits, there should be full gingival contact with the porcelain (*right*), which provides for optimum gingival health.

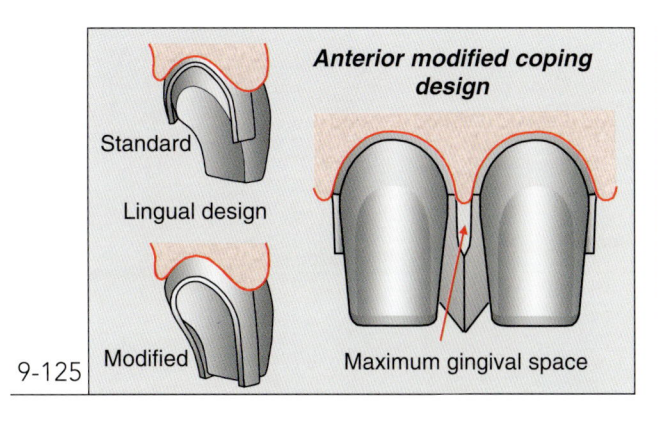

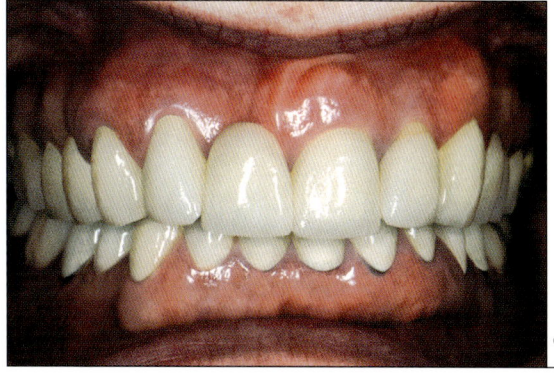

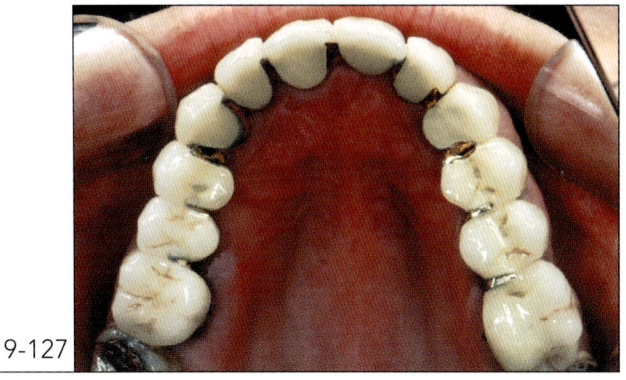

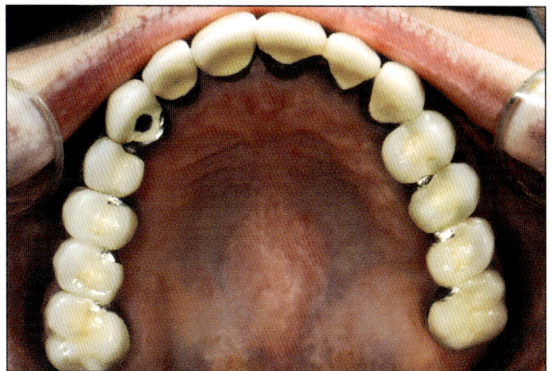

Modified Coping Design for Anterior Teeth

Modified lingual coping design

The standard lingual coping design provides minimum lingual bulk and gingival location of the connecting (soldering) strut (Fig 9-125, *upper left*). The modified configuration provides increased linguogingival bulk and occlusal location of the connecting (soldering) strut (*lower left*). From the labial view, the connecting strut is extended occlusally, slightly beyond the incisal edges of the coping (*right*). This configuration provides maximum gingival space, as well as improved esthetics due to the gingival taper (Fig 9-126).

Clinical cases

The anterior and posterior proximal connecting struts can be seen in the 8-year postoperative occlusal view shown in Fig 9-127 of the patient described in detail in chapter 3 (see Figs 3-23 to 3-56). Note that from the occlusal view, the porcelain lingual height of contour conceals the gingivolingual gold configuration. Figure 9-128 illustrates a 41-year postoperative occlusal view of a patient with the modified coping design.

In the author's opinion, the secret to longevity of extensive prostheses lies in the clinical perfection of the occlusion. No improvement in design, no matter how meritorious, can overcome defective occlusion.[17,18]

Summary

There are many clinical considerations associated with the fabrication of an extensive prosthesis, such as rotating versus nonrotating configuration of the abutments, abutment reangulation, anterior single-tooth restorations, impression accuracy, provisional and permanent cementation, and coping design. Prosthodontic success, particularly with implant-supported prostheses, depends on the careful completion of a series of critical steps. The clinical procedures are very technique sensitive; therefore, success lies in the details.

Acknowledgments

Figures 9-113 to 9-125 and portions of the text related to coping designs for porcelain-fused-to-metal restorations were adapted from an article appearing in *Journal of Prosthetic Dentistry* by Weinberg[7] with permission from Mosby, Inc.

References

1. Weinberg LA. The biomechanics of force distribution in implant-supported prostheses. Int J Oral Maxillofac Implants 1993;8:19–31.
2. Lewis S, Beumer J, Moy P, Hornburg W. The "UCLA" abutment. Int J Oral Maxillofac Implants 1988; 3:183–189.
3. Andersson B, Odman P, Lindvall AM, Brånemark Pl. Cemented single crowns on osseointegrated implants after 5 years: Results from a prospective study on CeraOne. Int J Prosthodont 1998;11: 212–218.
4. Kastenbaum FB. Achieving ideal esthetics in osseointegrated prostheses. I. Multiple units. Int J Periodontics Restorative Dent 1992;12:153–159.
5. Kastenbaum FB. Achieving ideal esthetics in osseointegrated prostheses. II. The single unit: Int J Periodontics Restorative Dent 1992;12:500–507.
6. Hsu CC, Millstein PL, Stein RS. A comparative analysis of the accuracy of implant transfer techniques. J Prosthet Dent 1993;69:588–593.
7. Weinberg LA. A new design for porcelain-fused-to-metal prostheses. J Prosthet Dent 1967;17:178–194.
8. Shell JS, Neilsen JP. Study of the bond between gold alloys and porcelain. J Dent Res 1962;41: 1424–1437.
9. Hoffman EJ. How to utilize porcelain fused to gold as a crown and bridge material. Dent Clin North Am 1965;57–64.
10. Mumford G. The porcelain fused to metal restoration. Dent Clin North Am 1965;241–249.
11. Ryge G. Current American research on porcelain-fused-to-metal restorations. Int Dent J 1965;15: 385–392.
12. Johnston JF, Dykema RW, Mumford G, Phillips RW. Construction and assembly of porcelain veneer gold crowns and pontics. J Prosthet Dent 1962;12:1125–1137.
13. Weinberg LA. Atlas of Crown and Bridge Prosthodontics. St Louis: Mosby, 1965:278.
14. Berliner A. Clinical Periodontology, Dynamics and Treatment. A Biologic Approach to Practice. New York: Park, 1953:91–93.
15. Schweitzer JM. Gold copings for problematic teeth. J Prosthet Dent 1960;10:163–166.
16. Stein RS. Pontic-residual ridge relationship: A research report. J Prosthet Dent 1966;16:251–285.
17. Schuyler CH. Correction of occlusal disharmony of the natural dentition. N Y State Dent J 1947;13: 445–462.
18. Weinberg LA. Rationale and technique for occlusal equilibration. J Prosthet Dent 1964;14:74–86.

10 Occlusion and Centric Relation Evaluation

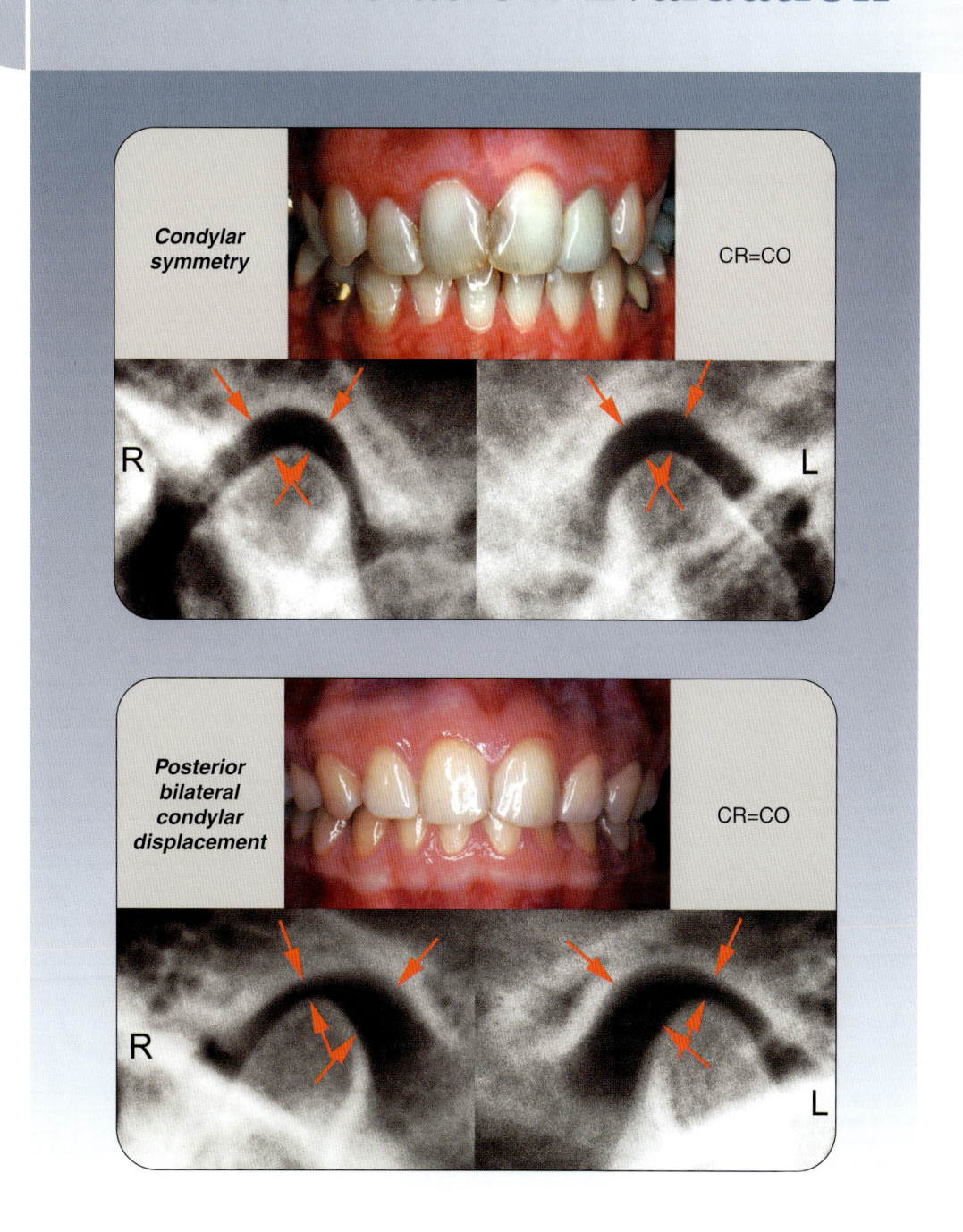

Condylar symmetry

CR=CO

R L

Posterior bilateral condylar displacement

CR=CO

R L

Occlusion and centric relation have always been controversial topics.[1] In the past there were strongly conflicting concepts of where centric relation is, how to record it, and what occlusal form is best for the patient. Each concept was associated with a specific articulator specially designed to produce the desired occlusion.

The current state of the art is almost complete confusion. In a recent survey of seven dental schools, it was found that no consensus on the definition of centric relation was possible.[2] Similarly, a literature review of 300 scientific papers found that centric relation still remains one of the most controversial issues in prosthodontics and orthodontics.[3] To resolve this dilemma, it has been suggested that the existing maximum occlusion (centric occlusion) should be provided when the patient requires quadrant restoration, and the classic concept of centric relation (ie, the most retruded, unstrained position) should be used when complete-arch restoration is required.[4] However, in the author's opinion, this is a hazardous oversimplification. To provide a wider perspective of treatment, it is useful to review some of the highlights of the past great debate on occlusion.

Summary of Major Concepts of Occlusion

Origins of gnathology

The first concepts of occlusion were introduced in the late 1920s by Gysi and Clapp[5] and Hanau,[6] who developed the first articulators to construct complete dentures. The concept of centric relation had its origin in the need to find a jaw position that was replicable. As restorative dentistry became more popular, particularly for complete-arch restorations, the requirements for occlusion, and thus articulators, became more precise. Many clinicians began to passionately study the movement of the mandible in order to develop three-dimensional articulators capable of reproducing that movement in the laboratory, with the ultimate goal of clinically achieving an occlusal anatomy in harmony with physiologic movement.[7-10] This study and instrumentation became known as *gnathology*.

To accomplish the above, it was essential to replicate the starting position of the condyles in the fossae. Gnathologists tattooed the skin on each side of the patient's head with a dot to represent the hinge axis position of the mandible,[7] which became a vital part of the process of recording and transferring three-dimensional records. The waxing-up process and the construction of complete-mouth gnathologic restorations was so arduous that provisional gold and acrylic veneers became an integral part of the process. The original studies of McCullum,[7] Stuart,[8] Stallard,[9] and more recently Granger,[10] although controversial in their time, contributed greatly to the interest and understanding of occlusion, articulators, and restorative dentistry.

Canine-protected articulation

In a study of 80 Native Americans, D'Amico[11] claimed that the ideal occlusion contained a canine-protected articulation, also known as *cuspid rise* or *cuspid-protected occlusion*. However, in a cinematic evaluation of dental students with no history of orthodontics or occlusal adjustment, the author reported that within 3 mm of lateral excursion, canine-protected articulation was not clinically significant.[12] A study of wear facets supported this conclusion.[13]

Lateral Bennett shift

The three-dimensional extraoral gnathologic tracings recorded the degree and timing of the lateral Bennett shift and reproduced it on the three-dimensional articulators.[7-10] However, some clinicians claimed the lateral Bennett shift was an artifact produced by manipulation of the mandible to obtain the external tracings. Landa[14] and Isaacson[15] found that the lateral Bennett shift of the working condyle did not exist. The present author reported that the use of the lateral Bennett shift on a semi-adjustable articulator for fixed prostheses resulted in posterior occlusal opening (negative error) during lateral working-side movements.[16] Furthermore, the elimination of lateral Bennett shift on the instrument produced harmonious posterior contact during lateral working-side excursions,[16] as described in chapter 2 (see Figs 2-9 to 2-12).

Centric relation

Research papers written in the late 1960s and early 1970s by Grasso and Sharry,[17] Kantor et al,[18] Calagna et al,[19] and Celenza[20] evaluated the effect of four different factors (time, method, neuromuscular deconditioning, and muscle tone) on the accuracy of centric relation. In all cases, centric relation was found to be an *area*, in the range of ± 0.4 mm, rather than a constant point.[17-20] However, for any three-dimensional record to be replicable, and thus valid, it must have a specific finite starting point (hinge axis tattoo). As a result, many different concepts of centric relation have been developed in an attempt to provide clinical replicability.

Centric relation was first conceived as the most retruded position of the condyles in the fossae from which lateral movements can be made at a given vertical dimension. Later modifications of this concept defined centric relation as the most retruded, *unstrained* position, then the posteriormost, uppermost position, and finally the "bracing position" of the condyle against the superior anterior wall of the glenoid fossa.[21] Each concept was associated with specific clinical techniques. (The author's clinical approach is discussed in chapter 11.)

However, in the 50 years of literature describing where the condyles *should be* in centric relation, little radiographic evidence of *actual* condylar position has been provided. Moreover, there is a lack of radiographic evidence that any particular therapeutic clinical technique actually places the condyles in the planned position.

There are fundamental questions regarding condylar position and centric relation that need to be answered, such as: Is the actual condylar position in the fossae clinically significant? When the mandible is in the most retruded position of centric relation (by any definition), where are the condyles in the fossae? Should the condyles be in the middle of the fossae when the mandible is in centric relation? Does condylar position in the fossae affect function? Has the literature provided us with a basis to judge whether condylar position in the fossae is of any importance at all?

In 1970, the author began a study on centric relation using temporomandibular joint (TMJ) radiographs[22,23] that related the actual position of the condyles in the fossae to the clinical description of the occlusion. These research data spanned 21 years and more than 30 scientific papers in an effort to establish a valid basis for diagnosis and clinical treatment procedures.[22-53] However, before the results of this research can be presented in detail, a clear description of the terminology is required.

Terminology

Centric relation

Centric relation is the most retruded, unstrained condylar position in the glenoid fossae at a specific vertical dimension from which lateral movements can be made (Fig 10-1).

Centric relation deflective contact

A *centric relation deflective contact* prevents the mandibular teeth from fully contacting the maxillary teeth while the mandible moves in hinge closure and the condyles are in centric relation. With shallow cusps this causes a modest increase in vertical dimension (Fig 10-2), whereas steep cusps result in an exaggerated increase in vertical dimension (Fig 10-3).

Deflective slide to centric occlusion

In *deflective slide to centric occlusion*, the mandible slides forward and upward, with or without a lateral component, to the acquired centric occlusion to provide maximum occlusal contact. With shallow cuspal anatomy, the condyles must translate into an eccentric position to provide maximum occlusion. This causes a mild decrease in vertical dimension (Fig 10-4). With steep cuspal anatomy, the condyles may rotate in centric relation without discernible translation, resulting in an exaggerated decrease in vertical dimension (Fig 10-5).

A deflective contact in centric relation and the resultant slide into centric occlusion may or may not cause condylar translation. It depends on the degree of vertical dimension change that takes place during the linear slide to centric occlusion. When the vertical dimension change is small relative to the forward linear slide (shallow cusps; see Figs 10-2 and 10-4), then the condyles (and mandible) should be expected to translate forward. When the opposite is true, ie, the vertical dimension change is exaggerated compared to the forward linear slide (steep cusps; see Figs 10-3 and 10-5), then the condyles (and mandible) can be expected to rotate in a hinge motion without discernable anterior condylar translation. In summary, with a given degree of linear deflective slide, it is the proportion of vertical dimension change (ie, cuspal anatomy) that determines if the condyles will translate or rotate.

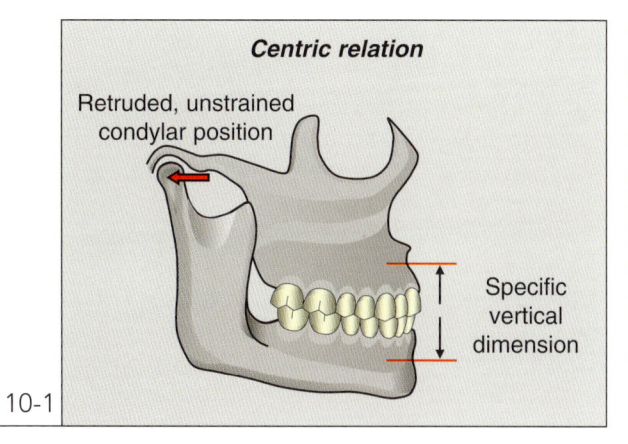

Terminology

10-1 Centric relation — Retruded, unstrained condylar position; Specific vertical dimension

10-2 Centric relation deflective contact (shallow cusps) — Condyles in centric relation; Hinge closure; Increase in vertical dimension

10-3 Centric relation deflective contact (steep cusps) — Condyles in centric relation; Hinge closure; Exaggerated increase in vertical dimension

10-4 Defective slide to centric occlusion (shallow cusps) — Condyles in eccentric position; Forward and upward slide; Mild decrease in vertical dimension

10-5 Defective slide to centric occlusion (steep cusps) — Condyles rotate in centric relation; Slide and hinge closure equal; Exaggerated decrease in vertical dimension

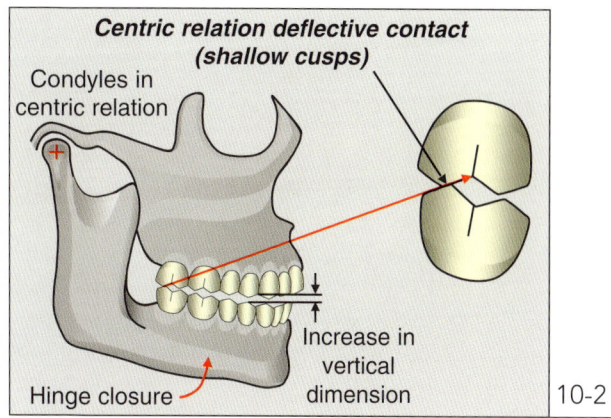

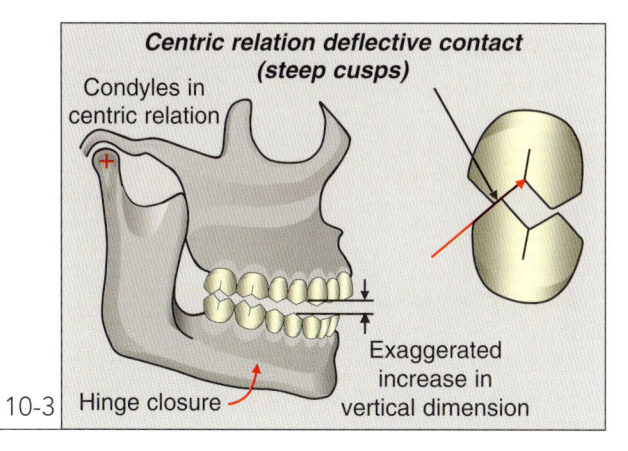

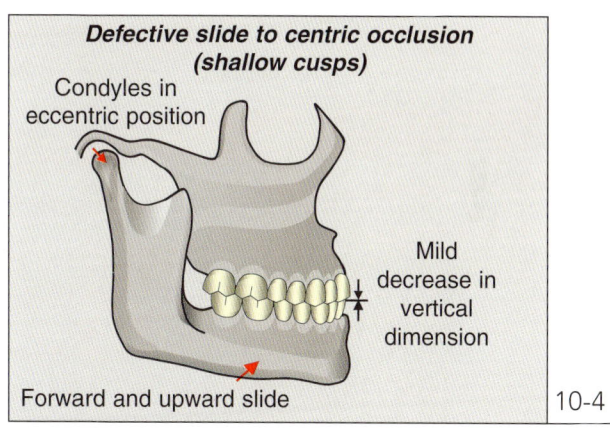

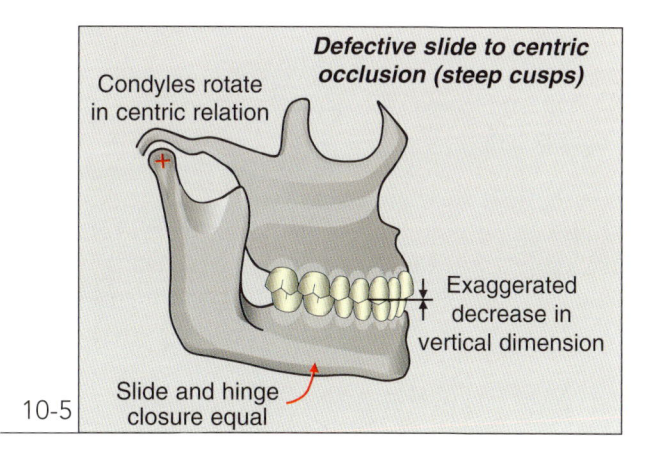

TMJ Radiographic Techniques

The subject of TMJ imaging remains controversial[54]; however, it is beyond the scope of this text to present all viewpoints on the issue. Instead, while the author respectfully acknowledges the many variations in opinion, this text details the scientific basis of the author's clinical opinion derived from his own work and that of others who have demonstrated similar results. It must be emphasized that the following discussion of TMJ radiographs, condylar position, and occlusion is directed toward the refinement of the definition of centric relation for prosthodontic purposes in this text, and not for the diagnosis and treatment of temporomandibular dysfunction (TMD)–related pain.

All TMJ radiographs, regardless of the imaging technique used (lateral transcranial, tomography, computerized tomography [CT] scan, or magnetic resonance imaging [MRI]), should be obtained with the teeth in centric occlusion (Fig 10-6). Centric occlusion is used rather than centric relation, because it is a constant position, without physiologic variation, and does not require vertical dimension change, records, or variable impression techniques. The clinical intraoral findings can be related to this standard for evaluation.

Lateral transcranial TMJ radiographs

The lateral transcranial TMJ radiographic technique was chosen for the author's investigations[22-53] because it is an inexpensive in-office procedure that facilitates control and confirmation of the jaw position (centric occlusion) while the radiograph is obtained (Fig 10-7).[23] Techniques used outside the dental office would not provide a reliable jaw position unless the dental clinician or a knowledgeable assistant was present. A simple TMJ head positioner was designed[23] and tested for replicability on a skull. The TMJ radiographs were replicable within ± 0.2 mm in a statistically valid study.[22]

A simple in-office TMJ radiographic technique also provides immediate access for treatment planning and verification. The accurate three-dimensional aiming facilitates the placement of a narrow lead diaphragm, which reduces the final radiograph to 2.5 inches in diameter.[23] The narrow beam markedly reduces background fogging and increases contrast in the final radiograph (Fig 10-8). There also is a major reduction in radiation to the surrounding soft tissue and bone. Moreover, the controlled TMJ radiographic technique facilitates minor corrective changes in head position in case of unwanted superimposition of bone onto the image of the joint space.[23,26]

Landmarks on TMJ radiographs

The auditory meatus (AM), which is circular and radiolucent, helps to immediately identify the posterior portion of the TMJ radiograph (see Fig 10-8). Anterior to the auditory meatus is the petrotympanic fissure, through which the anterior tympanic artery passes to the interior of the tympanum. (Posterior displacement of the soft tissue, rather than the condyle itself, could interfere with the blood supply to the ear, contributing to symptoms originally suggested by Costen in 1934.[55]) The head of the condyle and fossa should be clearly distinguishable without superimposition of the diagonal radiopaque petrous portion of the tempororal bone (see Fig 10-8, PPT).

Other landmarks shown in Fig 10-8 include the tuberosity (T), which is the anterior limit of normal movement, and the anterior joint space (AJS) and posterior joint space (PJS), which are used to determine condylar position clinically, as discussed later in this chapter.

TMJ Radiographic Techniques

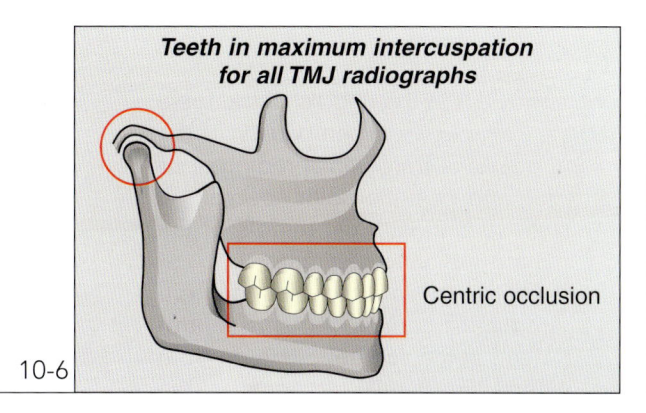

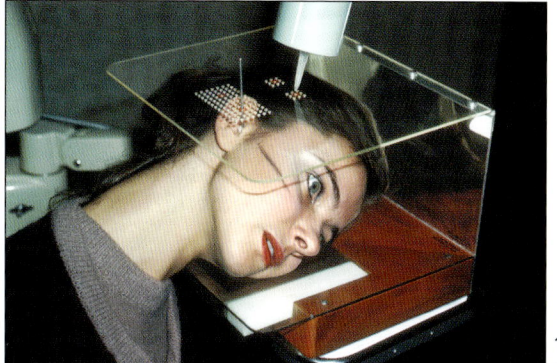

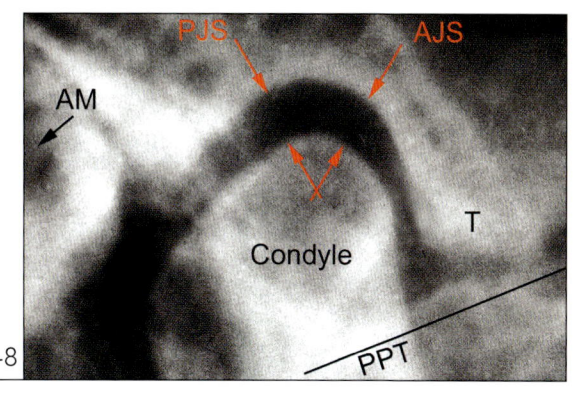

10-6 Teeth in maximum intercuspation for all TMJ radiographs — Centric occlusion

10-7

10-8 AM, PJS, AJS, Condyle, T, PPT

Anatomic and functional considerations

The superior portion of the fossa is in the shape of an arc, the diameter of which varies depending on the individual. It is relatively constant throughout adult life and extremely symmetrical because in normal function only the anterior wall of the fossa is weight bearing, while the superior portion is protected by the thickened posterior (soft tissue) portion of the disc. Otherwise, a quantitative bone loss similar to that occasionally observed at the tuberosity might occur in the superior portion of the fossa, causing a communication with the midcranial fossa, which could result in death. Clinical observations of thousands of TMJ radiographs over a period 40 years confirm the consistency and symmetry of the superior portion of the fossa.[22–53]

Determining condylar position

An untrained eye could easily identify whether a condyle is in the middle of the fossa or displaced to one end or the other. This process is a simple visual comparison of the joint spaces. In 1970, the replicability (± 0.2 mm) of lateral transcranial radiographs was established by measuring the superior, anterior, and posterior joint spaces.[22] A template was created to orient the radiograph itself, starting with the middle of the symmetrical superior portion of the fossae, to eliminate subjective estimates.

The measurement of a joint space on a radiograph, as well as a comparison of different imaging methods relative to the actual anatomic joint space, remains controversial.[54] Early experiments with 0.010-inch wire placed in the sagittal plane on both fossa and condylar surfaces indicated that with lateral transcranial radiographs, the entire joint space has a tendency to decrease proportionately as the sagittal plane is moved toward the medial; however, the medial border position showed marked variations.[26] In the author's opinion, the most important factor is the condylar position within the fossae relative to the occlusion, rather than the physical dimension of the joint spaces, which is subject to the proportional distortion factor associated with the particular technique used (transcranial, tomography, CT scan, or MRI).

The original research on the replicability of lateral TMJ radiographs used a 10.5-mm template for measurement.[22] This limited the distortion caused by physiologic bone changes of the anterior portion of the condyle and the corresponding fossa. The conflicting results in the literature related to the comparison of different techniques can be attributed to a lack of standardization of measuring points for the anterior and posterior joint spaces (Fig 10-9).

Condylar concentricity and anterior and posterior displacement

For clinical purposes, a simple visual procedure is effective for determining condylar position. First, the anterior joint space is measured by dropping a visual perpendicular from the superiormost point of the anterior slope of the fossa to the condyle (see Fig 10-9). The same procedure then is used at the posterior slope of the fossa to find the posterior joint space. The condyle is said to be concentrically located in the fossa when the posterior and anterior joint spaces are equal (see Fig 10-9). When the posterior joint space (PJS) is smaller than the anterior joint space (AJS), the condyle is displaced posteriorly (Fig 10-10). Anterior condylar displacement is evident when the anterior joint space is decreased compared to the posterior joint space (Fig 10-11). A scientific study would require at least 14 times enlargement, a template system for orientation,[22] and a measurement process to compare values, as discussed previously.

Superior condylar displacement

Superior condylar displacement is a clinical entity first described by Gerber[56] in which there is significantly reduced joint space on one side (Fig 10-12, R) compared to the other (L). Unless pain exists on the reduced joint space side, the radiographic findings could be attributed to anatomic asymmetry. A clinical test procedure devised in 1975 demonstrated that a true (painful) superiorly displaced condyle could be moved inferiorly, thus reducing pain symptoms almost immediately.[29] On the other hand, an anatomic asymmetrical (reduced) joint space without pain symptoms cannot be moved inferiorly in the fossa against the muscle strap in a conscious patient.[29] Moreover, powerful muscle relaxants provided to a patient requiring intubation prior to general anesthesia cause the mandible to drop vertically out of the fossae. Thus, this clinical test becomes a practical diagnostic tool.

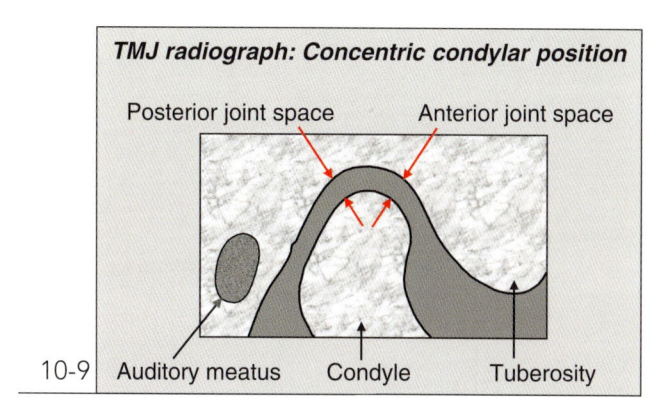

Fig 10-9 TMJ radiograph: Concentric condylar position. Posterior joint space, Anterior joint space, Auditory meatus, Condyle, Tuberosity.

Fig 10-10 TMJ radiograph: Posterior condylar displacement. Decreased PJS, Increased AJS, Auditory meatus, Condyle, Tuberosity.

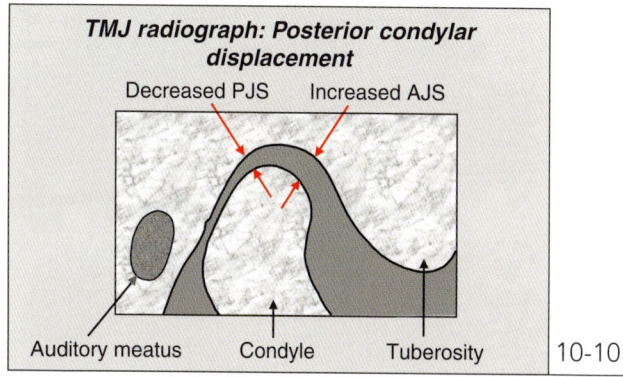

Fig 10-11 TMJ radiograph: Anterior condylar displacement. Increased PJS, Decreased AJS, Auditory meatus, Condyle, Tuberosity.

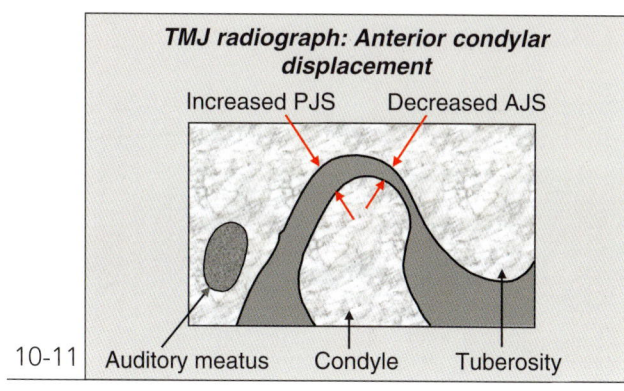

Fig 10-12 Right and left TMJ radiographs: Superior condylar displacement. Reduced joint space, Normal joint space.

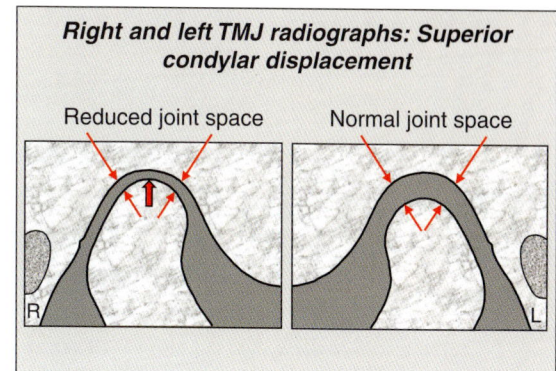

Unilateral loss in vertical dimension

It is important to point out that the mandible can lose vertical dimension unilaterally, such as during the process of complete-arch restorative dentistry.[29] Unilateral superior condylar displacement can cause compression of nerve fibers in the periphery of the disc, producing pain. For this reason, Dr C. Schuyler (personal communication) recommended in 1951 that TMJ radiographs always be obtained before and after initiating complete-arch restorative procedures to serve as a reference. Today this practice is particularly important because it reduces the clinician's liability.

Table 10-1 Condylar positions in acute TMD patients*

Study	No. of patients	Posterior (%)	Concentric (%)	Anterior (%)	Reduced/Other (%)
Weinberg[38]	55	71	4	18	7
Mikhail and Rosen[58]	63	59	11	24	6
Weinberg and Lager[42]	138	53	11	27	9
Weinberg and Chastain[52]	220	50	15	30	5
All studies	476	54	12	27	6

*Adapted from Weinberg and Chastain[52] with permission from ADA Publishing.

Table 10-2 Condylar positions in asymptomatic control patients*

Study	No. of patients	Posterior (%)	Concentric (%)	Anterior (%)	Reduced/Other (%)
Madsen[59]	96	16	70	14	0
Palla[60]	61	22	64	7	7
Weinberg[38]	61	36	23	31	10
Mikhail and Rosen[58]	38	30	26	31	13
Rieder and Martinoff[61]	111	11	47	42	0
Weinberg and Chastain[52]	60	27	48	23	2
All studies	427	21	50	26	4

*Adapted from Weinberg and Chastain[52] with permission from ADA Publishing.

Condylar Position in the Fossa Relative to Occlusion

From 1970 to 1991, TMJ radiographs were obtained from patients who were asymptomatic, as well as from those with TMD-related pain, and the results reported.[22–53] Based on these data, it can be categorically stated, regardless of the method of TMJ imaging, that there is no absolute correlation between the occlusion intraorally and the actual position of the condyles in the fossae. There is, however, a statistically valid association of one particular condylar displacement (ie, posterior displacement) with TMD-related pain symptoms, and conversely, another condylar position (ie, concentricity) associated with an absence of symptoms (Tables 10-1 and 10-2). Therefore, these data, as well as the pertinent literature, provide guidelines for establishing clear definitions of what is normal (functional) and what is abnormal (dysfunctional) to aid in diagnosis and treatment.

Condylar Position in the Fossa Relative to Occlusion

Condylar symmetry — CR=CO
R / L
10-13

Posterior bilateral condylar displacement — CR=CO
R / L
10-14

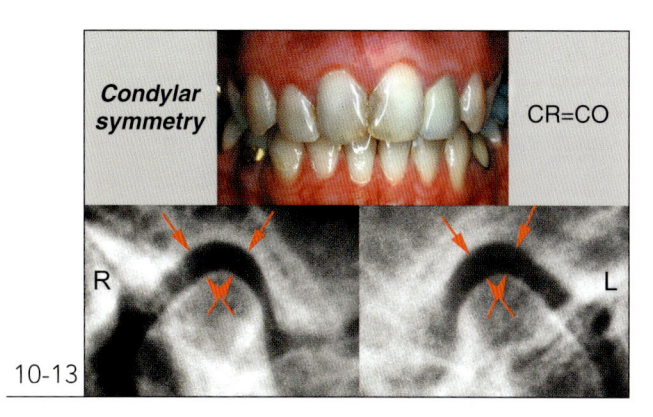

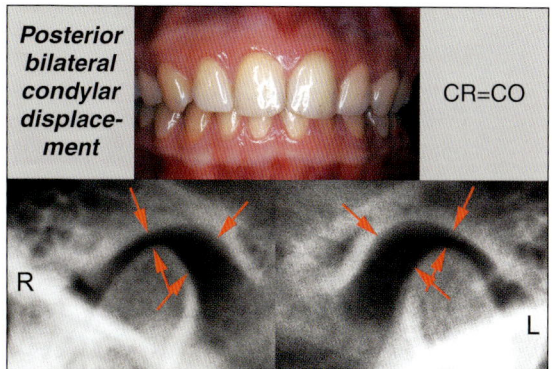

Right superior condylar displacement — CR=CO
R / L
10-15

Clinical examples

The following patients have clinically equal centric relation (CR) and centric occlusion (CO) but different condylar positions radiographically. Figure 10-13 illustrates a patient with both condyles concentrically located in the fossae, while the patient in Fig 10-14 has severe bilateral posterior condylar displacement. It is important to emphasize that the degree of condylar displacement does not necessarily indicate the degree of clinical dysfunction and/or pain. For example, the patient in Fig 10-14 has a long history of orthodontics and no TMD-related pain. (Gill[57] has demonstrated that there are relatively few stretch receptors in the lateral pterygoid muscles, which could explain these findings.) On the other hand, the patient in Fig 10-15 has right superior condylar displacement with TMD-related pain on that side. (The right condyle was subsequently moved inferiorly, and the pain was relieved almost immediately.[29])

Summary of research

Valid statistical sampling, as well as data gathered from several clinicians using different methods, is required to establish criteria for what is functional and what is dysfunctional relative to the actual condylar position in the fossae, as determined by TMJ imaging. Tables 10-1 and 10-2 present data gathered from seven different clinicians reporting on patients with acute TMD symptoms and a control group of asymptomatic patients. Lateral transcranial radiographs with the teeth in the maximum (centric) occlusion were obtained to determine condylar position. In the acute TMD group, 54% of patients had posterior condylar displacement, while only 12% had concentrically located condyles, a statistically significant difference.[13] In contrast, only 21% of the control patients had posterior condylar displacement, while 50% had condyles in concentric position.

Rieder and Martinoff[61] focused on severity of symptoms in 926 patients, comparing bilateral concentric condylar positions with nonconcentric condylar positions, rather than specific condylar displacements. The severity of symptoms was significantly higher in patients with nonconcentric condylar variations compared with those having bilateral condylar concentricity.[61]

Summary of findings

Combining the above data, condylar nonconcentricity was found to be a statistically significant factor in TMD symptoms in 1,829 acute TMD patients and controls. This does not mean, however, that condylar displacement is *pathognomonic* for TMD symptoms, but it does provide guidelines for determining a new definition of centric relation that includes joint imaging.

TMJ imaging controversy

Tomograms versus transcranial TMJ radiographs

The data reported above have been controversial because some clinicians express the opinion that the transcranial radiographs are not accurate, despite the statistically valid study that showed that these radiographs are replicable within ± 0.2 mm.[22] Moreover, Mongini's studies[62] showed that transcranial radiographs compared favorably with tomograms, and Pullinger et al[63] reported results similar to those found with transcranial radiographs in a tomographic study of 66 patients with TMD: 57% had posterior condylar displacement, 35% had concentrically located condyles, and 8% had anteriorly displaced condyles. The findings of a tomographic study[64] of 25 asymptomatic TMD patients were also similar to those of the transcranial radiographic studies, ie, more condylar concentricity (57%) and less posterior (27%) and anterior (16%) condylar displacement.

TMJ imaging using advanced technology

Most advanced imaging technologies (ie, CT scan and MRI) have been devoted to the diagnosis and treatment of internal disc derangements.[65] Similarly, research on condylar position in the fossae, as determined by arthrography, has been reported mainly in relation to internal disc derangement rather than occlusion per se.[66] It has generally been recognized that each imaging technique has inherent strengths and limitations.[67] However, although the MRI is noninvasive and unchallenged in its excellent diagnostic validity for certain conditions, there is an absence of MRI studies relating condylar positions in the fossae to clinical TMD-related pain; therefore, the validity of its use in such studies is unknown.[68] In summary, there has not been sufficient use of advanced TMJ imaging to provide data relating condylar position in the fossae to occlusion in functional and dysfunctional patients. However, it is likely that such use would help solve the problem of centric relation.

Research conflicts

Research on condylar position relative to occlusion using radiographic evidence remains controversial. For example, condylar position (the joint space) has been shown to vary at different sagittal locations within the TMJ.[69] The author placed 0.01-inch wire on the condyle and fossa in the sagittal plane in four locations using lateral transcranial radiographs.[26] The following conclusions can be drawn from the findings: *(1)* The lateral third of the condyle and fossa are recorded using this technique; *(2)* the joint spaces varied in size in various sagittal planes; *(3)* the joint space tended to be larger laterally and diminished medially; and *(4)* the condylar position within the fossa (ie, anterior, concentric, or posterior) was similar in all planes except the medial border position, in which it varied widely.[26] Knoernschild et al[54] measured impressions of the joint spaces as compared to corrected and uncorrected tomographic projections and lateral transcranial radiographs. Only corrected tomographic projections reflected the actual measured joint spaces.[54]

Conclusions

Some of the conflicting reports can be attributed to the lack of a standard measuring system. The most important factor is condylar position in the fossa, not specific measurement values at one sagittal plane compared with those taken at another. Most of the early research reports are based on evidence from lateral transcranial radiographs and tomograms, and there is general agreement between the two imaging systems.

Clinical implications

There is clear evidence of a statistically significant higher incidence of posterior condylar displacement in patients with acute TMD-related pain than in those without pain.[52] On the other hand, condylar displacement does exist in patients without symptoms, but to a statistically significant lesser degree. These facts indicate several conclusions: *(1)* Condylar displacement in and of itself is not pathognomonic for TMD; *(2)* condylar displacement is an *etiologic factor* in TMD, which is a multicausal disorder; *(3)* a new definition of centric relation relating the actual condylar position in the fossae (via TMJ imaging) with the clinical occlusal findings is indicated; and *(4)* condylar position in the fossae should be included in the diagnosis and treatment planning for complete-arch restorations when treating asymptomatic patients, as well as patients with TMD-related pain. (The diagnosis and treatment of TMD-related pain is beyond the scope of this text; see the literature[22-53] for more information.)

New Definition of Centric Relation

Centric relation equal to centric occlusion

Functional centric relation
When centric relation and centric occlusion are equal and the condyles are positioned symmetrically in the middle of the fossae (Fig 10-16), centric relation is functional and should be used for restorative procedures.[24,25,27–53]

Dysfunctional centric relation
When centric relation and centric occlusion are equal and one or both condyles are retruded (see Fig 10-14), restorative procedures in centric relation are hazardous. If TMD symptoms are present, the patient should not be restored in centric relation until the pain is eliminated.[32,33] If there are no TMD symptoms, the patient can be restored with a "long centric," as originally described by Mann and Pankey,[70] to prevent locking the patient into a posteriorly displaced condylar position. This can be easily accomplished on an articulator,[71] as described in chapter 2 (see Figs 2-14 to 2-18). For any new restorative prostheses, the patient should undergo a 2-month clinical trial in the planned occlusion before the final prosthesis is constructed.[32]

It is important to note that all condyles do not necessarily belong in the exact middle of the fossa bilaterally. When there is a dysfunctional centric relation without pain, however, the clinician should be aware that there is the potential for acute TMD-related pain as a result of treatment. Superior condylar displacement may require diagnostic procedures[29] before the initiation of treatment. If there is pain on the superior displaced side (see Fig 10-15, R) the patient should be treated by a clinician who is familiar with the treatment requirements.[29]

Deflective slide to centric occlusion

It should be remembered that all TMJ radiographs are obtained in maximum (centric) occlusion. Therefore, if there is a deflective slide to centric occlusion, the TMJ radiographs reveal where the condyles are at the end of the deflective slide, which is centric occlusion and not centric relation. In that case, centric relation cannot be evaluated directly from TMJ radiographs. The only time an evaluation of centric relation can be made directly from TMJ radiographs is when centric relation and centric occlusion are equal (see Figs 10-13 to 10-16).

When there is a deflective slide to centric occlusion, the assessment of centric relation requires a reverse evaluation process. For example, if the intraoral displacement is similar to the anterior condylar displacement seen in the TMJ radiographs, then the centric relation is functional. In this case, removal of the deflective slide will reposition the condyles posteriorly and concentrically in the fossae and therefore is recommended. Conversely, if the intraoral displacement does not resemble the condylar displacement seen in the TMJ radiographs, then the centric relation is dysfunctional, and the deflective slide should not be removed.

When constructing complete-mouth prostheses, these data indicate when to remove centric relation deflective contacts and when to maintain them because they are protective against possible TMD-related pain after the prosthesis is placed. A few practical cases are presented in the following sections to illustrate this diagnostic process.

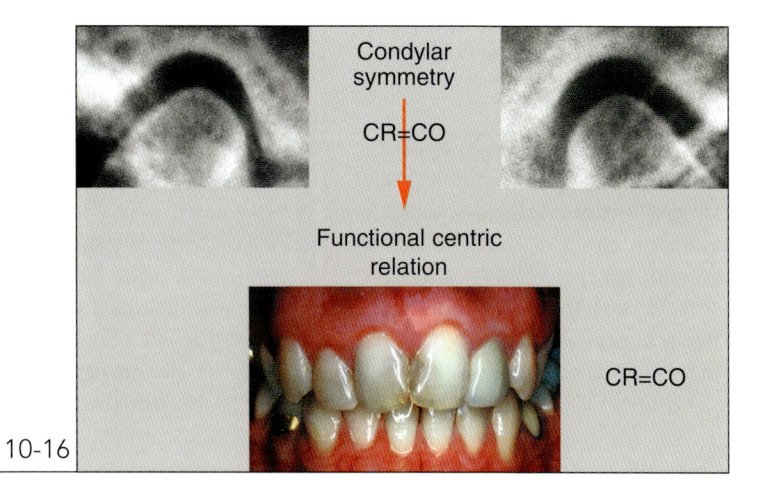

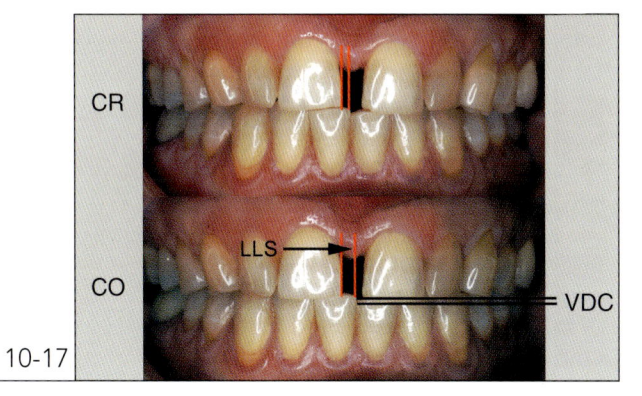

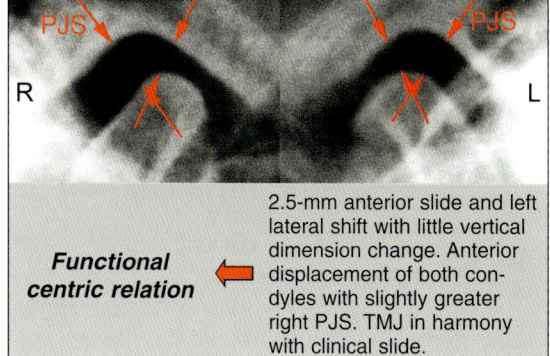

Functional centric relation with deflective slide and lateral shift

Figure 10-17 (*top*) shows a patient in centric relation closure lightly touching a posterior deflective contact. The center line of the mandibular central incisors is marked in red. As the patient closes to centric occlusion (*bottom*), the mandible slides forward 2.5 mm with minimal vertical dimension change (VDC) and a slight left lateral shift (LLS).

Both condyles are displaced anteriorly, as expected with a 2.5-mm linear shift with minimal vertical dimension change (see Figs 10-2 and 10-4). Because of the left lateral shift, the anterior displacement of the right condyle should be slightly greater than that of the left condyle. The TMJ radiographs (Fig 10-18) are in harmony with the clinical occlusal findings; therefore, the patient's centric relation is functional, and the deflective slide can be safely corrected.

If the patient had TMD symptoms, or if a complete-arch prosthesis were required in a patient without TMD symptoms, the author's recommendation would be removal of centric relation deflective contacts to provide harmony between centric relation and centric occlusion. Postoperative TMJ radiographs would show the condyles concentrically placed in the middle of the fossae. (This is discussed in more detail later in the chapter.)

Dysfunctional centric relation with deflective slide and lateral shift

Figure 10-19 (*top*) shows a patient in centric relation closure lightly touching a posterior deflective contact. As the patient slides to centric occlusion (*bottom*), the movement is almost entirely lateral toward the patient's right side (RLS) with modest vertical dimension change (VDC). Since the deflective slide is practically a right lateral excursion with no discernable anterior component, the right TMJ radiograph (Fig 10-20, R) would be expected to demonstrate a slightly reduced posterior joint space (PJS). After a lateral shift to the patient's right side, the left condyle should be anteriorly displaced in the fossa equal to the linear distance of the right lateral side shift. However, the left TMJ radiograph (see Fig 10-20, L) demonstrates a reduced posterior joint space (PJS), indicating posterior condylar displacement *after* the lateral shift to the opposite side. The intraoral lateral side shift is not in harmony with the TMJ radiographs; therefore, the centric relation is dysfunctional and the deflective contacts are protective, ie, removal of the centric relation deflective contacts would cause further posterior condylar displacement on the left side, which is likely to result in TMD-related pain.

Removal of centric relation deflective contacts

The existence of a deflective slide to centric occlusion does not in itself indicate that the deflective contacts should be removed to bring about a harmony between centric relation and centric occlusion, regardless of the size of the planned restoration. Removal of centric relation deflective contacts should only be accomplished after TMJ imaging and diagnosis of the centric relation as functional (see Figs 10-17 and 10-18), ie, when TMJ imaging shows a correlation between occlusal and condylar displacement and removing the deflective contacts therefore would reposition the condyles symmetrically in both fossae. If removal of the deflective contacts would reposition the condyles asymmetrically in the fossae as determined by TMJ imaging, ie, if the centric relation is dysfunctional, the deflective contacts are *protective* and should be maintained.

The patient in Fig 10-17 demonstrated functional centric relation with a deflective slide to centric occlusion. In such cases, the clinician may choose to perform quadrant restoration using the existing centric occlusion. However, complete-mouth restoration should be initiated only after the centric relation deflective contacts are removed to harmonize centric relation and centric occlusion (see chapter 11). A suitable clinical trial should precede tooth preparation.

Centric relation is illustrated before treatment in Fig 10-21 (*top*). Note the very slight increase in vertical dimension (VDI) as well as the location of the center line (CLB). After occlusal adjustment to remove the deflective contacts, centric relation and centric occlusion are equal, which provides maximum occlusion (*bottom*). Note that the center line (CLA) remains in the same vertical plane, indicating that the left lateral shift has been eliminated.

TMJ radiographs of the right side before and after treatment are shown in Fig 10-22. As noted earlier, the patient demonstrated anterior bilateral condylar displacement, with the right condyle displaced to a slightly greater degree than the left (see Fig 10-18), as evidenced by the exaggerated posterior joint space (see Fig 10-22, PJSB). After removal of the deflective occlusal contacts, the posterior joint space is markedly reduced (see Fig 10-22, PJSA) and the condyle more centrally located in the fossa.

TMJ radiographs of the left side before and after treatment are shown in Fig 10-23. Before treatment, the left side TMJ radiograph demonstrates exaggerated posterior

New Definition of Centric Relation

Fig 10-19 (CR / CO / VDC / RLS)

Fig 10-20 Dysfunctional centric relation — Left posterior condylar displacement not in harmony with right clinical slide. (PJS)

Fig 10-21 (VDI / CR=CO / CLB / CLA / CR befor / CR after)

Fig 10-22 Right TMJ before — Exaggerated posterior joint space (PJSB). Right TMJ after — Posterior joint space reduced after occlusal adjustment (PJSA).

Fig 10-23 Left TMJ before — Enlarged posterior joint space (PJSB). Left TMJ after — Posterior joint space reduced after occlusal adjustment (PJSA).

Fig 10-24 Right TMJ after / Left TMJ after — After occlusal adjustment bilateral condylar position is more symmetrical and concentric. (PJSA)

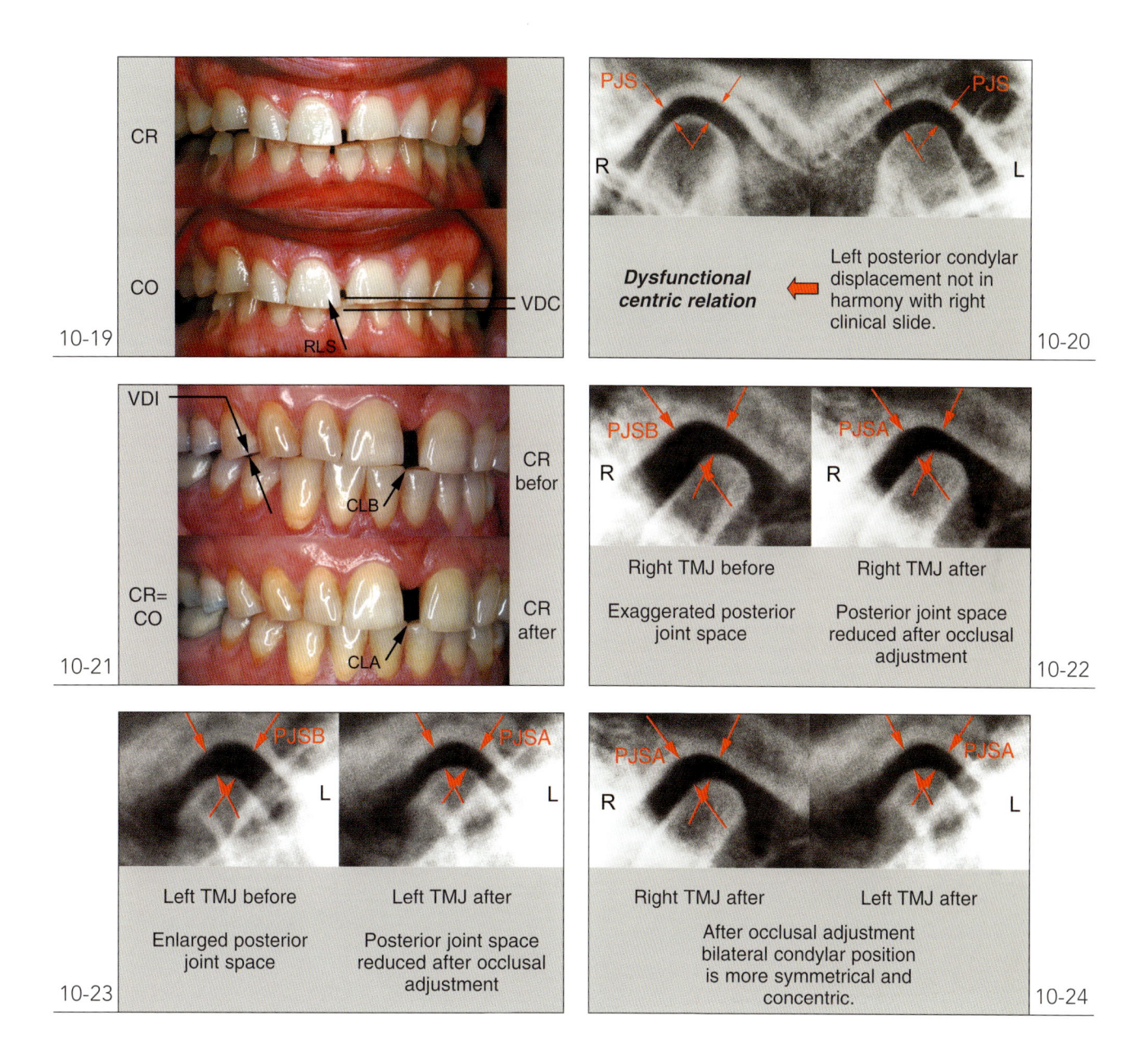

joint space (see Fig 10-23, PJSB). After occlusal adjustment, the posterior joint space is reduced (see Fig 10-23, PJSA) and the condyle is centrally located in the fossa. Figure 10-24 shows the right and left postoperative TMJ radiographs. Bilateral condylar position is more symmetrical and concentric compared with the preoperative TMJ radiographs (see Fig 10-18).

Note, however, that the right postoperative TMJ radiograph (see Fig 10-24, R) reveals that the condyle is not *exactly* in the middle of the fossa, which illustrates an important point: Condylar repositioning should not be approached as a strict geometric mechanical process. Sometimes the degree of improvement shown between the before and after radiographs (see Fig 10-22) is the maximum that can be accomplished with a given patient. In the end, it is the comfort of the patient that is the final criteria; therefore, an 8-week trial period should always be provided to confirm the physiologic acceptance of any given occlusal change before final restorations are placed.

Summary

A new definition of centric relation that includes the actual position of the condyles in the fossae (determined through joint imaging) in relation to the occlusion should be developed.[24,25,27–53] Statistically valid evidence has shown that condylar symmetry in both fossae has a far greater incidence of patient comfort and function than anterior or posterior displacement of one or both condyles.[24–53,58–64] The controversy over various methods of joint imaging not withstanding, the confusion over centric relation[2,3,69,72] as it relates to prosthodontics could be eliminated with more research on the relationship between occlusion and condylar position in the fossae using different imaging modalities.

It can be concluded clinically that the deflective slide to centric occlusion should be corrected only when the centric relation is functional, ie, when TMJ imaging shows a correlation between the occlusal displacement and the condylar displacement. When such a correlation is not found, the centric relation is dysfunctional and the deflective contacts are usually protective and therefore should be maintained.

References

1. Weinberg LA. A visualized technique of occlusal equilibration. J Dent Med 1952;7:9–15,18–25.
2. Jasinevicius TR, Yellowitz JA, Vaughan GG, Brooks ES, Baughan LW, Theiss LB. Centric relation definitions taught in 7 dental schools: Results of faculty and student surveys. J Prosthet Dent 2000;9:87–94.
3. Keshvad A, Winstanley RB. An appraisal of the literature on centric relation. Part I. J Oral Rehabil 2000;27:823–833.
4. Wilson J, Nairn RI. Condylar repositioning in mandiblar retrusion. J Prosthet Dent 2000;84:612–616.
5. Gysi A, Clapp GW. Practical application of research results in denture construction (mandibular movements). J Am Dent Assoc 1929;16:199–223.
6. Hanau RL. Full Denture Prosthesis, ed 4. Buffalo: Hanau Engineering, 1930:39.
7. McCullum BB. Fundamentals involved in prescribing restorative remedies. D Items Interest 1939;61:522–535,641–648,724–736,852–856,942–950.
8. Stuart CE, Stallard H. Principles involved in restoring occlusion to natural teeth. J Prosthet Dent 1960;10:304–313.
9. Stallard H. Dental articulation as an orthodontic aim. J Am Dent Assoc Dent Cosmos 1937;24:348–376.
10. Granger ER, Lucia V, Hudson W, Celenza F, Pruden W Jr. Hinge axis committee research report. Presented to the New York Academy of Prosthodontists, 1959.
11. D'Amico A. The canine teeth—Normal functional relation of the natural teeth of man. J South Calif State Dent Assoc 1958;26:6–23,49–60,127–142,175–182,194–208,239–241.
12. Weinberg LA. A cinematic study of centric and eccentric occlusions. J Prosthet Dent 1964;14:290–293.
13. Weinberg LA. The prevalence of tooth contact in eccentric movements of the jaw: Its clinical implications. J Am Dent Assoc 1961;62:403–406.
14. Landa J. Critical analysis of the Bennett movement. J Prosthet Dent 1958;8:709–726.
15. Isaacson D. A clinical study of the Bennett movement. J Prosthet Dent 1958;8:841–849.
16. Weinberg LA. An evaluation of basic articulators and their concepts. J Prosthet Dent 1963;13:622–644, 645–663,873–888,1038–1054.
17. Grasso J, Sharry J. The duplicability of arrow-point tracing in dentulous subjects. J Prosthet Dent 1968;20:106–115.
18. Kantor M, Silverman S, Garfinkel L. Centric relation recording techniques: A comparative investigation. J Prosthet Dent 1972;28:593–600.
19. Calagna L, Silverman S, Garfinkel L. Influence of neuromuscular conditioning on centric relation registrations. J Prosthet Dent 1973;30:598–604.
20. Celenza FV. The centric position: Replacement and character. J Prosthet Dent 1973;30:591–598.
21. Dawson PE. Evaluation, Diagnosis, and Treatment of Occlusal Problems. St Louis: Mosby, 1974.
22. Weinberg LA. An evaluation of duplicability of temporomandibular joint radiographs. J Prosthet Dent 1970;24:512–541.
23. Weinberg LA. Technique for temporomandibular joint radiographs. J Prosthet Dent 1972;28:284–308.
24. Weinberg LA. Correlation of temporomandibular dysfunction with radiographic findings. J Prosthet Dent 1972;28:519–539.

References

25. Weinberg LA. Temporomandibular joint function and its effect on centric relation. J Prosthet Dent 1973;30:176–195.
26. Weinberg LA. What we really see in a TMJ radiograph. J Prosthet Dent 1973;30:898–913.
27. Weinberg LA. Temporomandibular dysfunctional profile: A patient-oriented approach. J Prosthet Dent 1974;32:312–325.
28. Weinberg LA. Radiographic investigations into temporomandibular joint function. J Prosthet Dent 1975;33:672–688.
29. Weinberg LA. Superior condylar displacement: Its diagnosis and treatment. J Prosthet Dent 1975;34:59–76.
30. Weinberg LA. Anterior condylar displacement: Its diagnosis and treatment. J Prosthet Dent 1975;34:195–207.
31. Weinberg LA. Temporomandibular joint function and its effect on concepts of occlusion. J Prosthet Dent 1976;35:553–566.
32. Weinberg LA. Posterior bilateral condylar displacement: Its diagnosis and treatment. J Prosthet Dent 1976;36:426–440.
33. Weinberg LA. Posterior unilateral condylar displacement: Its diagnosis and treatment. J Prosthet Dent 1977;37:559–569.
34. Weinberg LA. An evaluation of stress in TMJ dysfunction pain syndrome. J Prosthet Dent 1977;38:192–207.
35. Weinberg LA. Treatment prosthesis in TMJ dysfunction pain syndrome. J Prosthet Dent 1978;39:654–669.
36. Weinberg LA. An evaluation of asymmetry in TMJ radiography. J Prosthet Dent 1978;40:315–323.
37. Weinberg LA. An evaluation of occlusal factors in TMJ dysfunctional pain syndrome. J Prosthet Dent 1979;41:198–208.
38. Weinberg LA. The role of condylar position in TMJ dysfunctional pain syndrome. J Prosthet Dent 1979;41:636–643.
39. Weinberg LA. The etiology, diagnosis, and treatment of TMJ dysfunction-pain syndrome. Part I: Etiology. J Prosthet Dent 1979;42:654–664.
40. Weinberg LA. The etiology, diagnosis, and treatment of TMJ dysfunction-pain syndrome. Part II: Differential diagnosis. J Prosthet Dent 1980;43:58–70.
41. Weinberg LA. The etiology, diagnosis, and treatment of TMJ dysfunction-pain syndrome. Part III: Treatment. J Prosthet Dent 1980;43:186–196.
42. Weinberg LA, Lager L. Clinical report on the etiology and diagnosis of TMJ dysfunction pain syndrome. J Prosthet Dent 1980;44:642–653.
43. Weinberg LA. Vertical dimension: A research and clinical analysis. J Prosthet Dent 1982;47:290–302.
44. Weinberg LA. The role of stress, occlusion and condylar position in TMJ dysfunction pain. J Prosthet Dent 1983;49:532–545.
45. Weinberg LA. Definitive prosthodontic therapy for TMJ patients. Part I: Anterior and posterior condylar displacement. J Prosthet Dent 1983;50:544–557.
46. Weinberg LA. Definitive prosthodontic therapy for TMJ patients. Part II: Posterior and superior condylar displacement. J Prosthet Dent 1983;50:690–699.
47. Weinberg LA. Practical evaluation of the lateral TMJ radiograph. J Prosthet Dent 1984;54:676–685.
48. Weinberg LA. A conceptual overview of the state of the art of TMJ dysfunction pain. N Y State Dent J 1987;53:18–24.
49. Weinberg LA. An overview of the TMJ controversy. Compend Contin Educ Dent 1987;8:420,422,424–425.
50. Weinberg LA. Malpractice prevention: New problems require new solutions. N Y State Dent J 1988;54:18–21.
51. Weinberg LA. Optimum temporomandibular joint condyle position in clinical practice. Int J Periodontics Restorative Dent 1985;1:11–27.
52. Weinberg LA, Chastain J. New TMJ clinical data and its implication on diagnosis and treatment. J Am Dent Assoc 1990;120:305–311.
53. Weinberg LA. The role of muscle deconditioning for occlusal corrective procedures. J Prosthet Dent 1991;66:250–255.
54. Knoernschild KL, Aquilino SA, Ruprecht A. Transcranial radiography and linear tomography: A comparative study. J Prosthet Dent 1991;66:239–250.
55. Costen JB. Syndrome of ear and sinus symptoms dependent on disturbed function of the temporomandibular joint. Ann Otol Rhinol Laryngol 1934;43:1–15.
56. Gerber V. Kiefergelenk und zahnolljusion. Dtsch Zahnarztl Z 1971;26:119–141.
57. Gill HI. Neuromuscular spindles in human lateral pterygoid muscle. J Anat 1971;109:157–167.
58. Mikhail MG, Rosen H. The validity of temporomandibular joint radiographs using the head positioner. J Prosthet Dent 1979;42:441–446.
59. Madsen B. Normal variations in anatomy, condylar movements, and arthrosis frequency of the temporomandibular joints. Acta Radiol Diagn (Stockh) 1966;4:273–288.

60. Palla S. Eine studie uber die kondylenposition in rontgenbild. SSO Schweiz Monatsschr Zahnheilkd 1977;87:304.
61. Rieder CE, Martinoff JT. Comparison of the multiphasic dysfunction profile with lateral transcranial radiographs. J Prosthet Dent 1984;52:572–580.
62. Mongini F. The importance of radiography in diagnosis of TMJ dysfunctions. A comparative evaluation of transcranial radiographs and serial tomography. J Prosthet Dent 1981;45:186–198.
63. Pullinger AG, Solberg WK, Hollender L, Guichet D. Tomographic analysis of mandibular condyle position in diagnostic subgroups of temporomandibular disorders. J Prosthet Dent 1986;55:723–729.
64. Blaschke DD, Blaschke TJ. Normal TMJ bony relationships in centric occlusion. J Dent Res 1981;60:98–104.
65. Larheim TA. Current trends in temporomandibular joint imaging. Oral Surg Oral Med Oral Pathol Oral Radiol Endod 1995;80:555–576.
66. Ren YF, Isberg A, Westesson PL. Condyle position in the temporomandibular joint. Oral Surg Oral Med Oral Pathol Oral Radiol Endod 1995;80:101–107.
67. Brooks SL, Brand JW, Gibbs SJ, et al. Imaging of the temporomandibular joint. Oral Surg Oral Med Oral Pathol Oral Radiol Endod 1997;83:609–618.
68. Dixon CD. Radiographic diagnosis of temporomandibular disorders. Semin Orthod 1995;1:207–221.
69. Aquilino SA, Matteson SR, Holland GA, Phillips C. Evaluation of condylar position from temporomandibular joint radiographs. J Prosthet Dent 1985;53:88–97.
70. Mann A, Pankey L. Oral rehabilitation II. Reconstruction of the upper teeth using a functionally generated path technique. J Prosthet Dent 1960;10:151–162.
71. Weinberg LA. Therapeutic biomechanics concepts and clinical procedures to reduce implant loading. Part I. J Oral Implantol 2001;27:293–301.
72. Becker CM, Kaiser DA, Schwalm C. Mandibular centricity: Centric relation. J Prosthet Dent 2000;83:158–160.

11 Clinical Techniques for Occlusal Adjustment

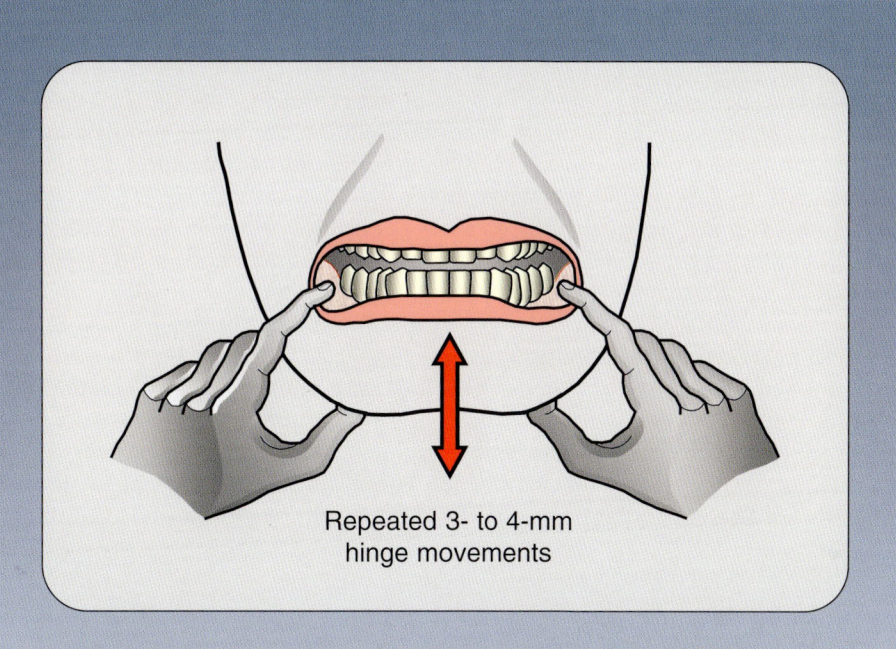

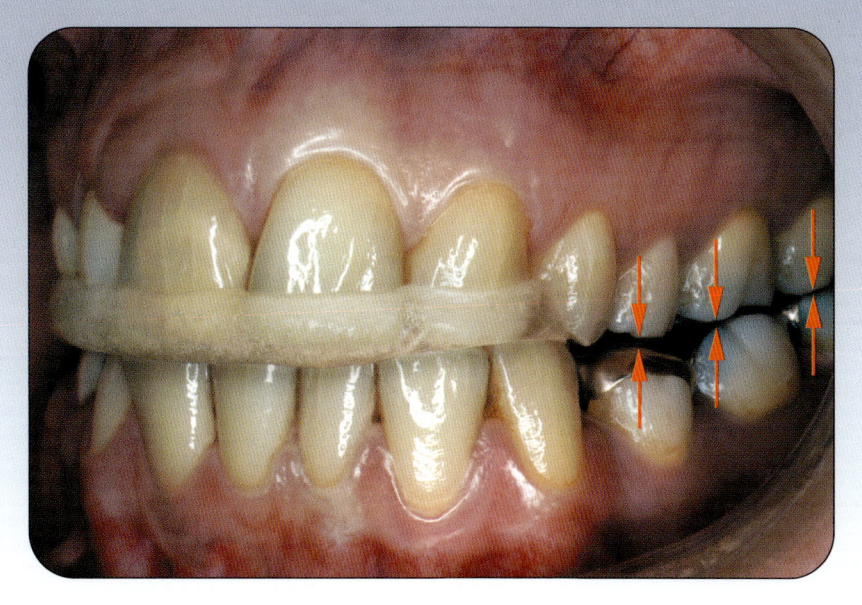

Repeated 3- to 4-mm hinge movements

This chapter describes clinical techniques for the correction of a deflective slide to centric occlusion (elimination of centric relation deflective contacts) and traditional occlusal equilibration.[1] Of the two clinical entities, the elimination of centric relation deflective contacts is by far the more difficult because the patient's muscles are programmed to close the mandible into maximum occlusion, ie, acquired centric occlusion.

Correction of Deflective Slide to Centric Occlusion

There are several challenges involved in the elimination of centric relation deflective contacts: *(1)* observation and diagnosis of the three-dimensional characteristics of the deflective slide into centric occlusion, *(2)* muscle deprogramming before and during clinical procedures, *(3)* color marking of the deflective contacts, and *(4)* successful removal of the deflections until centric relation and centric occlusion are equal.

The first requirement for removal of centric relation deflective contacts is observation of the three-dimensional direction of the mandibular deviation. Of particular importance is the lateral shift that takes place with the anterior slide. The next step is to determine which occlusal surfaces are responsible for the anterior slide and the lateral deviation; the technique presented in this chapter allows the clinician to immediately eliminate half of the possible involved surfaces.

Removal of centric relation deflective contacts will usually require several office visits, and muscle deprogramming must be repeated 24 hours before each of the appointments. At each clinical visit, the surfaces are marked with articulating paper while the patient is in controlled hinge closure, aided by the chairside muscle deprogramming technique. This technique isolates the first deflective contact during light closure. The offending guiding incline is adjusted and the process continued until all the deflective contacts are removed and centric relation and centric occlusion are equal.

Guiding inclines for mandibular deviation

Anterior mandibular deviation
The maxilla is stabilized while the mandible moves in a three-dimensional motion resembling an inverted mortar and pestle (Fig 11-1, A), with the guiding inclines of the maxillary teeth serving as the mortar. In deflective protrusive movement, only the mesial cusp inclines of the maxillary posterior teeth direct anterior mandibular deflective movement (see Fig 11-1, B). This includes the lingual inclines of the maxillary anterior teeth that provide anterior and lateral incisal guidance to voluntary movement (see Fig 11-1, C). Therefore, the distal maxillary cusp inclines are eliminated as possible causes of the anterior mandibular shift.

Posterior mandibular deviation
Posterior mandibular deviation of centric relation rarely occurs and is caused by the distal inclines of the posterior maxillary teeth and/or the maxillary anterior teeth. Diagnosis and treatment follow the same procedures as those used for anterior mandibular deflective slide to centric occlusion.

Lateral mandibular deviation
Normal lateral mandibular movement Before considering the lateral component of the deflective slide to centric occlusion, it is necessary to review the normal guiding inclines for lateral mandibular movement. The maxillary guiding inclines for right

Correction of Deflective Slide to Centric Occlusion

Fig 11-1 Guiding inclines for mandibular deviation. Maxillary mesial cusp inclines. (A) Motion / Guiding incline. (B) Anterior mandibular shift. (C) Anterior and lateral incisal guidance.

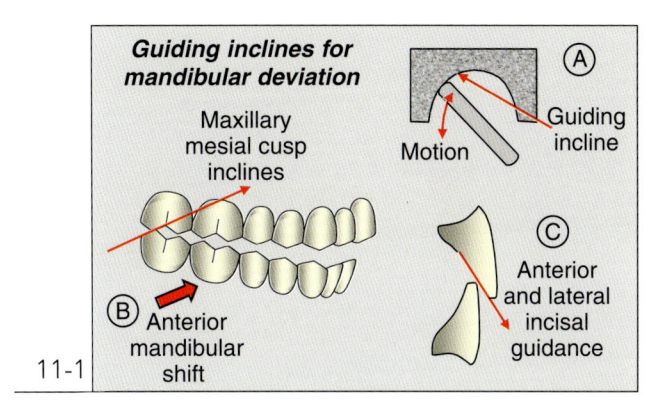

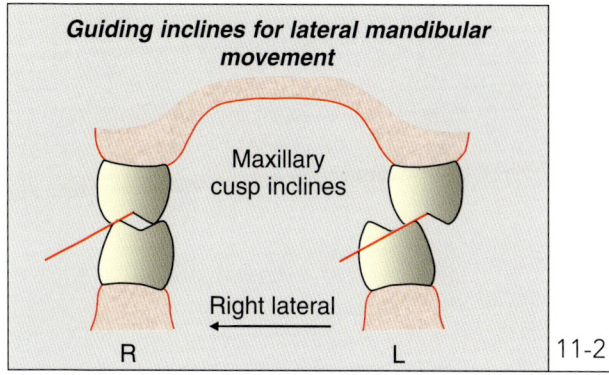

Fig 11-2 Guiding inclines for lateral mandibular movement. Maxillary cusp inclines. Right lateral.

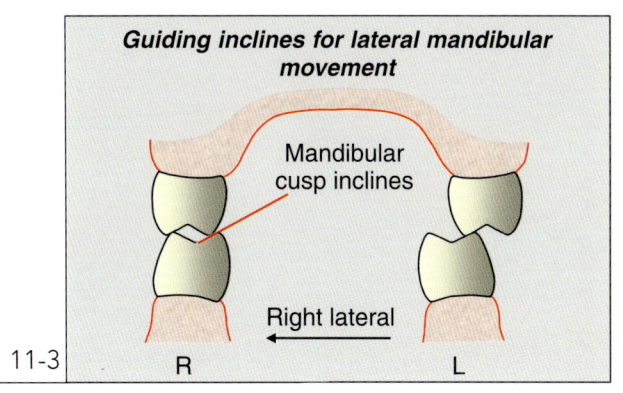

Fig 11-3 Guiding inclines for lateral mandibular movement. Mandibular cusp inclines. Right lateral.

Fig 11-4 Mechanism of centric relation deflective slide. Right side. Buccal. Centric relation deflective contact on cusp incline. Direction of mandibular shift. Shift into centric occlusion.

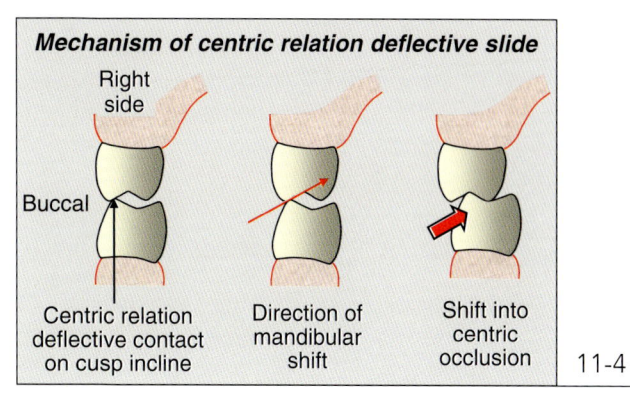

working-side mandibular movement are the buccal cusp inclines on the patient's right side and the lingual cusp inclines on the patient's left side (Fig 11-2). These are the familiar working and nonworking guiding inclines of the maxilla. The mandibular guiding inclines for right lateral mandibular movement are the right lingual cusp inclines (Fig 11-3).

Mechanism of a lateral deflective slide It should be remembered that the preceding description was for *normal* lateral movement starting from the central fossa in centric occlusion and moving laterally in eccentric excursion. By definition, a centric relation deflective contact is caused by a cusp contact occurring on a cusp incline rather than in a fossa during mandibular hinge closure (Fig 11-4, *left*). Such a centric relation deflective contact on an incline plane is biomechanically unstable because only one or two teeth in the whole arch are in contact. Vertical closing force biomechanically requires the mandible to slide to maximum (centric) occlusion to provide stability.

Direction of a lateral deflective slide The direction of a centric relation deflective slide on an incline plane is toward the fossa (see Fig 11-4, *center*). This will produce a lateral shift into centric occlusion (see Fig 11-4, *right*). Without visual aid, this process and its correction are difficult to imagine three-dimensionally. The diagnosis of the direction of the lateral deflective slide is simplified by drawing (on the bracket table) first the occlusal deflective relationship and then a line on the cusp incline with an arrow at the top of the line. That arrow will indicate the direction in which the mandible will slide into centric occlusion, regardless of the occlusal relationship.

For example, if the existing buccolingual occlusal contact in centric relation is as shown in Fig 11-5, lines are drawn on the guiding inclines with arrows at the top of each line as described above. Occlusal contact on any of those inclines will cause lateral deviation of the mandible in the direction of the arrows. Even cross-occlusion contact is simple to diagnose using this method (Fig 11-6). The lines are drawn on the guiding inclines with arrows placed on top of each line, indicating right mandibular deflective slide.

Diagnosis of a lateral deflective slide Suppose a centric relation lateral deflective slide occurs to the patient's left. To determine which cusp inclines are responsible, the familiar diagram of a working- and nonworking-side type of relationship is drawn (Fig 11-7). Lines are drawn on the possible guiding inclines with arrows at the top. Only these inclines could induce the deflective slide to the patient's left. That eliminates 50% of the possible cusp inclines that could cause left mandibular shift. In case the patient has a cross occlusion on the left side, the same process is repeated on that side (Fig 11-8). It is confirmed that only the maxillary lingual cusp incline and mandibular buccal cusp incline could induce a left lateral mandibular deflective slide.

Clinical procedures for correction of deflective slide

Centric relation hinge closure

When a patient has a centric relation deflective slide to centric occlusion, the proprioceptors[2] in the joint capsule[3–6] and muscle spindles[7–9] contribute to the rest position of the mandible, while the periodontal pressoreceptors[10–12] and proprioceptors in the oral mucosa[13,14] contribute to the acquired centric occlusion. The clinical objective for diagnosis and correction requires the patient to close in the pure hinge motion of centric relation. The clinician's clinical technique,[15,16] as well as time[17,18] and muscle tone,[19] affect hinge closure. The patient can be trained to reproduce hinge closure by using posterior bilateral stimulation (Fig 11-9).[20] This is accomplished without any posterior pressure by the clinician.

Pre-office muscle deprogramming

Long-term experience indicates that attempting to immediately overcome muscle programming chairside by pushing the mandible posteriorly is both time consuming and ineffectual. Instead, muscle deprogramming should involve two phases: 24-hour pre-office deprogramming and chairside deprogramming. Muscle deprogramming[21] carried out 24 hours prior to clinical visits has been shown to overcome reflex closure into acquired centric occlusion. The larger the linear deflective slide the more essential this pre-office deprogramming is.

The pre-office deprogramming is best accomplished with a simple maxillary posterior disocclusion prosthesis that covers only the anterior teeth (IA) and limits the posterior opening to 1 mm (Fig 11-10).[22] The lingual acrylic contact area should provide a continuous horizontal stop (*arrows*), which encourages neutral muscle deprogramming (Fig 11-11). No wrought clasps or labial wires are necessary for retention. The use of clasps usually increases the vertical dimension excessively and may interfere with the speaking space and trigger clenching.[22] This process of muscle deprogramming is repeated 24 hours before each clinical visit and is considered *pre-office muscle deprogramming* as differentiated from *chairside deprogramming*, which is subsequently discussed.

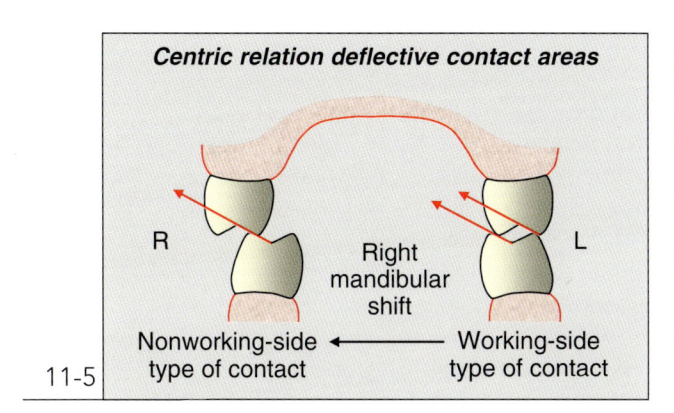

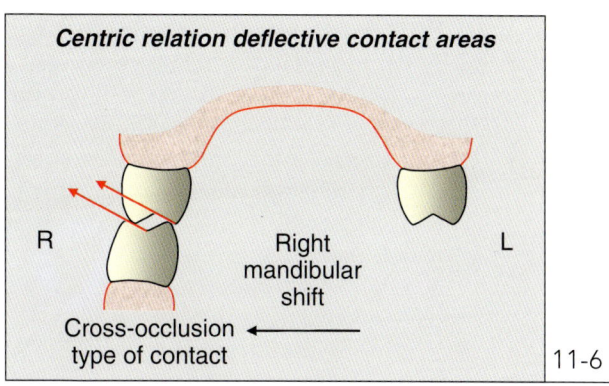

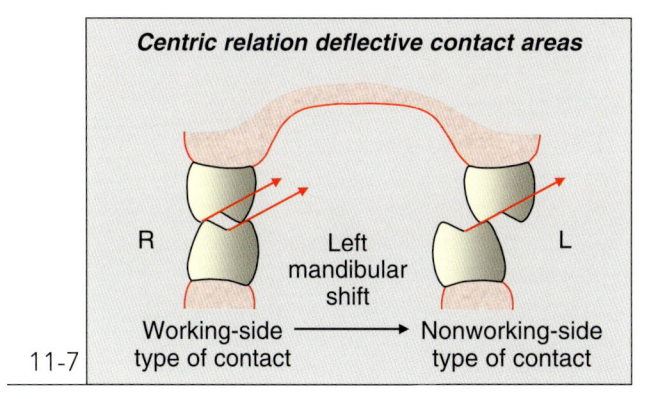

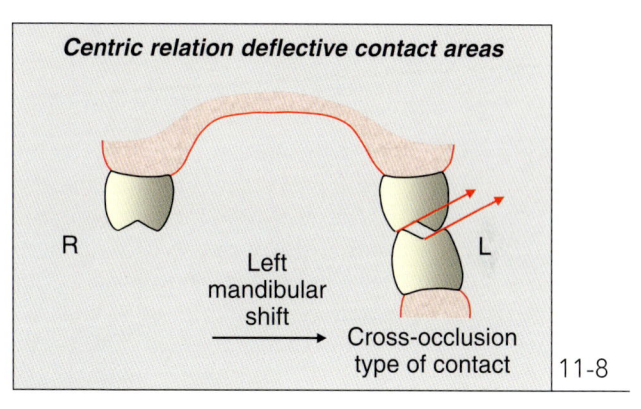

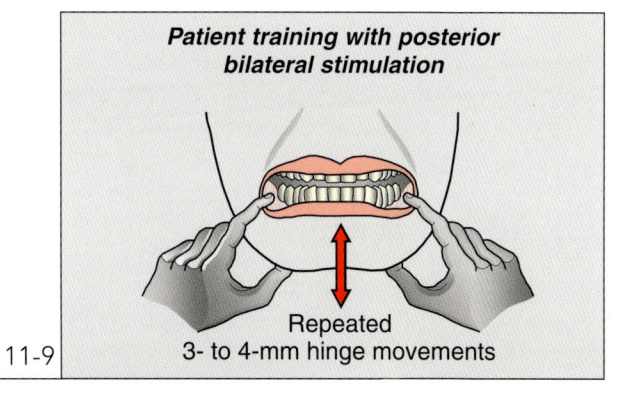

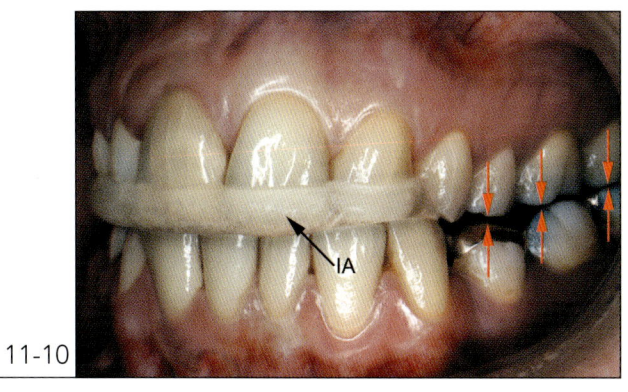

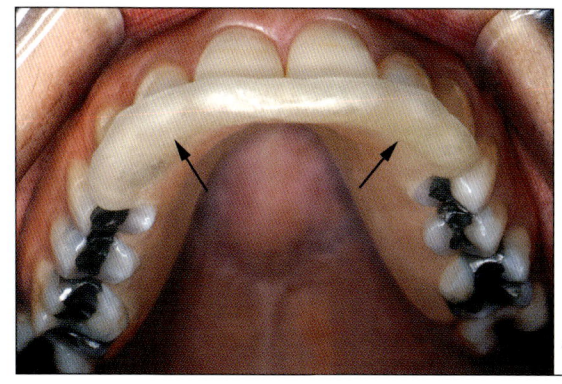

Correction of Deflective Slide to Centric Occlusion

11-5 Centric relation deflective contact areas
R — Nonworking-side type of contact ← Working-side type of contact — L
Right mandibular shift

11-6 Centric relation deflective contact areas
R — Cross-occlusion type of contact ← L
Right mandibular shift

11-7 Centric relation deflective contact areas
R — Working-side type of contact → Nonworking-side type of contact — L
Left mandibular shift

11-8 Centric relation deflective contact areas
R — Left mandibular shift → Cross-occlusion type of contact — L

11-9 Patient training with posterior bilateral stimulation
Repeated 3- to 4-mm hinge movements

11-10 IA

11-11

205

11 Clinical Techniques for Occlusal Adjustment

Clinical adjustment diagnostic procedure
The centric relation deflective contact of the patient in Fig 11-12 is identified by repeated hinge closure of 3 to 4 mm generated by gentle posterior bilateral stimulation (see Fig 11-9). The mandibular center line is indicated by the red line in Fig 11-12 (*top*). As the patient slides anteriorly into centric occlusion (CO) the vertical dimension change (VDC) is minimal, and a left lateral shift (LLS) is observed (see Fig 11-12, *bottom*).

Since there is an anterior centric relation deflective slide to centric occlusion, only the mesial posterior maxillary cusp inclines can be involved, thus eliminating all maxillary distal cusp inclines (Fig 11-13, *left*). However, this is an oversimplification because the mesial cusp inclines also have a potential lateral component (see Figs 11-5 to 11-8) that must be identified before correction (see Fig 11-13, *right*). The left lateral shift has only three possible sources: the right maxillary buccal cusp inclines, the right mandibular lingual cusp inclines, and the left maxillary lingual cusp inclines (Fig 11-14).

Occlusal adjustment of centric relation deflective contacts
The clinical procedure for the adjustment of centric relation deflective contacts requires a dynamic process involving many intraoral marking and occlusal correction procedures. This process is more physiologically complicated than obtaining a static centric relation record. The clinical correction procedure is facilitated by 24-hour pre-office muscle deprogramming as well as proactive chairside deprogramming throughout the corrective procedure. The teeth should not be permitted to occlude in the acquired centric occlusion from the time the patient enters the office until the corrective treatment has been completed. Otherwise, the 24-hour muscle deprogramming would be negated and centric relation hinge closure would become more difficult. The importance of this should be explained to the patient before the corrective process has begun. Between visits the disocclusion prosthesis is only used 24 hours before the next office visit, when the whole process is repeated.

Chairside muscle deprogramming

History of chairside muscle deprogramming
Lucia[23] introduced the Lucia Jig to allow chairside deprogramming of the muscles as an alternative to the long-term pre-office deprogramming previously described (see Figs 11-10 and 11-11). To facilitate a centric relation record, Lucia suggested a slight lingual (incisal) incline on the jig that would guide the mandible into the most retruded position. Long[24] recommended placing leaf gauges (thin acrylic strips) between the maxillary and mandibular central incisors during closure until the posterior teeth were disoccluded, as an aid to occlusal adjustment of centric relation deflective contacts.

Chairside muscle deprogramming procedures
The first step is to record the linear distance of the deflective slide, the vertical dimension change, and the degree of any existing lateral component. The three-dimensional character of the slide into centric occlusion usually increases substantially with 24-hour muscle deprogramming. Posterior bilateral stimulation always should be used for centric relation hinge closure (see Fig 11-9) to locate the centric relation deflective contact. It is best to re-seat the disocclusion prosthesis for a few minutes to confirm the muscle deprogramming.

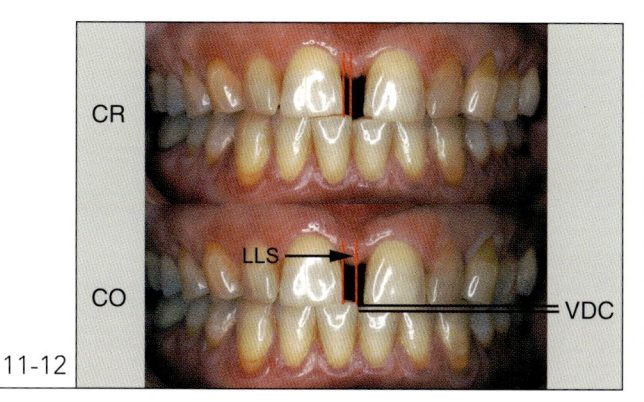

Correction of Deflective Slide to Centric Occlusion

11-12

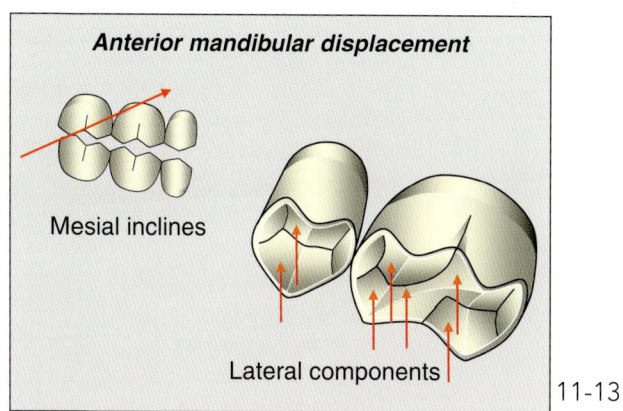

CR

CO — LLS — VDC

11-13 Anterior mandibular displacement

Mesial inclines

Lateral components

11-14 Centric relation deflective areas

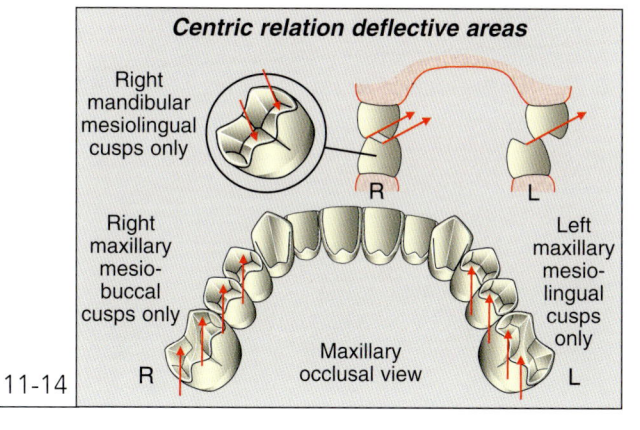

Right mandibular mesiolingual cusps only

Right maxillary mesiobuccal cusps only

Left maxillary mesiolingual cusps only

Maxillary occlusal view

R   L

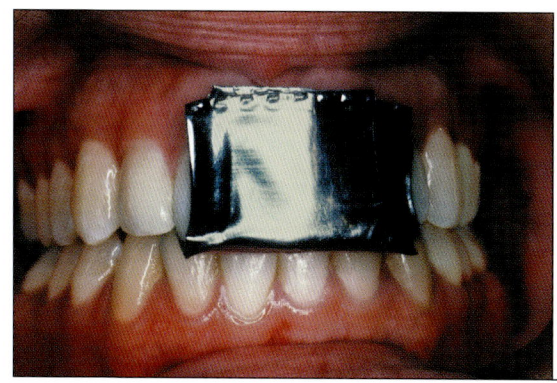

11-15

Presterilized lead tinfoil strips (from dental radiographs) are made available before the disocclusion prosthesis is removed from the mouth. Each sheet of lead foil is positioned over the maxillary incisors and burnished in place with the fingers (Fig 11-15). The patient is guided into closure with posterior bilateral stimulation, thus flattening the lead foil in the lingual incisal contact area. The patient is instructed not to close or swallow autonomically. (It is best to place a saliva ejector between the teeth during any pause in treatment.) This is extremely important to prevent instantaneous regression back into the lifelong muscle programming of the acquired centric occlusion. Additional sheets of lead foil are placed over the maxillary incisors until the posterior teeth are disoccluded. The technique of posterior disocclusion described here, a clinical adaptation of the work of Lucia[23] and Long,[24] greatly simplifies the corrective process.

Occlusal adjustment procedures

While removing one piece of the lead foil at a time, bilateral posterior stimulation is used until only one deflective cusp occludes. The patient's tactile sense aids in identifying the maxillary tooth involved. The area is dried thoroughly, and thin red articulating paper (Bausch 40μ Micro-Thin; Bausch Articulating Papers, Nashua, NH) is placed manually (without an articulating paper holder) over the mandibular teeth to prevent unilateral proprioception and to facilitate bilateral posterior stimulation hinge closure. The deflective contact is marked and identified using the procedure previously outlined (see Figs 11-1 to 11-8).

Pure anterior deflective slide, without a lateral component, will produce a mark on a maxillary mesial incline without any buccolingual inclination. However, there often is a lateral deflective slide, which, in this case, is toward the patient's left side, as evidenced by the mark produced on the buccal cusp incline of a right molar (Fig 11-16, *left*). The author prefers to first adjust the incline only slightly with a round diamond stone, then confirm the location by having the patient close very slowly and lightly using posterior bilateral stimulation and report whether they can feel "a difference." Since only one tooth occludes (because of the incisal lead foil), the patient has no difficulty in confirming whether the minimal adjustment made a difference. Once this is confirmed, the same deflective surface is given a therapeutic correction (see Fig 11-16, *center*). Clinical experience with this procedure produces efficiency.

Therapeutic correction

The objective of a therapeutic correction is to create a new cusp-to-fossa relationship, lateral to the original fossa, that produces stability (see Fig 11-16, *right*). Therefore, a therapeutic correction is intended to change the incline to a fossa, which requires more extensive removal of enamel (or restoration) than the customary occlusal adjustment associated with classic occlusal equilibration. The first incline correction usually requires the most severe removal of tooth structure; this will diminish in degree as the deflective slide decreases and centric relation is approached.

After each therapeutic correction, posterior bilateral stimulation hinge closure is used to test the effectiveness of the adjustment. The patient might report that contact has diminished or relocated to the opposite side, which indicates that the adjustment removed that particular deflective incline. However, removal of one deflective incline will not eliminate the deflective slide into centric occlusion. Once one incline is adjusted, a similar deflective slide will take place, but with a slightly diminished linear degree. The adjustment location will relocate laterally and anteroposteriorly to the original correction.

As with any new clinical procedure, the first treatment process will seem interminable, as will the correction of a deflective slide. Experience will soon facilitate a clinical relationship between the degree of linear slide, and particularly the vertical dimension change, and the amount of tooth structure removal required to correct each deflective contact. For instance, when the occlusion has flat inclines, each occlusal correction should be less severe. Similarly, as the deflective slide is reduced by the corrective grinding, the amount of each successive correction is usually diminished.

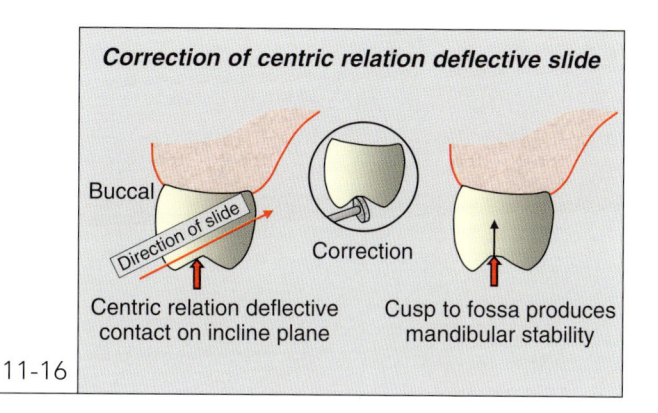

11-16 *Correction of centric relation deflective slide.* Centric relation deflective contact on incline plane; cusp to fossa produces mandibular stability.

Elimination of deflective slide

Although the deflective slide has been eliminated and centric relation and centric occlusion have been harmonized, there will not be even distribution of the occlusal contacts throughout the arch. Eccentric mandibular movements also will need to be evaluated and most often corrected with traditional occlusal equilibration.

Traditional Occlusal Equilibration

Brief history

There are many different clinical procedures for occlusal correction as a result of the long-standing debate over occlusal objectives. Four schools of thought have developed over the years based on the following approaches: *(1)* bilateral balanced occlusion, *(2)* unilateral (working-side) contact, *(3)* canine-protected articulation, and *(4)* the physiologic concept.

The concept of bilateral balance for the occlusion originated in the prevention of denture tipping.[25] The concept was then applied with ultimate exactness to certain gnathologic concepts.[26] Schuyler[1] was the first to describe the technique of occlusal equilibration illustrated in this text. Box,[27] Miller,[28] and Sorrin[29] emphasized the need for the distribution of stress to the periodontal structures of the natural teeth. Jankelson[30] showed evidence that teeth did not meet in occlusion except during deglutition. Yurkstas and Emerson[31] demonstrated that during mastication with artificial denture teeth, there was considerable occlusal contact on the working side and almost always on the nonworking side. Using miniature electronic devices in complete dentures, Brewer and Hudson[32] reported findings that supported those of Yurkstas and Emerson.[31] Brewer and Hudson[32] maintained that nonworking-side occlusion in the natural dentition is destructive to the periodontal structures, a theory that was confirmed mathematically.[33] Unilateral (working-side) contact was based on the concept of even distribution of occlusal forces for periodontal health. D'Amico[34] advocated a canine-protected articulation, a concept that became popular within the gnathologic school of thought.

The present author reported findings[35–37] contradictory to this concept and prefers unilateral group function for tooth-supported prostheses, which efficiently distributes the forces of masticatory and nonmasticatory function. With this brief history as a background, the traditional occlusal equilibration technique is described in the following sections.

11 Clinical Techniques for Occlusal Adjustment

Preliminary correction

Esthetics and tooth-to-tooth anatomic relationships

Any incisors extending beyond the smile line are reshaped to improve esthetics and ensure future harmonious eccentric mandibular excursions (Fig 11-17, *left*). Uneven marginal ridges should be adjusted to prevent food impaction (see Fig 11-17, *right*). Often a tooth in malposition, such as linguoversion (see Fig 11-17, *center*), can induce food impaction as a result of the uneven levels of the marginal ridges of the adjacent occlusal surfaces.

Even if the marginal ridges are even, a sharp cusp that precisely articulates between two adjacent teeth can form a plunger cusp that results in food impaction (Fig 11-18, *left*). The sharp point of the cusp can be rounded off without eliminating centric occlusal contact.

Good study casts show prominent wear facets, and their location indicates the excursion in which they are created.[37,38] If there are only a few wear facets, the opposing guiding inclines may require occlusal adjustment in eccentric excursions. To increase chewing efficiency, the flattened areas should be rounded without interfering with centric occlusion contacts (*arrows*) at the cusp height (see Fig 11-18, *right*).

Centric occlusion correction

A cusp that is hyperocclusal in centric occlusion can be relieved by corrective grinding on either the cusp height or the fossa (Fig 11-19, *left, red arrow*). The determining factor is how the cusp functions in eccentric (working-side) occlusion (see Fig 11-19, *right*). In this case, there is working-side harmony; therefore, the fossa is corrected to avoid interfering with working-side contact. On the other hand, when a similar cusp is hyperocclusal in centric occlusion (Fig 11-20, *left, red arrow*) and working-side occlusion (see Fig 11-20, *right, red arrow*), the cusp should be adjusted to remove the original hyperocclusion in centric occlusion.

Clinical technique

A clinician can immediately judge when any particular tooth is in hyperocclusion compared to the other teeth in that quadrant using 0.0005-inch-thick Mylar strips (Occlusal Registration Strips; Artus, Englewood, NJ). The patient is instructed to occlude and resist the lateral pull on the Mylar strip (Fig 11-21). This is repeated on the adjacent teeth in the quadrant (Fig 11-22). In this way the clinician is able to discern exactly which tooth is in hyperocclusion without aid from the patient. This is particularly important because many procedures require local anesthesia, which negates the patient's tactile senses.

Vertical occlusal pressure refinement

The vertical pressure on each tooth can be selectively refined using pressure-sensitive Mylar ribbon (Bausch 8μ). Because the Mylar ribbons are sensitive and easy to use, the preliminary phase can be accomplished in a few minutes. Such extremely accurate occlusal adjustment allows application of the new technique of therapeutic differential loading[28] when tooth- and implant-supported prostheses are provided in the same arch. (See chapter 5 for discussion and intraoral techniques.)

Traditional Occlusal Equilibration

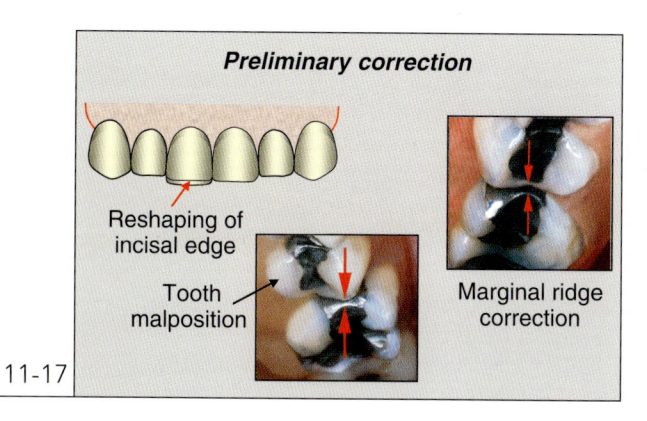

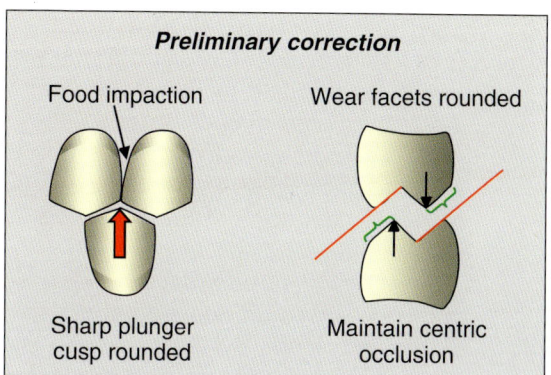

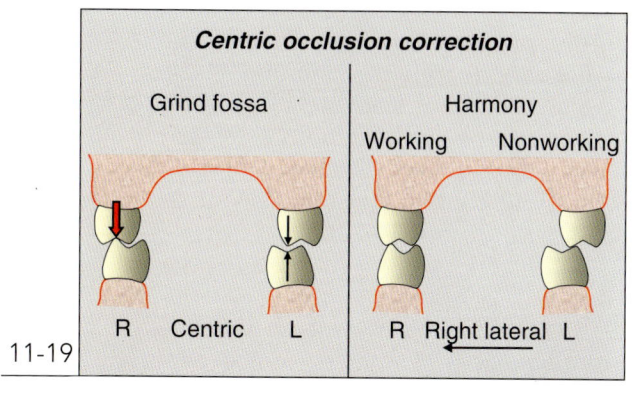

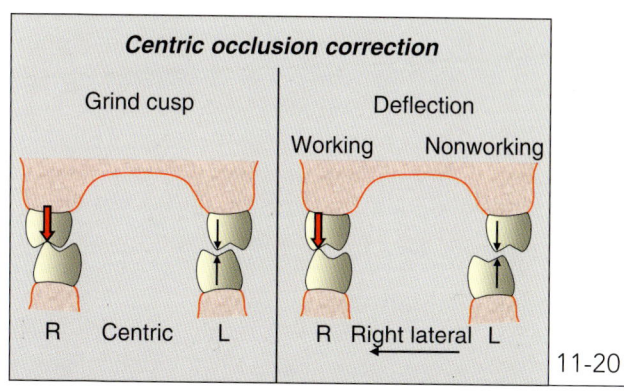

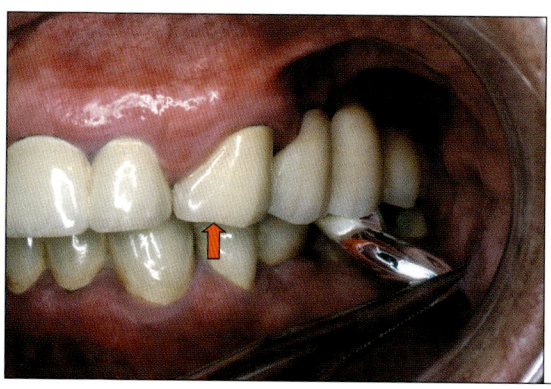

11-17 Preliminary correction
- Reshaping of incisal edge
- Tooth malposition
- Marginal ridge correction

11-18 Preliminary correction
- Food impaction — Sharp plunger cusp rounded
- Wear facets rounded — Maintain centric occlusion

11-19 Centric occlusion correction
- Grind fossa — R Centric L
- Harmony — Working Nonworking — R Right lateral L

11-20 Centric occlusion correction
- Grind cusp — R Centric L
- Deflection — Working Nonworking — R Right lateral L

11-21

11-22

211

Marking and occlusal adjustment

Articulating paper that smudges should be avoided. The initial articulating paper should be thin and mark relatively easily (ie, Bausch 40µ Micro-Thin). (Note that all articulating papers mark better on a dry surface.) The hyperoccluded tooth is adjusted with a round diamond stone as indicated by the articulating paper, and Mylar strips are used to evaluate the result (see Figs 11-21 and 11-22). The corrective grinding is repeated until none of the occluding surfaces permits lateral passage of the Mylar strip.

Next, Mylar ribbon (Bausch 8µ), which is 8 µm thick, comes in a roll, and has a marking surface on one side and a shiny surface on the other, is precut into 4- to 5-inch-long strips by the chairside assistant. The ribbon is then folded with the marking surface exposed and placed between the teeth using an articulating paper holder. The occlusal surfaces must be *completely dry* (Fig 11-23) and the patient must close forcefully 3 to 4 times in order for the pressure-indicating ribbon to be effective. The pressure-sensitive ribbon leaves a very discrete marking (Fig 11-24, *arrows*) compared with the larger, less discrete marking of standard articulating paper (see Fig 11-24, *circles*). The degree of adjustment at this stage is extremely small and undetectable by the patient's tactile senses. The Mylar (0.0005-inch) strips are then placed between all the teeth in the arch to confirm that they cannot be pulled from between the occluded teeth (see Figs 11-21 and 11-22).

Palpation

The index finger is lightly placed on the buccal aspect of the maxillary teeth while the patient taps the teeth together. There will be differences in vibration as the periodontal membrane permits slight movement in response to hyperocclusal contact. This is most palpable on unsplinted anterior maxillary teeth. The incline planes of anterior centric contact due to the vertical overlap causes micromovement of the maxillary anterior teeth that is very easy to diagnose with palpation. The effect is diminished when these teeth are splinted, and it is not effective at all when implants are used because of the stiffness of the osseointegrated interface.

The preceding methods are undetectable by the patient's tactile senses, which is acceptable since tactile senses are different for each patient. Moreover, when a new restoration is seated on a natural tooth, the patient has no instant tactile reference and thus can give the clinician erroneous information regarding which tooth is "high." Therefore, the techniques presented above provide a very rapid and scientific approach to the adjustment of the occlusion, which often is thought to be in the realm of artistic skill or indescribable "touch and feel" therapy that cannot be easily taught or quantified.

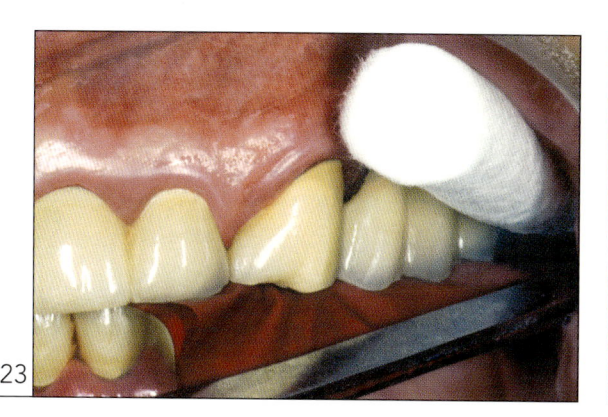

Traditional Occlusal Equilibration

11-23

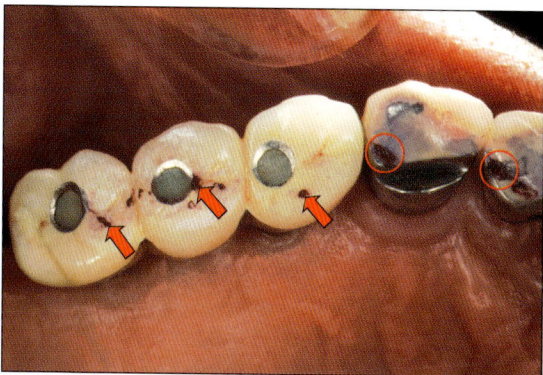

11-24

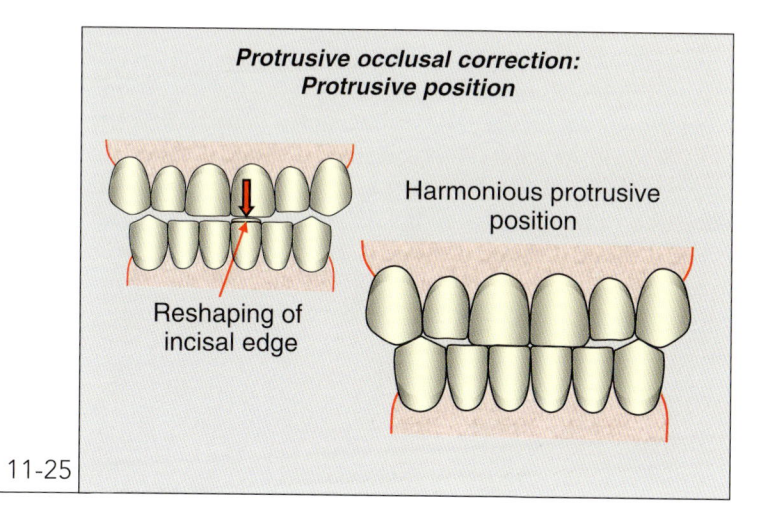

Protrusive occlusal correction: Protrusive position

Reshaping of incisal edge

Harmonious protrusive position

11-25

Protrusive occlusal correction

Protrusive position

The first step in protrusive occlusal adjustment is to establish the static relationship of the protrusive position. Any elongated maxillary incisors were shortened for esthetics during preliminary grinding (see Fig 11-16, *left*); therefore, any premature contact of a mandibular incisor with a maxillary incisor is corrected by shortening the mandibular incisor (Fig 11-25, *left*). This process establishes a harmonious protrusive position (see Fig 11-25, *right*). The mandibular tooth will not elongate because functional protrusive movements will provide sufficient contact.

Protrusive excursion

The condylar inclination, posterior cusp inclines, and incisal guidance must be in harmony in order to provide harmonious protrusive mandibular excursions. When the mandible slides forward in protrusive excursion, any deflective contact on the distal acute incline (A) of a maxillary posterior tooth can cause an anterior opening, preventing anterior incisal contact (Fig 11-26). The offending posterior distal incline is marked, using a two-color marking system to prevent removal of centric occlusal contact, and reduced. With this procedure, protrusive excursion can provide a harmonious protrusive condylar path (H), posterior distal cusp inclines, and incisal guidance (Fig 11-27).

Protrusive excursion biomechanics

As protrusive excursion takes place, occlusal force (O) from the mandibular incisors produces a resultant lateral force (LF) perpendicular to the lingual inclination (Fig 11-28, *left*). Before occlusal adjustment, occlusal contact of the lingual surfaces of the maxillary anterior teeth will vary during protrusive excursive movements, resulting in various biomechanic effects. For example, if a protrusive excursion on the left canine is concentrated on the mesial half of the lingual incline, a mild rotational force will be produced (Fig 11-28, *right*). The left central incisor has no protrusive force distribution except from centric occlusion (CO). The right central incisor exhibits protrusive excursion contact along the right marginal ridge, which will produce a severe rotational force. The objective of protrusive excursion is to provide even contact on all the maxillary anterior teeth to the extent practical (Fig 11-29).

Working-side occlusal correction

Maxillary buccal cusp incline

The working-side correction is one of the more simple occlusal adjustments using the two-color marking system. The working-side guiding inclines (maxillary buccal cusp incline [I] and mandibular lingual cusp incline [II]) are shown in Fig 11-30 (*left*). A more acute maxillary buccal cusp incline (see Fig 11-30, *right*, AI) will be in hyperocclusion during right lateral movement (Fig 11-31, *left*, *red arrow*). Centric occlusion is marked in blue while the working-side excursion is marked in red (see Fig 11-31, *right*). Corrective grinding is accomplished on the maxillary buccal cusp incline without affecting centric occlusion.

Mandibular lingual cusp incline

A more acute mandibular lingual cusp incline (II) will be in hyperocclusion during right lateral movement (Fig 11-32, *left*, *red arrow*). Centric occlusion is marked in blue and lateral excursion in red, and the mandibular lingual cusp incline is corrected (see Fig 11-32, *right*, *red arrow*). The two-color marking system facilitates preservation of centric contact when corrective grinding is accomplished on the mandibular lingual cusp incline.

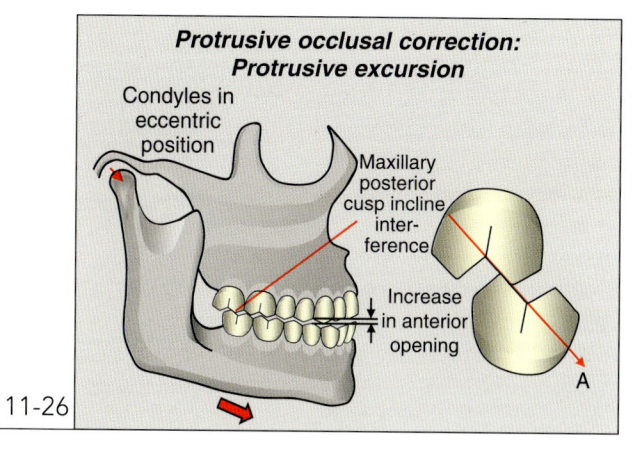

Traditional Occlusal Equilibration

11-26 Protrusive occlusal correction: Protrusive excursion — Condyles in eccentric position; Maxillary posterior cusp incline interference; Increase in anterior opening; A

11-27 Protrusive occlusal correction: Protrusive excursion — Condyles in eccentric position; Maxillary posterior cusp incline adjustment; Harmonious protrusive excursion; H, A

11-28 Protrusive excursion biomechanics — LF; O; Mild rotational force; Severe rotational force; CO; No protrusive force distribution

11-29 Protrusive excursion biomechanics — CO; Protrusive excursion; Centric occlusion maintained; Harmonious protrusive inclines distribute forces

11-30 Working-side correction — Working-side guiding inclines I, II; AI; R Right lateral L; Working / Nonworking; R Centric L

11-31 Working-side correction — Guiding inclines; Working / Nonworking; I; AI; R Right lateral L; Corrective grinding; Centric contact maintained

11-32 Working-side correction — Guiding inclines; Working / Nonworking; II; R Right lateral L; Corrective grinding: Lingual cusp incline; Centric contact maintained

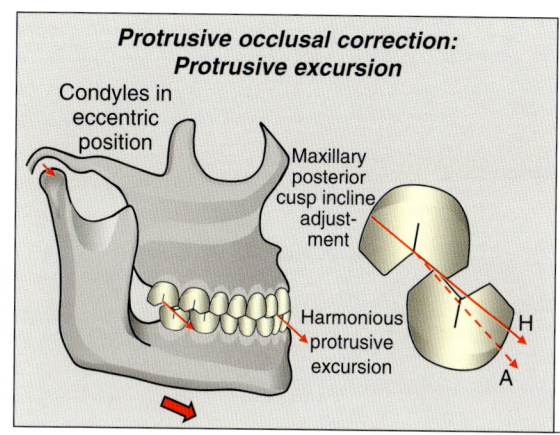

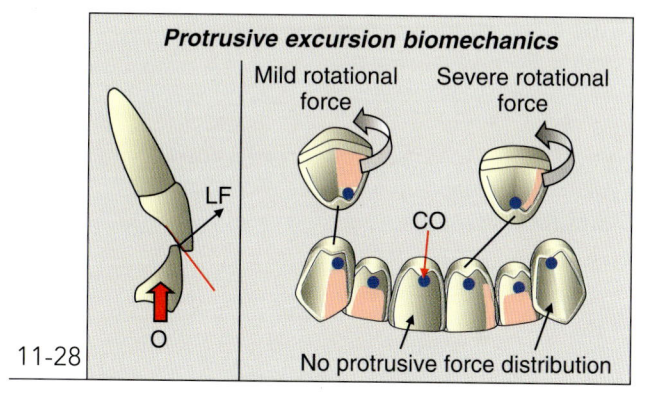

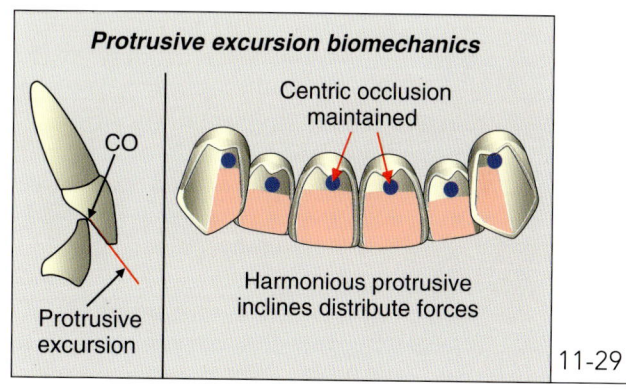

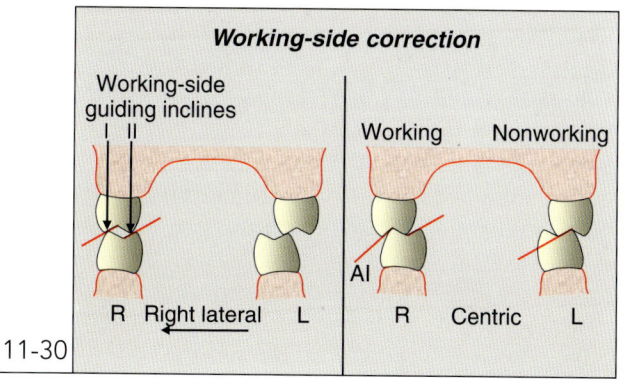

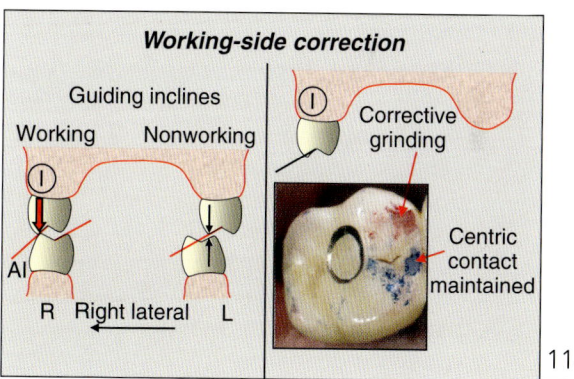

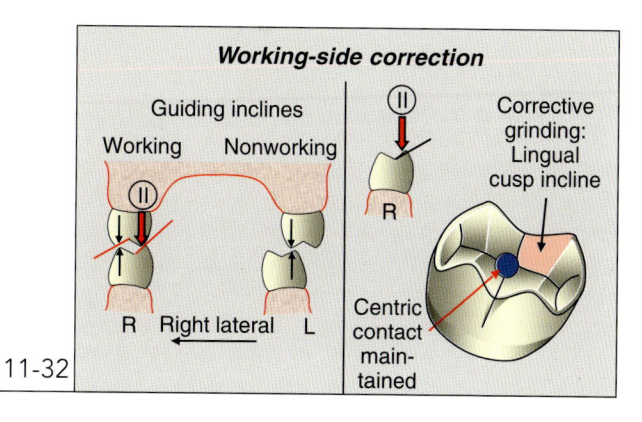

215

Nonworking-side occlusal correction

Figure 11-33 illustrates the guiding inclines for right lateral excursion with the nonworking guiding incline (AI) more acute than the others. The maxillary left lingual cusp incline interferes with harmonious right lateral excursion (see Fig 11-33, *right, red arrow*). The nonworking-side interference cusp inclines (Fig 11-34, *left, red arrow*), namely the maxillary lingual and mandibular buccal cusp inclines, maintain centric occlusion (see Fig 11-34, *right*).

Figure 11-35 illustrates the right lateral incline relationship (*top*) and the two-color marking system on the left side of the maxillary arch when centric occlusion and bilateral movements are made (*bottom*). The centric contacts are in blue, the eccentric in red. The red marking on the buccal cusp incline of the molar indicates working-side contact and the red marking on the lingual cusp incline of the second premolar records nonworking-side contact. As demonstrated in Fig 11-34 (*right*), the maxillary lingual and mandibular buccal cusps both maintain centric contact (*black arrows*); therefore, the clinician must determine which cusp should be adjusted.

Correction of the maxillary lingual cusp

The nonworking-side interference is demonstrated in Fig 11-36 (*left, red arrow*). When there is good centric occlusal contact of the mandibular buccal cusp with the maxillary fossa (*right, top*), corrective grinding is accomplished on the maxillary lingual cusp incline (*right, bottom*).

Correction of the mandibular buccal cusp

Nonworking-side interference is shown again in Fig 11-37 (*left*) for orientation. When the mandibular buccal cusp is not functioning in centric occlusion (*right, top*), all corrective grinding is done on the mandibular buccal cusp incline (*right, bottom*).

Incorrect adjustment of nonworking-side interference

Adjustment of nonworking-side interferences is critical because a mistake in diagnosis will result in the elimination of centric contact (Fig 11-38). Once centric contact is eliminated, the teeth that are out of occlusion will move occlusally to produce functional stimuli, which usually are the same as the original nonworking-side interferences. The rules are: *(1)* Never grind both maxillary lingual and mandibular buccal cusp inclines; *(2)* if there is good centric mandibular buccal cusp contact in the maxillary fossa, then all correction is done on the maxillary lingual cusp incline; and *(3)* if there is poor centric mandibular buccal cusp contact in the maxillary fossa, then all corrective grinding is done on the mandibular buccal cusp incline, and the maxillary lingual cusp and mandibular fossa maintain centric occlusion.

Reconfirmation of centric occlusion contact

After all the occlusal corrections are completed, reconfirmation of centric occlusion with the Mylar (0.0005-inch) occlusion strips is recommended. The clinician should not be able to pull the strips through any centric contact (see Fig 11-21). Pressure-sensitive 8-μm Mylar ribbon is used (only with completely dry occlusal surfaces) to provide sharply delineated markings if correction is needed (Fig 11-39, *top*). Palpation on the maxillary teeth is effective only with tooth-supported prostheses, unless the implant-supported prosthesis is in the mandibular arch. After each adjustment visit, all corrected teeth should be thoroughly polished with an abrasive rubber wheel (see Fig 11-39, *bottom*).

Traditional Occlusal Equilibration

11-33 Nonworking-side correction

11-34 Nonworking-side correction

11-35

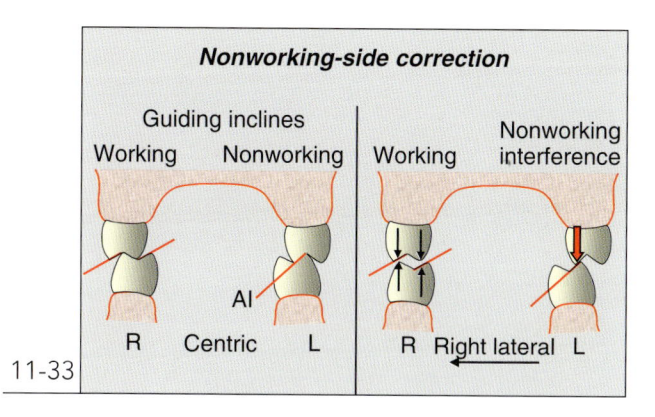

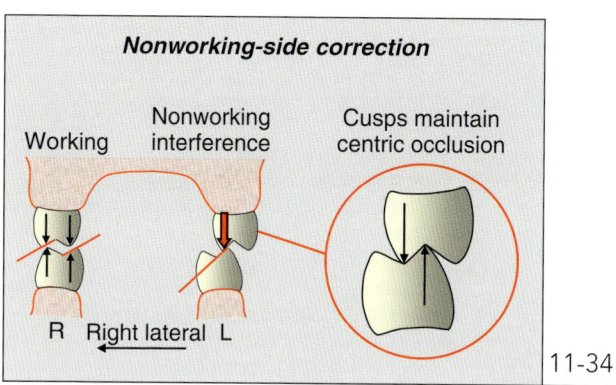

11-36 Nonworking-side correction

11-37 Nonworking-side correction

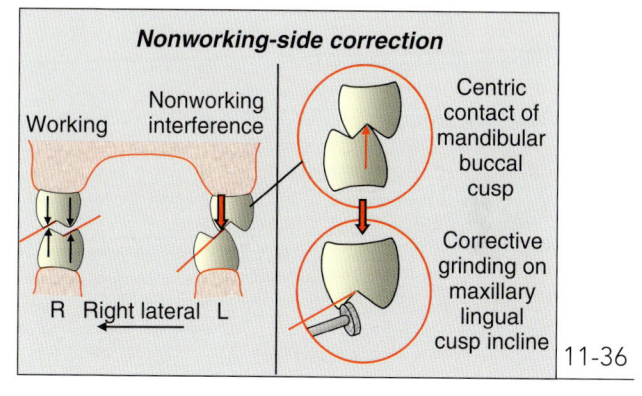

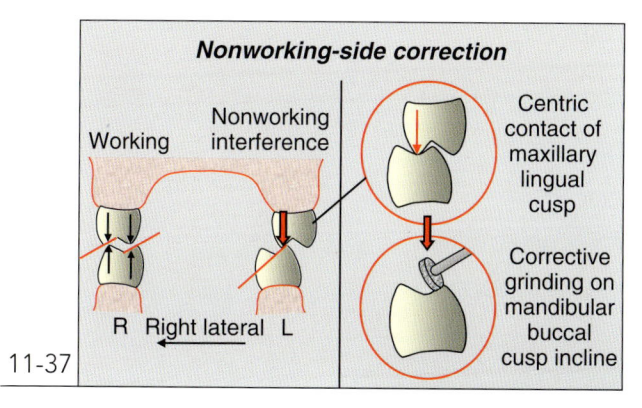

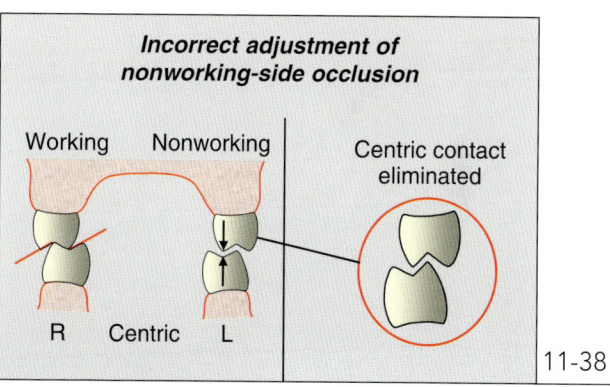

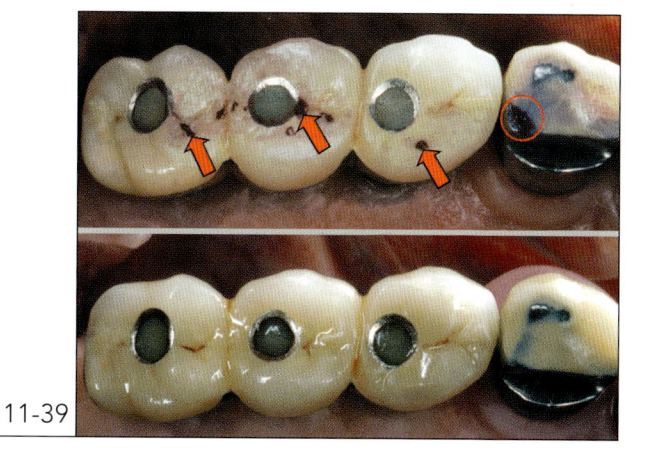

11-38 Incorrect adjustment of nonworking-side occlusion

11-39

217

References

1. Schuyler CH. Correction of occlusal disharmony of the natural dentition. N Y State Dent J 1947;13: 445–462.
2. Ransjö J, Thilander B. Perception of mandibular position in cases of temporomandibular joint disorders. Odontol Tidskr 1969;71:134.
3. Weinberg LA. Vertical dimension: A research and clinical analysis. J Prosthet Dent 1982;47:290–302.
4. Thilander B. Innervation of the temporomandibular joint capsule in man. Trans R Sch Dent Stockh Umea 1961;7:1–67.
5. Kawamura Y, Majima T, Kato I. Physiologic role of deep mechanoreceptor in temporomandibular joint capsule [in Japanese]. J Osaka Univ Dent Sch 1967;7:63–76.
6. Greenfield BE, Wyke BD. Reflex innervation of the temporomandibular joint. Nature 1966;211:940.
7. Sherrington CS. The Integrative Action of the Nervous System. New Haven: Yale Univ Press, 1952.
8. Szentagothai J. Anatomical considerations of monosynaptic reflex arcs. J Neurophysiol 1948;11:445.
9. Kawamura Y, Majima T. Temporomandibular joint's sensory mechanisms controlling activities of the jaw muscles. J Dent Res 1964;43:150.
10. Corbin KB, Harrison F. Functions of the mesencephalic root of the fifth cranial nerve. J Neurophysiol 1940;3:423.
11. Atwood DA. A cephalometric study of the clinical rest position of the mandible. Part III: Clinical factors related to variability of the clinical rest position following removal of occlusal contacts. J Prosthet Dent 1956;8:698–708.
12. Thompson JR. The rest position of the mandible and its significance to dental science. J Am Dent Assoc 1946;33:151–180.
13. Brill N. Reflexes, registrations, and prosthetic dentistry. J Prosthet Dent 1957;7:341–360.
14. Berry DC, Wilkie JK. Lips and tongue behavior in relation to prosthetics. Dent Pract Dent Rec 1961;11: 334–340.
15. Kantor M, Silverman S, Garfinkel L. Centric relation recording techniques: A comparative investigation. J Prosthet Dent 1972;28:593–600.
16. Kabcenell JL. Effect of clinical procedures on mandibular position. J Prosthet Dent 1964;14:266–278.
17. Grasso J, Sharry J. The duplicability of arrow-point tracing in dentulous subjects. J Prosthet Dent 1968; 20:106–115.
18. Shafagh I, Yoder J, Thayer K. Diurnal variance of centric relation position. J Prosthet Dent 1975;34: 574–582.
19. Celenza FV. The centric position: Replacement and character. J Prosthet Dent 1973;30:591–598.
20. Silverman SI. Oral Physiology. St Louis: Mosby, 1961:338–339.
21. Calagna L, Silverman S, Garfinkel L. Influence of neuromuscular conditioning on centric relation registrations. J Prosthet Dent 1973;30:598–604.
22. Weinberg LA. The role of muscle deconditioning for occlusal corrective procedures. J Prosthet Dent 1991;66:250–255.
23. Lucia VO. Modern Gnathological Concepts. St Louis: Mosby, 1961:610.
24. Long JH. Locating centric relation with a leaf gauge. J Prosthet Dent 1973;29:608–610.
25. Swenson MG. Complete Dentures, ed 4. St Louis: Mosby, 1959:256–272.
26. McCullum BB. Fundamentals involved in prescribing restorative remedies. D Items Interest 1939;61: 522–535,641–648,724–736,852–856,942–950.
27. Box HK. Traumatic occlusion and traumatogenic occlusion. Oral Health 1930;20:642–646.
28. Miller SC. Textbook of Periodontia, ed 3. Philadelphia: Blakiston, 1950:343–384.
29. Sorrin S. Traumatic occlusion: Its detection and correction. Dent Dig 1934;40:170–173,202–208.
30. Jankelson B. Physiology of human dental occlusion. J Am Dent Assoc 1955;50:664–680.
31. Yurkstas AA, Emerson WH. Study of tooth contact during mastication with artificial dentures. J Prosthet Dent 1954;4:168–174.
32. Brewer AA, Hudson DC. Application of miniaturized electronic devices to the study of tooth contact in complete dentures. A progress report. J Prosthet Dent 1961;11:62–72.
33. Weinberg LA. Force distribution in mastication, clenching, and bruxism. Dent Dig 1957;63:58–61, 116–120.
34. D'Amico A. The canine teeth—Normal functional relation of the natural teeth of man. J South Calif State Dent Assoc 1958;26: 6–23,49–60,127–142,175–182,194–208,239–241.
35. Weinberg LA. Occlusal equilibration in eccentric positions. N Y State Dent J 1957;23:310–312.
36. Weinberg LA. The prevalence of tooth contact in eccentric movements of the jaw: Its clinical implications. J Am Dent Assoc 1961;62:403–406.
37. Weinberg LA. A cinematic study of centric and eccentric occlusions. J Prosthet Dent 1964;14:290–293.
38. Weinberg LA. Diagnosis of facets in occlusal equilibration. J Am Dent Assoc 1956;52:26–35.

Index

Page numbers followed by "f" denote figures; those followed by "t" denote tables

A

Abutment
  CeraOne
    with ceramometal coping, 162, 163f
    design of, 160, 161f
    with modified access channel, 164, 164f
    nontorque bone-implant interface procedure, 162, 162f
    posterior, 162, 163f
  design of, 151f, 152
  EsthetiCone, 165f, 165–166
  gingival depth and, 168, 168f
  implants as, 60
  impression copings, 167, 167f
  nonrotating configuration of, 145, 145f
  prefabricated angulated, 150, 151f
  seating of, 172, 173f
  selection criteria and process, 166–168, 167f
  standard, disadvantages of, 155, 155f
  titanium, 155, 155f
  types of, 143, 143f
  UCLA
    anterior, 156, 157f
    custom-reangulated, 152–153, 153f, 156, 157f
    in multiple implant–supported fixed prostheses, 159f, 168, 174
    posterior, 152–154, 153f–154f
    summary of, 158
    without reangulation, 154, 156, 157f
Abutment screws
  design of, 142–143, 143f
  tightness of, 170–171
Acrylic lingual index, 29f
Anterior full-crown preparation
  esthetic objectives of, 6
  esthetic refinements of, 11–12
  framework finishing, 10, 11f
  metal finish lines, 10, 10f
  modified chamfer, 9, 9f
  parallelism, 8, 9f, 11
  tooth preparation for, 8, 9f
Anterior maxillary bone loss, 74–76, 75f
Articulator. *See* Semi-adjustable articulator

B

Bennett angle, 14, 15f
Biomechanics
  reactive, 74, 75f
  therapeutic. *See* Therapeutic biomechanics

Bone loss
  anterior maxillary, 74–76, 75f
  posterior mandible, 72, 73f
  posterior maxillary, 73f, 73–74

C

Canine-protected articulation, 20, 182
Centric occlusion
  correction of, 210–212
  deflective slide to. *See* Deflective slide to centric occlusion
  reconfirmation of contact, 216, 217f
  transfer record, 38–40, 39f
Centric relation
  definition of, 184
  deflective contacts. *See also* Deflective slide to centric occlusion
    description of, 184, 185f
    occlusal adjustment of, 206
    removal of, 196–197, 197f, 202
  dysfunctional
    definition of, 194
    with deflective slide and lateral shift, 196, 197f
  early studies of, 183
  functional
    definition of, 194, 195f
    with deflective slide and lateral shift, 195, 195f
  hinge closure, 204, 205f
  historical descriptions of, 183
  record, for maxillary complete-arch osseointegrated prostheses, 112, 113f
CeraOne abutment
  with ceramometal coping, 162, 163f
  design of, 160, 161f
  with modified access channel, 164, 164f
  nontorque bone-implant interface procedure, 162, 162f
  posterior, 162, 163f
Chairside muscle deprogramming, for deflective slide to centric occlusion, 206–207
Chamfer, 9, 9f
Chewing motion, 48, 49f
Clip bar overdenture. *See* Implant-supported clip bar overdenture; Tooth-supported clip bar overdenture
Combined prostheses
  diagnostic factors in, 60–62, 61f
  force distribution in, 56–57, 57f
Compound tube impressions, 36, 37f
Computed tomography
  for implant-supported clip bar overdenture, 126
  for three-dimensional guidance system
    cross-sectional image, 90, 91f
    need for, 86, 87f

219

Index

panoramic reformatted image, 90, 91f
procedure for, 88, 89f
reformatted images, 101, 101f
transaxial, 88, 90, 91f
Condylar position
 clinical implications of, 193
 concentricity, 188, 189f
 description of, 188
 displacement, 188, 189f, 191f, 193
 occlusion and, relationship between, 190–192, 191f
 posterior displacement, 191f, 193
 research of, 193
 studies of, 190t
 superior displacement, 188, 189f, 191f
Copings
 design of
  for anterior teeth, 179–180
  for porcelain-fused-to-metal restoration, 176–179
 square abutment copings, 110, 111f
 square impression copings
  accuracy of, 170, 171f
  nonrotating, 146, 147f
Corrugation, 176, 177f
Cross occlusion, 70, 71f
Cusp inclines
 buccal, 214, 215f
 implant loading and, 62, 69, 69f
 incisal guidance and, 16–18, 17f
 lingual, 214, 215f

D

Deflective slide to centric occlusion. See also Centric relation, deflective contacts
 correction methods
  centric relation hinge closure, 204, 205f
  chairside muscle deprogramming, 206–207
  guiding inclines for mandibular deviation, 202–204
  pre-office muscle deprogramming, 204, 205f
 description of, 184, 185f, 194
 elimination of, 209
 lateral, 203f, 203–204
Differential mobility, 56–59, 76
Differential occlusal adjustment, 76, 78, 79f

E

Esthetic planning
 corrections, 28, 29f
 impressions, 36, 37f
 laminate, 2–4, 3f
 provisional restorations, 30–31
 smile line, 28
 transfer of esthetic changes, 28, 29f, 34, 35f, 40, 41f
 vertical dimension. See Vertical dimension
EsthetiCone abutment, 165f, 165–166

F

Fixed-retrievable implant-supported prosthesis, 124, 125f
Force distribution
 in combined prostheses, 56–57, 57f
 factors that influence, 50–51, 51f
 in multiple-implant prostheses, 54–55, 55f
 in prostheses, 52, 53f
 in splinted natural teeth, 54, 55f
Full crowns, anterior. See Anterior full-crown preparation

G

Gingiva
 depth of, 168, 168f
 healing of, 168, 169f
 reproduction of, 169f, 169–170
Gnathology, 14, 182
Gold cylinders, nonrotating, 146, 147f
Group function articulation, 20
Guiding inclines, for mandibular deviation, 202–204, 203f

H

Hanau formula, 18
Horizontal fossae, 20, 21f
Hyperocclusion, 210, 211f

I

Implant(s)
 abutments. See Abutment
 anterior, 102, 103f
 apical offset, 62, 63f
 configuration of, 142
 divergence of, 148–150, 149f
 force distribution with, 51f, 51–52, 53f
 horizontal offset, 62, 63f
 nonrotating configuration of, 144
 posterior, 102, 103f
 reangulation of, 150
 staggered offset, 64, 64f
 three-dimensional guidance system for placement of. See Three-dimensional guidance system
Implant loading
 cross occlusion to reduce, 70, 71f, 82
 cusp inclination and, 69, 69f
 description of, 68
 maxillary complete-arch osseointegrated prosthesis, 108–109, 109f
 methods to decrease, 62, 63f, 68, 82
 modified occlusal anatomy and, 72, 73f
 physiologic variation and, 70–71, 71f
 sinus location and, 70, 71f
 therapeutic biomechanics for, 69–72
 therapeutic differential loading, 76, 77f
Implant-supported clip bar overdenture
 assemblage procedures, 134–136, 135f
 buccal strut fabrication, 128, 129f
 centric relation record, 132, 133f
 clip bar fabrication, 134
 computed tomography for, 126
 denture bases, 126
 diagnostic factors, 128, 129f
 final impression, 132, 133f
 insertion of, 138, 138f
 intraoral records, 128, 129f
 laboratory procedures, 132, 134
 master cast, 132, 133f
 mounting procedures, 128, 129f
 prosthesis completion, 136, 137f

provisional dentures, 126
soft tissue treatment, 130–132, 131f, 133f
surgery, 130, 131f
surgical guide for, 126, 127f
Implant-supported fixed prostheses
  provisional
    cementation of, 173
    esthetics of, 172, 173
    maxillary complete-arch, 108–115
    occlusion, 172, 173f
    vertical dimension, 172, 173f
  UCLA abutment for, 159f, 168, 174
Impression(s)
  compound tube, 36, 37f
  description of, 36
  maxillary complete-arch osseointegrated prosthesis, 110, 111f
Impression tray, 172, 173f
Incisal guidance, semi-adjustable articulator
  condylar relationship to, 16–18, 17f
  cusp inclines and, 16–18, 17f
  lateral, 16, 40–44
  for modified occlusal anatomy, 22
  protrusive, 16
  transfer of, 40, 41f
Incisal index, 114, 114f

J
Joint capsule receptors, 32

L
Laminate(s), 2–4, 3f
Laminate tooth preparation, 4–6, 5f
Lateral Bennett shift, 183
Lateral deflective slide, 203f, 203–204
Loading
  implant. See Implant loading
  therapeutic differential
    definition of, 76
    elements of, 76, 77f
    long-term, 79–80
Lucia Jig, 206, 207f

M
Magnetic resonance imaging, 192
Mandible
  condylar position. See Condylar position
  deviation of
    anterior, 202, 203f
    lateral, 202–203, 203f
    posterior, 202
  lingual cusp incline, 214, 215f
  physiologic movement of
    articulator imitation of, 15–16
    description of, 14, 15f
  posterior, 72, 73f
  vertical dimension of. See Vertical dimension
  working-side condylar movement, 14, 15f
Mandibular cross-arch splint, 54, 55f
Master impressions, 36, 37f

Maxilla
  bone loss
    anterior, 74–76, 75f
    posterior, 73f, 73–74
  buccal cusp incline, 214, 215f
Maxillary cross-arch splint, 54, 55f
Micromovement, 57
Micron movement, 57
Modified occlusal anatomy
  with existing restorations, 24
  implant loading and, 72, 73f
  incisal guidance for, 22
  occlusal harmony with, 22, 23f
  occlusal loading reduced using, 20, 21f
Multiple implant-supported fixed prostheses
  provisional
    cementation of, 173
    esthetics of, 172, 173
    maxillary complete-arch, 108–115
    occlusion, 172, 173f
    vertical dimension, 172, 173f
  UCLA abutment for, 159f, 168, 174
Muscle deprogramming, for deflective slide to centric occlusion
  chairside, 206–207
  pre-office, 204, 205f

N
Natural tooth intrusion
  long-term, 76–77, 77f
  prevention of, 80, 81f
Nonrotating abutments, 145, 145f
Nonworking side
  occlusal correction of, 216, 217f
  semi-adjustable articulator imitation of movement on, 16

O
Occlusal adjustment
  centric relation deflective contacts, 206
  differential, 76, 78, 79f
  protrusive, 213f, 213–214, 215f
  standard, 78, 79f
  therapeutic correction, 208, 209f
Occlusal correction
  centric, 210–212
  esthetics, 210, 211f
  history of, 209
  nonworking-side, 216, 217f
  preliminary, 210
  protrusive, 213f, 213–214, 215f
  tooth-to-tooth anatomic relationships, 210, 211f
  working-side, 214, 215f
Occlusal index, 4, 38, 39f, 134
Occlusal loading, 20, 21f
Occlusal pressure, 210
Occlusion
  concepts of, 182–183
  condylar position in fossa relative to, 190–192, 191f
  deflective slide to centric occlusion. See Deflective slide to centric occlusion
  historical descriptions of, 182

Index

marking of, 212
modified anatomy. *See* Modified occlusal anatomy
Osseointegrated prostheses
  bilateral, therapeutic biomechanics using, 80–82, 81f
  final, 174, 175f
  maxillary complete-arch
    centric relation mounting, 114, 114f
    centric relation record, 112, 113f
    construction of, 115, 115f
    design requirements, 108, 109f
    esthetic incisal index transfer, 114, 114f
    final, 116–118, 117f
    impression procedure, 110, 111f
    progressive loading of, 108–109, 109f
    provisional, 108–115
    verification jig, 112, 113f
Osteotomy
  full-length, 98, 99f
  pilot, 98, 99f
  widening of, 98–100, 99f
Overdenture. *See* Implant-supported clip bar overdenture; Tooth-supported clip bar overdenture

P

Parallelism, in anterior full-crown preparation, 8, 9f
Physiologic rest position, 32
Pilot osteotomy, 98, 99f
Plaster labial flange, 38
Pontic, 178f, 178–179
Porcelain-fused-to-metal restoration, 176–179
Posterior mandibular bone loss, 72, 73f
Posterior maxillary bone loss, 73f, 73–74
Posterior teeth, 36, 37f
Prefabricated angulated abutment, 150, 151f
Pre-office muscle deprogramming, for deflective slide to centric occlusion, 204, 205f
Prostheses
  osseointegrated. *See* Osseointegrated prostheses
  provisional. *See* Provisional osseointegrated prosthesis
  retrievability of, 144, 145f
Protrusive occlusal correction, 213f, 213–214, 215f
Provisional osseointegrated prosthesis
  cementation of, 173
  esthetics of, 172, 173
  maxillary complete-arch, 108–115
  occlusion, 172, 173f
  vertical dimension, 172, 173f
Provisional restorations
  case study of, 30–31
  esthetic planning, 30–31
  maxillary study cast of, 31

R

Radiographs, temporomandibular joint. *See* Temporomandibular joint radiographs
Reactive biomechanics, 74, 75f
Remounting records, 42

S

Semi-adjustable articulator
  canine protection, 20
  cusp inclines, 16–18, 17f
  group function, 20
  incisal guidance
    condylar relationship to, 16–18, 17f
    cusp inclines and, 16–18, 17f
    lateral, 16
    for modified occlusal anatomy, 22
    protrusive, 16
  mandibular movement imitated using
    description of, 14–16, 15f
    nonworking-side, 16
    working-side, 16, 18
  modified occlusal anatomy
    with existing restorations, 24
    incisal guidance for, 22
    occlusal harmony with, 22, 23f
    occlusal loading reduced using, 20, 21f
  modified settings, 18, 19f
  nonworking-side
    contact, 20
    movement of, 16
  normal settings, 18, 19f
  protrusive guidance, 22
  settings of, 18, 19f
  uses of, 14
Single-stage surgery, 150
Smile line, 28
Solder joint, 178, 178f
Speaking space, 32, 33f
Splinted natural teeth, force distribution in, 54, 55f
Square abutment copings, 110, 111f
Square impression copings
  accuracy of, 170, 171f
  nonrotating, 146, 147f
Superior condylar displacement, 188, 189f
Surgery
  implant-supported clip bar overdenture, 130, 131f
  single-stage, 150

T

Tapered impression copings, 170, 171f
Temporomandibular joint radiographs
  anatomic considerations, 187
  condylar position
    clinical implications of, 193
    concentricity, 188, 189f
    description of, 188
    displacement, 188, 189f, 191f, 193
    occlusion and, relationship between, 190–192, 191f
    posterior displacement, 191f, 193
    research of, 193
    studies of, 190t
    superior displacement, 188, 189f, 191f
  deflective slide to centric occlusion effects, 194
  description of, 186
  functional considerations, 187
  landmarks on, 186, 187f
  lateral transcranial, 186, 187f
  replicability of, 188
  tomograms vs, 192
  vertical dimension losses, 189

Terminal implants, 62
Therapeutic biomechanics
  for anterior maxillary bone loss, 74–76, 75f
  bilateral osseointegrated prostheses using, 80–82, 81f
  description of, 49, 68, 69f
  for posterior mandibular bone loss, 72, 73f
  for posterior maxillary bone loss, 73f, 73–74
Therapeutic differential loading
  definition of, 76
  elements of, 76, 77f
  long-term, 79–80
Three-dimensional guidance system, for implant placement
  anterior restorations, 102, 103f
  computed tomography scan
    cross-sectional image, 90, 91f
    need for, 86, 87f
    panoramic reformatted image, 90, 91f
    procedure for, 88, 89f
    reformatted images, 101, 101f
    transaxial, 88, 90, 91f
  description of, 86
  diagnostic planning, 90, 91f
  implant orientation transfer
    to cast, 92–95
    to surgical guide, 96, 97f
  in vivo results of, 101, 101f
  osteotomy
    full-length, 98, 99f
    pilot, 98, 99f
    widening of, 98–100, 99f
  posterior restorations, 102, 103f
  procedure
    osteotomy, 98–100, 99f
    recommendations, 100
  radiographic guide, 88, 89f
  surgical guide, 92–97
  vertical orientation pins, 88

Tomography
  computed. *See* Computed tomography
  transcranial temporomandibular joint radiographs vs, 192
Tooth preparation
  anterior full-crown preparation, 8, 9f
  laminate, 4–6, 5f
Tooth-supported clip bar overdenture, 122–124, 123f–124f

U

UCLA abutment
  anterior, 156, 157f
  custom-reangulated, 152–153, 153f, 156, 157f
  in multiple implant–supported fixed prostheses, 159f, 168
  posterior, 152–154, 153f–154f
  summary of, 158
  without reangulation, 154, 156, 157f
U-pin attachment, for preventing natural tooth intrusion, 80, 81f

V

Verification jig, 112, 113f
Vertical dimension
  description of, 32
  loss of, 189
  physiologic rest position, 32
  posterior teeth, 36, 37f
  procedure for increasing, 34–36, 35f
  speaking space, 32, 33f

W

Waxups, 42, 43f
Working side
  occlusal correction, 214, 215f
  semi-adjustable articulator imitation of movement on, 16, 18